SVEC
2010
05

The Temperamental nude: class, medicine and representation in eighteenth-century France

SVEC (formerly known as *Studies on Voltaire and the Eighteenth Century*) is dedicated to eighteenth-century research. *SVEC* welcomes work across a broad range of disciplines and critical methodologies.

www.voltaire.ox.ac.uk

The Temperamental nude: class, medicine and representation in eighteenth-century France

TONY HALLIDAY

VOLTAIRE FOUNDATION
OXFORD
2010

ISBN 978 0 7294 0994 0
ISSN 0435-2866

The Voltaire Foundation is a department of the University of Oxford. It furthers the University's objective of excellence in research, scholarship and education by publishing worldwide.

Voltaire Foundation
99 Banbury Road
Oxford OX2 6JX, UK
www.voltaire.ox.ac.uk

A catalogue record for this book is available from the British Library

Art history / cultural history / history of ideas
Histoire de l'art / histoire culturelle / histoire des idées

Cover illustration: Jacques-Louis David, *Oath of the tennis court*, oil on canvas (unfinished), Versailles, Musée nationale du château: dépôt Cabinet des Dessins du Louvre, MV 5841.

Mixed Sources
Product group from well-managed forests, and other controlled sources
www.fsc.org Cert no. TT-COC-002706
© 1996 Forest Stewardship Council
FSC

FSC (the Forest Stewardship Council) is an independent organization established to promote responsible management of the world's forests.

This book is printed on acid-free paper

Printed in the UK by Page Bros (Norwich) Ltd

Contents

List of illustrations vii
Preface xi
Acknowledgements xiii

Introduction 1
1. The natural order 7
2. The labour of love 17
3. Temperament and the body 51
4. Temperament and the ideal: ancient and modern 89
5. The citizen body: the politics of abstraction 121
6. A body one and indivisible: Jacobin representations of the people 155
7. The labels of Hercules: representing the body after Thermidor 189
8. The trouble with Tatius: David's *Sabines* and the end of public art 221

Bibliography 237
Index 253

List of illustrations

Figure 1: Thomas Bewick, *Vignette of green woodpecker*, woodcut by Thomas Bewick in *History of British birds*, Newcastle, 1797, vol.1, p.141 (Photograph © Richard Wrigley). 12

Figure 2: Thomas Bewick, *Vignette of wood pigeon or stock dove*, woodcut by Thomas Bewick in *History of British birds*, Newcastle, 1797, vol.1, p.271 (Photograph © Richard Wrigley). 13

Figure 3: Nicolas Poussin, *Summer, or Ruth and Boaz*, oil on canvas, Musée du Louvre, Paris, Inv. 7304 (Photograph © Réunion des Musées Nationaux / Jean-Gilles Berizzi). 18

Figure 4: Edmé Bouchardon, *Love making himself a bow from the club of Hercules*, marble, 1750, Musée du Louvre, Paris, MR 1761 (Photograph © Richard Wrigley). 19

Figure 5: Hendrik Goltzius, *The Farnese Hercules*, engraving, *c.*1592 (Photograph © Creative Commons). 24

Figure 6: *Apollo Belvedere*, marble, Musei Vaticani, Rome (Photograph © WKnight94 / Creative Commons). 25

Figure 7: Giovanni Domenico Campiglia, *Statue of Venus with a dolphin, The Medici Venus*, drawing, red chalk, *c.* 1730, National Gallery of Scotland, Edinburgh (Photograph © Lady Murray of Henderland Gift 1860 as memorial of her husband, Lord Murray of Henderland). 26

Figure 8: *Belvedere Antinous*, marble, Musei Vaticani, Rome (Photograph © F. Bucher / Creative Commons). 27

Figure 9: *Borghese gladiator*, marble, Musée du Louvre, Paris, Inv. 224 (Photograph © Jastrow / Creative Commons). 28

Figure 10: Desjardins (Martin van den Bogaert), *Spain* (sanguine), bronze, Musée du Louvre, Paris, RF 4407 (Photograph © Richard Wrigley). 60

Figure 11: Desjardins (Martin van den Bogaert), *Holland* (bilious temperament), bronze, Musée du Louvre, Paris, RF 4410 (Photograph © Richard Wrigley). 60

Figure 12: Desjardins (Martin van den Bogaert), *Brandenburg* (phlegmatic), bronze, Musée du Louvre, Paris, RF 4409 (Photograph © Richard Wrigley). 61

Figure 13: Desjardins (Martin van den Bogaert), *Holy Roman Empire* (melancholy), bronze, Musée du Louvre, Paris, RF 4408 (Photograph © Richard Wrigley). 61

Figure 14: Daniel Chodowiecki, *Les Adieux de Calas à sa famille*, etching, 1768, British Museum, London (Photograph © Trustees of the British Museum). 82

Figure 15: Jean-Baptiste Delafosse after Louis Carmontelle, *La Malheureuse famille Calas*, etching and engraving, British Museum, London (Photograph © Trustees of the British Museum). 83

Figure 16: Polyclitus, *Doryphoros*, bronze copy, *c.* 450-40 B.C., Götaplatsen, Göteborg, Sweden (© Rolf Broberg / Creative Commons). 92

Figure 17: Polyclitus, *Diadumenos*, National Archaeological Museum of Athens (Photograph © Creative Commons). 93

Figure 18: *Laocoön*, marble, Musei Vaticani, Rome (Wikipedia Commons © Creative Commons). 101

Figure 19: Leonardo da Vinci, *Vitruvian man*, drawing (Wikipedia Commons © Creative Commons). 104

Figure 20: *Belvedere torso*, marble, Musei Vaticani, Rome (Wikipedia Commons © Creative Commons). 109

Figure 21: Jean-Baptiste Pigalle, *Monument to Louis XV*, bronze, 1765, Rheims (Photograph © Frédérique Desbuissons). 112

Figure 22: Albrecht Dürer, *Melancholia I*, engraving, British Museum, London (Photograph © Trustees of the British Museum). 118

Figure 23: Jean-Baptiste Pigalle, *Le Citoyen*, terracotta, 1758, Musée des beaux-arts, Orléans (Photograph © Musée des beaux-arts, Orléans). 119

Figure 24: Anonymous, *Le Réveil du Tiers État* ('Awakening of the Third Estate'), coloured etching, 1674, De Vinck Collection, Bibliothèque nationale de France, Paris, Qb 14 juillet 1789, M 98807 (Photograph © BnF). 133

Figure 25: William Hogarth, *Rake's progress: Bedlam*, oil on canvas, 1733-34, Sir John Soane's Museum, London (Photograph © Sir John Soane's Museum). 135

Figure 26: Anonymous, 'tôt tôt tôt / battez chaud...', coloured etching, 1789, De Vinck Collection 2072, Bibliothèque nationale de France, Paris, Qb1 25 août 1789 (Photograph © BnF). 136

Figure 27: Jacques-Louis David, *Oath of the tennis court*, pen and brown ink, with black ink, heightening and pencil, Versailles, Musée nationale du château: on deposit from Cabinet des Dessins du Louvre, RF 1914, MV 8409 (Photograph © Réunion des Musées Nationaux). 138

Figure 28: Jacques-Louis David, *Oath of the tennis court*, oil on canvas (unfinished), Versailles, Musée nationale du château: dépôt Cabinet des Dessins du Louvre, MV 5841 (Photograph © Réunion des Musées Nationaux). 140

Figure 29: Clodion, *Montesquieu*, marble, Salon de 1783, Musée du Louvre, Paris (Photograph © Réunion des Musées Nationaux). 144

Figure 30: Jean-Guillaume Moitte, *Cassini*, marble, 1810, Observatoire, Paris (Plaster at 1789 Salon) (Photograph © Home Page du Mathouriste). 146

Figure 31: Pierre Julien, *Poussin*, marble, Musée du Louvre, Paris, RF 2984 (Photograph © Richard Wrigley). 147

Figure 32: Nicolas Poussin, *Testament of Eudamidas*, oil on canvas, *c.* 1643-1644, Statens Museum for Kunst, Copenhagen (Photograph © SMK Foto). 148

Figure 33: Detail of *Oath of the tennis court*, Versailles (Photograph © Réunion des Musées Nationaux). 152

Figure 34: Antoine Denis Chaudet, *Le Charlatan politique, ou le léopard apprivoisé* ('The Political charlatan or the leopard tamed'), etching, first half of 1794, De Vinck Collection, vol.26, no. 4388, Département des arts graphiques, Bibliothèque nationale de France, Paris (Photograph © BnF). 159

Figure 35: Jacques-Louis David, *Triumph of the French people*, pencil, pen and ink, grey wash, Département des arts graphiques, Musée du Louvre, Paris, Inv. RF 71 (Photograph © Réunion des Musées Nationaux). 160

Figure 36: Jacques-Louis David, *Triumph of the French people*, pencil and grey wash, 1794, Musée Carnavalet, Paris, Inv. I.E.D. 4856 (Photograph © Photothèque des Musées de la Ville de Paris (Briant)). 161

Figure 37: Jacques-Louis David, *The Death of Bara*, oil on canvas, 1794, Musée Calvet, Avignon (Photograph © Musée Calvet, Avignon). 169

Figure 38: Johan Tobias Sergel, *Othryades the Spartan dying*, terracotta, 1779, NM Sk 454 (Photograph © Nationalmuseum, Stockholm). 173

Figure 39: Pierre Julien, *Dying gladiator*, marble, 1779, morceau de réception, Musée du Louvre, Paris, RF 4623 (Photograph © Richard Wrigley). 174

Figure 40: *Dying Gaul*, marble, Musei Capitolini, Rome (Wikipedia Commons © Creative Commons). 175

Figure 41: Jean-Baptiste Stouf, *Dying Abel*, marble, 1785 morceau de réception, Musée du Louvre, Paris, MN 80 (Photograph © Richard Wrigley). 177

Figure 42: David II Teniers, *Acts of charity*, *c.* 1640, Musée du Louvre, Paris, Inv. 1879 (Photograph © Réunion des Musées Nationaux). 185

Figure 43: Jean-Guillaume Moitte, *Jean-Jacques Rousseau*, terracotta, 1790, Musée Carnavalet, Paris (Photograph © Musée Carnavalet, Paris). 194

Figure 44: François Masson, *Project for monument to Jean-Jacques Rousseau*, plaster, 1798-1799, Musée du Louvre, Paris, RF 1984 (Photograph © Réunion des Musées Nationaux). 195

Figure 45: Jacques-Louis David, *Intervention of the Sabine women*, oil on canvas, 1795-1799, Musée du Louvre, Paris, RF 3691 (Photograph © Réunion des Musées Nationaux). 222

Figure 46: Jacques-Louis David, *Intervention of the Sabine women*, pen, brown and black ink, pencil, grey wash and heightening, Musée du Louvre, Paris, Inv. 26.183 (Photograph © Réunion des Musées Nationaux). 231

Figure 47: A. L. Girodet, *Une Scène de déluge*, oil on canvas, 1806, Musée du Louvre, Paris, Inv. 4934 (Photograph © Réunion des Musées Nationaux / Hervé Lewandowski). 235

Preface

In 2006, as the issue of the *Oxford Art Journal* containing Tony's article 'The Trouble with Tatius' was going to press, I learnt of his sudden death.[1] In a note written for the issue at the time, I referred to the book which I knew he had been working on. Indeed, I clearly recalled him telling me in a characteristically understated way, that he had finished his book within the time granted by AHRC funded leave. With the help of Ian Purdie, Tony's executor, it was possible to find the computer files, and ascertain that they were indeed complete (notwithstanding the inevitability that Tony would have added to and adjusted the text in preparation for publication; certain notes suggest it could have been extended into the nineteenth century). With Ian's agreement, I resolved to find a publisher, determined that Tony's work should not be lost. Looking around for a publisher with the right range and scholarly distinction, Studies on Voltaire and the Eighteenth Century seemed an ideal place for the book to appear, and I am immensely grateful to Jonathan Mallinson for his willingness to have the manuscript reviewed, and to the reader(s) for their prompt recognition of the book's great merits.

The text is as Tony left it, with a tiny number of corrections and run-of-the-mill edits by way of co-ordination of content. The bibliography has not been updated – it gathers together the extensive range of works used by Tony. The primary labour has been to accumulate the illustrations. Their relatively large number seems to me crucial, as they bear out the success of the argument in linking medical and political theory, and art practice. The burgeoning scope of copyright-free images provided by enlightened institutions (such as the British Museum) and individuals – which Tony would surely have applauded – has made this immeasurably more straightforward.

With the publication of *Facing the public: portraiture in the aftermath of the French Revolution* (Manchester, 1999), Tony had established a reputation within art-historical studies as an authority on French revolutionary art, although it is a measure of his breadth of knowledge that his first article was on Mantegna's *Triumphs of Caesar*, developed from an undergraduate paper at the Courtauld Institute of Art.[2] His scholarship could be relied

1. For a tribute to Tony's life see the obituary by David Lomas, John McLean, Elizabeth Wilson in *The Guardian*, Friday 7 July 2006.
2. 'The literary sources of Mantegna's 'Triumphs of Caesar'', in *Annali della scuola normale superiore di Pisa* 24 (1994), p.337-96. Tony's other published work should be listed here:

on to bring in little-known but pertinent sources, and to harness them to a lucid, forceful argument. He was not afraid in his numerous reviews to cast a sceptical eye on theoretically over-self-confident and historically misinformed writing, while never indulging in polemic for its own sake. Having expanded the horizons of portraiture studies in general and of French revolutionary art in particular with *Facing the public*, this book provides a fascinating complement, in its analysis of the conceptualisation of another form of corporeal representation – the male nude. In its brilliant weaving together of art history, medical theory, politics, and Greek and Latin sources, it achieves a remarkable – and remarkably convincing – synthesis. It is all the more poignant that a book which itself is so complete should remind us of a life cut short.

Richard Wrigley

'Academic outsiders at the Paris salons of the Revolution: the case of drawings *à la manière noire*', *Oxford Art Journal* 21 (1998), p. 69-86; 'David's *Marat* as posthumous portrait', in *David's The Death of Marat*, ed. William Vaughan and Helen Weston (Cambridge, 2000), p.56-76; 'The embodiment of strength: depicting a general as a civil leader', in John Bonehill and Geoff Quilley ed., *Conflicting visions. War and visual culture in Britain and France c.1700-1830* (London, 2005), p.169-88; 'The Trouble with Tatius', *Oxford art journal* 29 (2006), p.197-211.

Acknowledgements

I would like to thank Ian Purdie, Tony's executor, for his unflagging support and enthusiasm, Jonathan Mallinson for opening the doors of Studies on Voltaire and the Eighteenth Century, and Lyn Roberts for being an ideal editorial collaborator. In the Department of Art History at Nottingham, Liz Jennings provided some timely assistance in grappling with computer files and print outs. Caroline de Lambertie and her colleagues in the photographic department of the Réunion des Musées Nationaux, who provided a significant proportion of the images, have been impeccably efficient. Frédéric Desbuissons generously provided an image of Pigalle's Rheims monument, Katie Scott and Emma Barker provided morale-boosting encouragement when the project seemed to be losing momentum. They will, I know, share with me and all of Tony's friends, a terrible sadness to see his superb scholarship appear posthumously.

Introduction

This book documents the refashioning of temperament theory in eighteenth-century Europe (primarily France) and its hitherto unrecognised consequences for visual representation, principally in painting and sculpture. For centuries, the doctrine of temperaments and the theory of humours were integral to Western medicine. They appeared to offer a 'common sense' interpretation of the natural world and the place of humanity within it. In particular, they provided credible explanations of individual difference among human beings. This system of knowledge was discredited by the scientific discoveries of the seventeenth century, but temperament theory was revived in a revised form a hundred years later, when it was redeployed to create a moral and physiological typology of social distinctions in general and of the labouring classes in particular.

This is a largely forgotten episode in the history of Western thought, but it had lasting effects on the way in which people envisaged the embodiment of human identity. The revival of temperament theory was the work of medical writers, notably Haller and Cabanis, but the impact of their ideas extended far beyond the sphere of medicine. They helped shape the views of Kant, Lavater and Diderot among others. In particular, they invested the representation of the human body in art with new significance. The male nude was central to the teaching and practice of art throughout this period. This was partly a consequence of moral and religious strictures on the use of the female model, but it also reflected a continuing belief in the centrality of man to the definition of human identity. The representation of the male nude in European – and especially French – painting and sculpture provides the point of reference for this book. Interest in reworkings of temperament theory was greatest in France, and was closely tied to the social and political culture of the revolutionary and immediately post-revolutionary period.

The Temperamental nude deals with issues – the representation of the male nude and the development of a discourse on class identity – which have attracted much attention in recent years, but it approaches them from a new perspective. It suggests that debates which appear to have been about class actually *were* about class, and not, for example, gender. Its central goal is to show how matters of artistic representation were closely connected to medical and political discourses throughout the later eighteenth century, most especially during the successive phases of the French Revolution.

In Chapter 1, 'The natural order', examples from the art and writings of Thomas Bewick are used to show how differently nature was interpreted in the eighteenth century and, in particular, how natural history viewed the working and the leisured body. For eighteenth-century European readers, non-human animals were vested with the identities of gentry and workers, and not, as for us, of male and female.

Chapter 2, 'The labour of love', looks at the representation of a labouring god – Bouchardon's statue of the god Love fashioning a bow from the club of Hercules – and at the reactions it provoked, especially from Diderot. Diderot's response reveals his ambivalence about the effects of the division of labour on individual human identity. This ambivalence impinged on areas of his output – aesthetic, philosophical and political – which are usually interpreted from other perspectives. On a broader level, it points to a widespread curiosity and unease in late eighteenth-century Europe about the relationship of character, occupation and appearance.

Chapter 3, 'Temperament and the body', argues for the continued importance of temperament theory for eighteenth-century thinking about the body and about identity. This significance is indeed manifest in the way such theory was updated during this period. Traditionally, human appearance and character had been linked and their differences explained in terms of temperament. The theory of the four humours on which the doctrine of temperament depended was largely rejected by early modern medicine. But it was not so easy to eliminate the need and habit of explaining human difference in terms of the visible outward signs of temperament. In the 1760s Haller reinterpreted difference of temperament as an effect of innate physiological constitution, not the more or less fluid balance of humours. At the same time, his addition of a fifth, 'muscular' temperament placed a new emphasis on what might now be interpreted as effects of occupation or habitus. This aspect was echoed in writings by two of Haller's admirers, Kant and Lavater. Both used temperament as a key to the differentiation of aesthetic response, which they interpreted as an index of moral character.

In Chapter 4, 'Temperament and the ideal: ancient and modern', the relationship is explored between antique notions of an ideal body and its applicability to modern artistic representation. The belief in a necessary connection between the classification and treatment of the body in medicine and its representation in art was part of temperament theory since the time of Galen, as was the idea of a canon of universal human perfection, embodied, it was believed, in a lost statue by the Greek sculptor Polyclitus. The very possibility of such an embodiment was treated with increasing scepticism in a culture preoccupied with immutable difference between human beings. Hostility to an ideal canon was particularly marked in the new fields of art history and criticism. This chapter closes with a discussion of an attempt by the eighteenth-century sculptor Pigalle to realise an ideal of universal manhood in contemporary terms.

Chapter 5, 'The citizen body: the politics of abstraction', discusses views as to what form was most appropriate and viable for the visual representation of the new citizen, and how these problems related to matters of political representation. More abstract notions of the 'people' were undermined by discomfort about the unacceptability of the rural and urban *peuple*, who were deemed unfit for active political responsibility, as indeed they had been beyond the pale when it came to the stylised pseudo-social repertoire of fine art. Jacques-Louis David's project, *The Tennis court oath*, illustrates the uneasy negotiation of this kind of impasse as it applied to the image of a transformative moment in the history of revolutionary representation, set against an analysis of the evolution of the discourse of political representation. David's choice between heroic nudity and *portraits historiés* exemplifies the unresolved matter of how, in 1790-1792, to depict the nature and practice of political representation.

Chapter 6, 'A body one and indivisible: Jacobin representations of the people', considers representations of the people, and the People, in Jacobin imagery and discourse. David's *Triumph of the French people* is discussed as a multi-faceted attempt to create an inclusive image of national, republican unity – combining different registers and iconographical ingredients. The composite nature of the image is related to the fragmentation of the fragile, notional unity imposed on the various meanings of the word *peuple*. David's *Bara* is presented as a resolved figure of Jacobin unifying rhetoric. His nudity is crucial to the pointed use of the language of high art to communicate with a collective audience – to display a message in elevated form and manner, thus distanced from the threatening violence of popular politics. The image is revisited via Alvar Gonzales-Palacios' observation that there may well be a link to Stouf's *Abel* (1785), but this is given greater resonance (consistent with the thrust of the book's argument), by drawing out the significance of the literary source, Salomon Gessner's poem, *Death of Abel*, in terms of the representation of an adolescent body, that is, that of the shepherd Abel, murdered by his agricultural labourer brother Cain. This comparison, redolent of a burgeoning aesthetic recognition of socio-physical differentiation, is part of a reading of *Bara* as a coherent projection of the erasure of social distinction in Jacobin rhetoric. The chapter closes with an account of the discussions amongst artists in the Société populaire et républicaine des arts about the portrayal of poor and labouring classes, in which arguments in favour of idealisation denounced ignoble particularisation with its implications of social divisiveness.

In discussing the image of the people after the fall of Jacobins, the core of Chapter 7, 'The labels of Hercules: representing the body after Thermidor', concerns the updated theory of the temperaments devised by P. G. Cabanis, the medical theorist and revolutionary politician, and prominent member of the new Institut national. This was the most substantial and influential reworking of Haller's temperament theory. Cabanis emphasised the role of two new temperaments, the cerebral and muscular. His doctrine provided a medical justification for rewriting the French democratic constitution following Napoleon's coup of 1799, in which Cabanis himself played a crucial role. The new ways of looking at body types had important consequences for the symbolic use made of the male nude during the French Revolution – in particular for attempts to embody nationhood in a figure representative of the citizenry as a whole, whether in official propaganda or caricature. Linked to this question is the history of projects to reintroduce an ancient Greek cult of the body, including the first and now forgotten attempt to revive the Olympic games in a modern context, in Paris – judged a failure for the disappointingly squalid social identities of the victors.

Chapter 8, 'The trouble with Tatius: David's *Sabines* and the end of public art', argues that David's *Intervention of the Sabine women* (1799) exemplifies Cabanis' views on temperament; more precisely, and crucially, that this connection was introduced quite late in the evolution of the picture. Such an assimilation of ideas therefore corresponds to David's willingness to draw on up-to-date fundamentally repressive political ideas. The exposition of the picture and its reception focuses on the differentiated representation of bodily types, with specific references to muscular development – a key link to Cabanis' new version of temperament theory. David needed to make the two main protagonists, Romulus and Tatius, naked in order to show the difference in temperaments as it was manifest in terms of their respective physiques, hence his changed design, dispensing with the armour and clothing previously depicted. When clothed, the figures, and their narrative role, had fitted into a thematic of reconciliation; naked, their physical differences were revealed for what they were, innate and irreconcilable. Heroic or ideal nudity (Romulus) is contrasted with something more akin to everyday nakedness (Tatius). Thus, the *Sabines* appeared to offer a new way of treating historical subjects, as much by its attention to the social and the physiological as by its adoption of what David claimed to be an authentically antique approach.

The interest of this proposed link is not only a new way of thinking about the representation of the body at the end of the eighteenth century, but to show how this is intimately rooted in a specific moment of revolutionary – soon to be post-revolutionary – ideology. David's accommodation is shown to be contingent on a combination of political and artistic circumstances which were rapidly superseded. David had embodied reason in Romulus and passion in Tatius, confident that his spectators would regard themselves as sufficiently cerebral to identify with Romulus. But, as the picture's reception demonstrates, only a few observers (notably Chaussard), in tune with David's implicit project, appreciated the politics of corporeal representation which David had pointedly articulated.

A comparison with Girodet's *Une Scène de déluge* (1806), which was preferred to David's *Sabines* in the 1810 *Prix Décennaux* competition, illustrates the dissatisfaction with the didactic function of art in post-revolutionary culture. The *Sabines*' 'defeat' signalled the end of an era of enlightened history painting, as too an era of enlightened democracy. In what it reveals about the problematic relationship between history painting and social purpose, the *Sabines*' fate was indeed a lesson for the artists of the succeeding century.

1. The natural order

In this chapter I want to look at two images of birds engraved on wood by Thomas Bewick at the end of the eighteenth century. In doing so I want to show that however similar nature may have looked two hundred years ago, it was experienced and interpreted in radically different ways. This was not merely because of the state of scientific knowledge. People's views of nature were bound up with how they made sense of their own existence in society. The way they saw animals and birds related to the way they saw themselves and each other as human beings. Then as now the moral presumptions underlying social judgements were expressed with often crude clarity in the context of natural history. That makes it a useful starting point for an inquiry into the evolution of ideas about human identity and appearance.

Eighteenth-century art often looks alien to twenty-first-century spectators. Much of its subject matter seems remote or bombastic, suggesting different preoccupations from our own. Representations of nature appear to provide a reassuring exception to this rule. For British spectators in particular, such art is perhaps typified by the wood engravings produced by the Tyneside publisher and naturalist Thomas Bewick. These take the form of vignettes – small, irregularly shaped images which fit easily into a page with accompanying text. Most of Bewick's vignettes record the appearance of individual birds and animals with extraordinary fidelity and deft skill. Others illustrate scenes of rural life whose Northumbrian settings are sometimes still identifiable. In our own ecologically minded age we often turn to nature in search of values which are stable and unchanging. It is reassuring to find images which suggest that people were doing the same thing two hundred years ago, and that what they saw was not that different from what we experience nowadays. Here at least is an eighteenth-century record of the everyday which strikes us as fresh and authentic. But how well-grounded is our conviction? Did people at the end of the eighteenth century really react to such images and to the idea of nature which they represent in the same way as we do? To what extent was Bewick's vision ours, and to what extent have we merely assimilated an alien vision from another age? How much, for one thing, does our reaction depend on the context in which we encounter Bewick's work in the here and now, and how different is that context from that envisaged by Bewick himself?

Bewick's vignettes have become familiar to many people who have little or no idea of when or why they were engraved. Modest in scale and lacking a defined frame, they can be made to look at home in a variety of contexts. In recent years, they have been appropriated to commercial uses in particular. They easily fit into larger compositions, such as those of labels, posters or newspaper advertisements. The wood engraving's sturdy and well-defined interplay of black and white stands up well to reproduction on all sorts of surfaces – crockery, textiles and plastic as well as paper. Their idiosyncratic combination of rural imagery and detailed observation with a neat, clean and easily recognisable manner have turned these little images into useful tools for packaging and selling not merely a wide range of consumer goods, but a particular version of Britishness. They help market mass-produced materials to a largely urban middle class stubbornly in love with its rustic antecedents.

All this is a far cry from how Bewick's work was sold to his contemporaries. They bought it because it looked unfamiliar and revolutionary, not traditional, and they bought it as part of a package – books on natural history designed to enlighten and instruct the reader about the world around them and their own place within it. The technique employed by Bewick, wood engraving, was largely his own invention. Its significance in the history of art and industry extended far beyond his own immediate output, important though that was. Its introduction proved to be one of the most immediately influential of all technical revolutions, earning its inventor international fame and fortune in his own lifetime. Bewick developed wood engraving, not as a means of recording a personal vision of nature, but as a solution to the problems of mechanical book illustration. In the eighteenth century most book illustrations took the form of line engravings printed from metal plates. Another technique, woodcutting, survived from an earlier age, but it was a crude affair, yielding clumsy illustrations used for the most part in cheap, ephemeral publications. Wood engraving employed harder and more closely grained wood than that used for woodcuts. Instead of cutting with the grain, like woodcutters, Bewick sawed the wood across the grain, creating a hard, smooth surface which could then be polished and cut using an engraver's burin. The delicacy and vigour of the crisp, detailed images which Bewick produced make them instantly recognisable. The effect of wood engraving was unmistakably different from that of the techniques which it was destined to replace – the crude if often forceful contrasts of the woodcut, or the fine-lined copperplate engraving. But wood engraving's characteristic strength of line was not merely for aesthetic effect. It was also an indication of what made this invention so momentous in the history of book production. In wood engraving, the wood is worked to produce raised lines on the block which take the ink. In this it differs from traditional engraving on metal, where the lines incised into the plate trap the ink, so as to print on paper pressed against them in the printing process. Wood engraving, by contrast, prints in the same way as metal type, in relief. The wood employed by Bewick was hard enough for his vignettes to be set up together with type and printed in the same action. This had not been possible in books using metal-engraved illustrations, where the printing of the illustrations, usually on separate pages, always entailed a separate process. Bewick's innovative use of wood engraving made the production of illustrated books easier and cheaper than ever before. It also changed the appearance of the illustrated page. Illustrations engraved on metal had usually occupied a page of their own, facing the printed text. Wood engraving allowed images to appear on the same page as the text – an unprecedented integration of image with text. It is in part for this reason that Bewick's vignettes lack formal framing devices – it enables them to melt into the text which surrounds them. It is of course this same lack of a defined frame which makes Bewick's images easy to adapt to other contexts and thus so useful to commercial designers today. But it was an effect designed originally with a view to tying images as closely as possible to the texts they were designed to illustrate. Wood engraving made possible the golden age of the nineteenth-century illustrated book – a development whose most spectacular results were realised chiefly in France and Germany rather than England.

The practical possibilities of Bewick's invention were particularly important to the inventor himself. These images were not created as the infinitely transferable icons of English rurality which they have since become, still less as signifiers of the 'good taste' hopefully conferred by purchase of the sort of comestibles they are now used to advertise. Not that Bewick was prejudiced against commerce. He himself produced advertising goods, such as trade cards and tickets. But his boldest ventures were in the form of books on which he worked as a naturalist and author and who was also his own illustrator and publisher. Wood engraving enabled him to combine textual description with visual representation in a series of educational books, a *General history of quadrupeds*, a *History of British birds* and *The Fables of Aesop, and others*. Bewick was a man of strong didactic views. His books were designed to instruct readers in the design and meaning of the natural world.[1] In this his writings

1. The literature on Bewick is extensive. A good introduction, with some bibliography, is in John Brewer, *The Pleasures of the imagination: English culture in the eighteenth century* (London, 1997), p.499-530, 687-88. On Bewick and book illustration, see 'The Romantic vignette and Thomas Bewick', in *Romanticism and realism: the mythology of nineteenth-century art*, ed. Charles Rosen and Henri Zerner (New York and London, 1984), p.71-96. On Bewick's moral vision, see John Brewer and Stella Tillyard, 'The moral vision of Thomas Bewick', in *The Transformation of political culture: England and Germany in the late eighteenth century*, ed. Eckhard Hellmuth (Oxford, 1990), p.375-408.

emulated those of the famous French naturalist Buffon, to whose *Natural history*, published originally between 1749 and 1767, Bewick's own books were indebted. Natural history inherited a Christian view of the world. Its initial purpose was to explain the ways of God to man. As Jacques Roger observed, 'when nature was eventually substituted for God, the religious purpose disappeared, but the moral lesson remained'.[2] The moral purpose of Bewick's *Quadrupeds* and his *Birds* was as no less overt than that of his later collection of *Fables*.

Restored to the context for which they were designed, Bewick's illustrations can be seen as the artist intended. This makes them exceptional in comparison with most eighteenth-century art, particularly book illustration, where artists usually operated on a publisher's or an author's instructions and rarely if ever registered a personal response to their allotted task. In an age of increased specialisation, Bewick – at once illustrator, author, publisher and printer – was something of an anachronism. By combining such disparate roles, however, he was able to realise a remarkable unity of vision – a unity which the subsequent piecemeal appropriation of his vignettes to other uses has shattered. The result of setting these familiar illustrations alongside the texts which they were originally designed to accompany can be surprising and even disconcerting. This is certainly the case with the two illustrations I now want to discuss. Here, the surprises lie not merely in what the texts tell us about their subjects but in what they imply about the way in which Bewick and his contemporaries interpreted the world of nature as a whole. Both illustrations appeared in the 'Land birds' volume of the *History of British birds*, first published in 1797. The first is a vignette of a green woodpecker (see fig.1, p.12).

Bewick prefaced his descriptions of individual birds of this type with some general observations on the woodpecker family:

> Their characters are striking, and their manners singular. [...] M. Buffon, with his usual warmth of imagination, thus describes the seemingly dull and solitary life of the Woodpecker: – 'Of all the birds which earn their subsistence by spoil, none leads a life so laborious and painful as the Woodpecker: nature has condemned it to incessant toil and slavery. While others freely employ their courage or address, and either shoot on rapid wing or lurk in close ambush, the Woodpecker is constrained to drag out an insipid existence in boring the bark and hard fibres of trees to extract its humble prey. Necessity never suffers any intermission of its labours, never grants an interval of sound repose; often during the night it sleeps in the same painful

2. 'The living world', in *The Ferment of knowledge*, ed. G.S. Rousseau and R. Porter (Cambridge, 1980), p.264. See more generally Jacques Roger, *Les Sciences de la vie dans la pensée française du XVIIIe siècle. La génération des animaux de Descartes à l'Encyclopédie* (Paris, 1963); Keith Thomas, *Man and the natural world: changing attitudes in England 1500-1800* (Oxford, 1983).

posture as in the fatigues of the day. It never shares the sports of the other inhabitants of the air, it joins not their vocal concerts, and its wild cries and saddening tones, while they disturb the silence of the forest, express constraint and effort. Its movements are quick, its gestures full of inquietude; its looks coarse and vulgar; it shuns all society, even that of its own kind; and when it is prompted to seek a companion, its appetite is not softened by delicacy of feeling.'[3]

The other illustration, Bewick's wood engraving of the *Wood pigeon or stock dove* (see fig.2, p.13), occupies a corresponding position in the section on 'birds of the dove kind', which is similarly prefaced by remarks on the character of doves in general – a character very unlike that of woodpecker:

> The various families which constitute this beautiful genus are distinguished by shades gradations so minute, as to exceed all description. Of these by much the larger portion are the willing attendants on man, and depend on his bounty, seldom leaving the dwellings provided for them, and only roaming abroad to seek amusement, or to procure subsistence [...]. It must be observed, however, that in these [dwellings] they live, rather as voluntary captives, or transient guests, than permanent or settled inhabitants, enjoying a considerable portion of that liberty they so much delight in [...]. Every where their manners are gentle and lively; they are fond of society, and the very emblem of connubial attachment; they are faithful to their mates, whom they solicit with the softest cooings, the tenderest caresses, and the most graceful movements. The exterior form of the Pigeon is beautiful and elegant.[4]

Bewick provided detailed descriptions of the birds' physical appearance which helped flesh out his characterisation of their lifestyles. Thus the woodpecker's bill ('large, strong and fitted for its employment') was well-suited to its way of life, as were its neck ('short and thick, and furnished with powerful muscles, which enable it to strike with such force as to be heard at a considerable distance'), and its toes ('armed with strong hooked claws, by which it clings firmly, and creeps up and down in all directions'). The bills of doves and pigeons were, by contrast, 'weak, straight and slender'. What chiefly distinguished birds of the dove kind was 'the great strength of their wings', not that of their necks or their toes. This, combined with 'the lightness of their bodies' produced 'amazing rapidity of flight', so that 'it is a matter of wonder that they should

3. Thomas Bewick, *History of British birds* (1797; Newcastle, 1804), vol.1, p.118-19. The term 'warmth of imagination' applied to Buffon in this passage should not be read as pejorative. The text is a slightly modified version of that given by Smellie in Buffon, *The Natural history of birds. From the French of the Count de Buffon* (W. Strahan and T. Cadell; London, 1793), vol.7, p.2-3. For Bewick and Smellie, see P. Davis and J. Holmes, 'Thomas Bewick (1753-1828), engraver and ornithologist', *Archives of natural history* 20 (1993), p.167-84 (173).

4. Davis and Holmes, 'Thomas Bewick', vol.1, p.276-67. Buffon's assessment of the character of doves is couched in similar terms. See Buffon, *Natural history*, vol.2, p.435, 461.

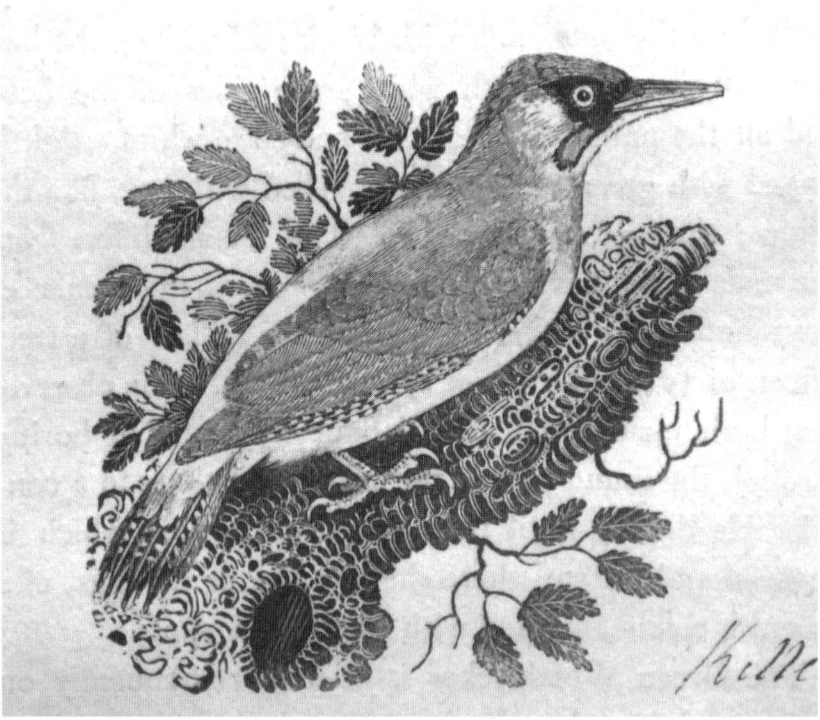

Figure 1: Thomas Bewick, *Vignette of green woodpecker*, woodcut by Thomas Bewick in *History of British birds*, Newcastle, 1797, vol.1, p.141.

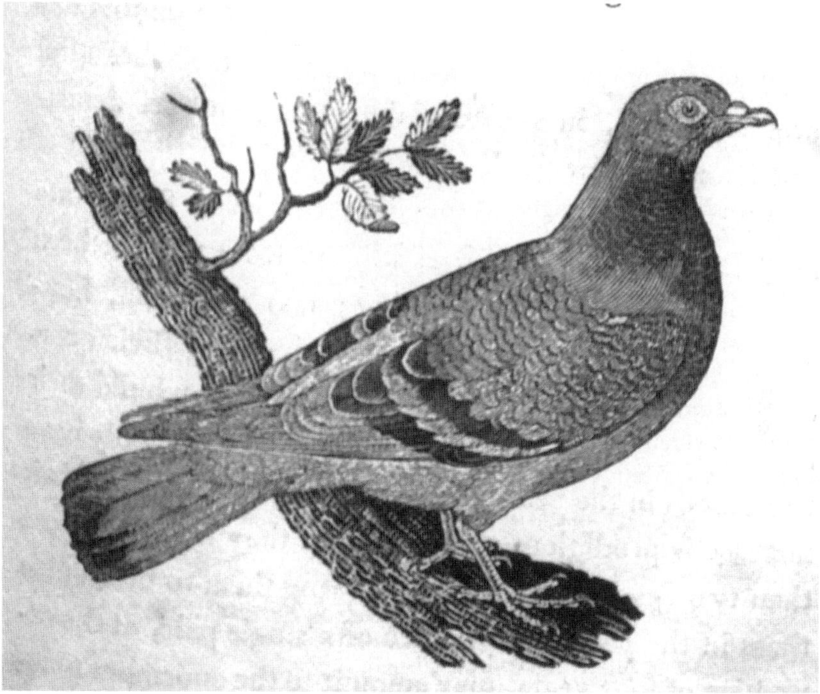

Figure 2: Thomas Bewick, *Vignette of wood pigeon or stock dove,* woodcut by Thomas Bewick in *History of British birds,* Newcastle, 1797, vol.1, p.271.

submit even to a partial kind of domestication, or occupy those tenements fitted up for the purpose of breeding and rearing their young'. If the woodpecker was formed for the servitude of labour, the dove was evidently the bird of freedom. Bewick's illustrations ably reinforce the interpretations given in his text. They possess an apparently artless objectivity, largely devoid of the overt anthropomorphism associated with the paintings of later animal artists such as Landseer, but this only serves to make their implied characterisations more plausible to a sympathetic reader. The woodpecker portrayed in Bewick's vignette inhabits the leafy recesses of an old, gnarled tree, the site of its labours and its refuge from the sight of men. The dove, by contrast, is set on an exposed branch, ready to soar. The form and use of the bill – both the woodpecker's powerful bill and the slender bill of the dove – were emphasised in Bewick's descriptions, and they are accorded equivalent prominence in the illustrations, silhouetted against the blank page, as indeed are the tips of the pigeon's wings at the point where they are made to interrupt the line of its back and tail. The woodpecker's toes, a mark of that bird's peculiar strength as the wings were of the dove's, are also emphasised, framed by the only patch of unbroken shadow in the composition.

Bewick's portrayals of animals are often admired for their accuracy of observation. Few would now want to say as much of the written descriptions for which they were designed. It is evident that human stereotypes of genteel and uncouth behaviour have been foisted onto two species of birds in a way that now seems contrived and crude. But it is not because we humans have ceased to interpret the lives of other animals in anthropomorphic terms that we see them that way. It is rather that the values according to which we construct our picture of nature have changed, both in relation to our own species and to others. It might seem distasteful to us that Buffon should have dismissed the physical labours necessary to a woodpecker's existence as 'toil and slavery'. Conversely, the dependence of the economically unproductive dove on human handouts would not endear it to twenty-first century observers, however genteel its home life. It might even come under pressure to retrain as a woodpecker in order to justify its existence. But we still project human values onto other animals, just as Bewick did. If we reject Bewick's stereotypes as descriptions of the natural world, that is in part because our points of reference have shifted. Bewick and Buffon referred the moral characters of birds to the ways in which they gained their livelihood. When twenty-first-century natural historians invite us to contemplate life in the nest – early on a Sunday evening, say, while watching a documentary on BBC 2 television – they do not portray a world of labour. We are shown instead a world of sex – albeit sex in its conventionally sanctioned human form, the nuclear family devoted to child rearing, with the occasional bout of infidelity on the side. The frequency with which such programmes treat the life of birds rather than that of other animals is perhaps attributable to the practice many birds have of coming together in pairs to breed and rear their young – a practice fortuitously similar to the way of life prescribed to human beings in contemporary Western societies. Even when television documentaries deal with animals which live in different social groupings, similarities to the social life of humans are created by attributing characteristic behaviour to gender identities – the footloose but sexually frustrated life of the young adult male excluded from the pack, for example, or the mother mindful of her errant young. Through the construction of such identities twenty-first-century spectators are invited to empathise with and make sense of alien lives whose inhumanity would otherwise bore or repel them. More to the point, they are also asked to recognise and thus accept as 'natural' the stereotypes which they themselves are called upon to act out.

But that is not how nature's realm looked to Bewick, Buffon and their contemporaries. For them, the habits which governed sexual mores were not grounded in gender identity. They were generated elsewhere. This was true of birds and animals, just as it was of humans. The woodpecker's labours were exhausting and brutalising. This meant that they could be complemented by no more than the occasional bout of hurried and casual sex, in which 'appetites' were unsoftened 'by delicacy of feeling'. The pleasure-loving dove, on the other hand, had the leisure to cultivate more refined emotional experiences. Its affective relations benefited as a result. Where David Attenborough was to see a world of mummies and daddies and the bird next door, Buffon and Bewick saw labourers and gentry. Eighteenth-century naturalists and their readers inhabited a society where social difference was celebrated, not dissimulated. Their interpretation of the effects of prolonged physical labour on the morale of the woodpecker derived, like their appreciation of the leisured life of the dove, from the way in which they viewed the organisation of human society and the formation of individual human identity. As a self-styled 'warm whig', Bewick subscribed to political views which differed in important respects from those of Buffon, a landed proprietor and entrepreneur. But the two men shared a faith in such core concepts as divine Providence, the beneficial effects of organised human labour and the inviolability of private property. As a result, they shared a perspective on the effects of labour and leisure whether on animals or on humans.[5]

5. For Bewick, see Brewer and Tillyard, 'Moral vision', p.387f. For Buffon, see Claude Blanckaert, 'La valeur de l'homme: l'idée de nature humaine chez Buffon', in *Buffon 88:*

The connection between occupation, character and appearance were as self-evident to Bewick and his readers as that between gender identity and behaviour to a twenty-first-century television audience. But what were the mechanisms which secured those links? How was lifestyle supposed to dictate not merely individual appearance but character as well? And why was occupation rather than, say, gender or gender orientation a determining factor in the process? As should by now be obvious, the answers to these questions must be sought, not in the natural history of birds, but in that of humans. It is time to turn this inquiry in the direction of our own species – to look at the human prototypes of Bewick's doves and woodpeckers – the leisured and the labouring members of the human race. It was among human beings that the patterns of daily life were seen to mould the bodies and the characters of individuals. But the self-evidence of such effects depended on the stability of the relations which secured them. What would happen if that stability were questioned?

---

actes du colloque international Paris-Montbard-Dijon, ed. J. Gayon et al. (Paris, 1992), p.583-600. For a comparison of their approach as natural historians, see Alex Potts, 'Natural order and the call of the wild: the politics of animal picturing', *Oxford art journal* 13 (1990), p.15 n.10.

2. The labour of love

Representations of people working were common enough in seventeenth- and eighteenth-century art, but only in so-called 'genre' painting – scenes of everyday low life. They did not figure greatly in history painting or sculpture – the sort of 'high art' which was likely to attract detailed critical scrutiny. If they were there at all, it was as an incidental presence – like the peasants labouring the fields in the background of Poussin's *Summer*, whose true narrative subject is the biblical encounter of Ruth and Boaz (fig.3, p.18).

Such art was geared to provide moral lessons for the great or at least the genteel. It rarely took as its subject acts of physical labour. The statue by the French sculptor Edmé Bouchardon which I want to look at now was therefore exceptional. This chapter will be chiefly concerned with the reaction to the statue of one man, the *philosophe* Denis Diderot. Diderot's response was unfavourable. His criticism centred on the strenuous and laborious character of the action depicted by the sculptor. That he took a negative view of the representation of such subject matter is surprising, given his own interest and expertise in the study of human labour, its organisation and representation. His comments on the statue are brief and enigmatic, but they touch on issues which appear time and again in his writing about the representation of the human body and about social relations in general. An investigation of the themes underlying Diderot's judgement in this case sheds light on the anxieties which informed his response and that of his contemporaries to representations of the human body, and in particular the working body, but which have generally been neglected by later commentators.

Bouchardon's unusual statue, which was completed in 1750, represents *Love making himself a bow from the club of Hercules* (fig.4, p.19).[1]

It was commissioned by the French Crown. The significance of the subject and of Bouchardon's decision to portray Love as an adolescent were explained in a letter to the press by one of the sculptor's principal supporters, the publisher and connoisseur P.-J. Mariette.[2] The sculp-

1. The best account of the statue and its history, to which my own is substantially indebted, is Katie Scott, 'Under the sign of Venus: the making and meaning of Bouchardon's *L'Amour* in the age of the French Rococo', in *Manifestations of Venus: art and sexuality*, ed. Caroline Arscott and Katie Scott (Manchester, 2000), p.69-89.
2. Published in May 1750 in the *Mercure*, it was reprinted as *LETTRE A M **** in (Anne-Claude-Phillipe Comte de) Caylus, *Vie d'Edmé Bouchardon, sculpteur du roi* (Paris, 1762), p.118-29.

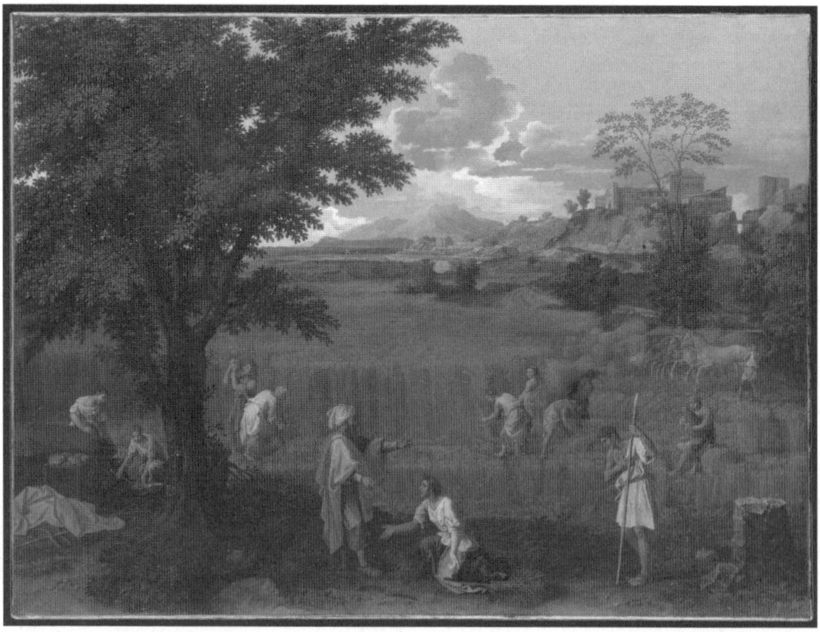

Figure 3: Nicolas Poussin, *Summer, or Ruth and Boaz*, oil on canvas, 118 × 160 cm, Musée du Louvre, Paris, Inv. 7304.

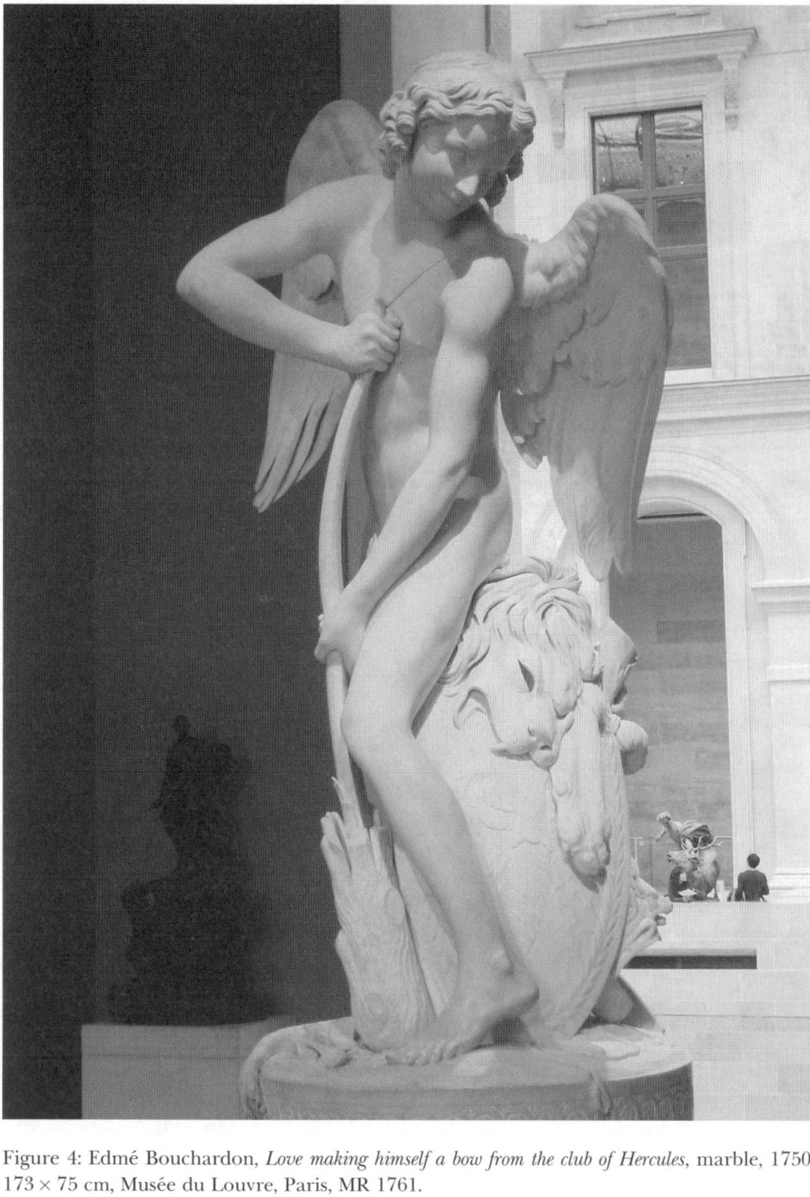

Figure 4: Edmé Bouchardon, *Love making himself a bow from the club of Hercules*, marble, 1750, 173 × 75 cm, Musée du Louvre, Paris, MR 1761.

ture's subject was allegorical. Its purpose was therefore not to illustrate an act of labour as such, but to provide a symbol of a more general, abstract truth couched in the vocabulary of Greek and Roman mythological symbolism – in this case, the power of love to subdue even the mighty. As was usual, Love was personified as a winged boy, Cupid, son of the goddess Venus. The Love depicted by Bouchardon has already defeated two other more venerable male gods – the deities who most typically embodied physical strength, Mars and Hercules. Love's victory is symbolised by the stump of living laurel behind him (ancient victors were crowned with laurel wreaths). Over the stump hang attributes of the vanquished gods – the skin of the Nemean lion, worn by Hercules following his victory over the lion itself, and Mars's shield and helmet. The young god has paused in the process of fashioning a bow from the club of Hercules with the aid of Mars's sword, which now lies temporarily at his feet. He is thereby transforming the arms of the two defeated gods into an instrument which will spread his own weapons – the arrows of desire – far and wide in the breasts of gods and humans. The sculpture is meticulously worked, with scrupulous attention to qualities of surface in the rendering of the god's flesh and his various accoutrements. The naturalistic gesture (he is testing the elasticity of the as yet partially carved bow) and the wood shavings lying at Love's feet further testify to the actuality of the undertaking in which he is engaged. It is his physical exertion as he pits his own strength against the resisting wood which provides the mainspring of the composition, playing off movement against equilibrium. Drawing on Leonardo da Vinci, contemporary art theory recognised two approaches to the composition of a figure in motion – the self-maintained balance of free-standing figures (*l'équilibre simple*) and the sort of composition in which a protagonist bore or resisted the weight of a foreign body, as in statues of Hercules wrestling with the giant Antaeus (*l'équilibre composé*).[3] Bouchardon's sculpture provides an instance of *l'équilibre composé* as Hercules' victor, Love, bends Hercules' club to his will. The spectator's attention is thereby directed to the narrative implied in the sculpture's subject – to causes and to consequences – to a degree which is unusual in the case of sculpture, a medium even less well equipped than painting to provide this sort of information, as Mariette pointed out.[4] The tension and torsion which result from the young god's action give this remarkable statue its overwhelming dynamism and restlessness. At the same time, the very virtuosity with which Bouchardon has represented the strenuous character of

3. C.-H. Watelet, *L'Art de peindre. Poème, avec des réflexions sur les différentes parties de la peinture* (Paris, 1761), p.97f. See Martial Guédron's discussion, *De Chair et de marbre: imiter et exprimer le nu en France, 1745-1815* (Paris, 2003), p.62.

4. In Caylus, *Lettre*, p.119.

Love's occupation inevitably pulls the statue's subject from the realm of the ideal towards that of the all too imaginably real. It draws the spectator's attention to the nature of the activity itself at the expense of its symbolic message. It is not surprising that Bouchardon's contemporaries found it difficult to read the statue as pure allegory.

That was not all. Bouchardon chose to represent Love as an adolescent, at an age when the youthful body was no longer that of a child, but had not fully acquired the rounded limbs and other stable characteristics of adulthood. This was unusual. Love was portrayed as an adolescent in representations of the story of his love affair with Psyche, but in other contexts he was more often personified by a more or less wayward and delinquent infant.[5] This was how he had been portrayed in poems by the ancient Greek poets Anacreon and Moschus which were well known and much imitated in later European literature and art. In the person of a toddler, Love was allowed to engage in more or less playful activities which invited allegorical interpretation. The behaviour attributed to him often involved voyeurism or conscious cruelty. But the infantilisation of Love prevented the moral impropriety of such actions from being taken too seriously. Babies were expected to be naughty. The choice of an adolescent to personify Love made the relationship of Bouchardon's statue to its ostensible subject more problematic. It involved depicting the young god at an age at which human males were often required to undertake similar acts of heavy labour, at least in the eighteenth century. The figure is of course winged, and is surrounded by mythological accoutrements such as the lion skin which serve in part to block any contemporary reference. But the emphasis on the awkward marks of transition in the boy god's body – the arms too thin, the feet disproportionately big for a fully formed adult male, as Cochin noted at the time[6] – were more appropriate to the representation of a human boy than to that of a deity, by definition immortal and unchanging.

5. Mariette in Caylus, *Lettre*, p.120. For Bouchardon's immediate source, a composition deriving from Parmigianino, see Scott, 'Under the sign', p.73. There are also numerous versions of an ancient statue attributed to Lysippus which represents an adolescent Eros stringing a bow. Of these, Bouchardon is most likely to have been familiar with that purchased by Benedict XIV in Rome in 1753 and now in the Museo Capitolino. The suggestion that the bow represented in the ancient statues was that of Hercules appears to be of later date than Bouchardon's statue. See H. Stuart Jones, ed., *A Catalogue of the ancient sculptures preserved in the municipal collections of Rome. The sculptures of the Museo Capitolino* (Oxford, 1912), p.87f; W. H. Roscher, *Ausführliches Lexikon der griechischen und römischen Mythologie* (Leipzig, 1886-1890), s.v. *Eros* (article by A. Furtwängler), vol.1, p.1362; C. Friederichs, *Amor mit dem Bogen des Herkules, Marmorstatue im Museum zu Berlin. Siebenundzwanzigstes Programm zum Winckelmannsfest der archäologischen Gesellschaft zu Berlin* (Berlin, 1867).

6. C.-N. Cochin in *Mémoires inédits de Charles-Nicolas Cochin sur le Comte de Caylus, Bouchardon, les Slodtz*, ed. C. Henry (Paris, 1880), p.105. Cochin was Secretary of the Royal Academy of Painting and Sculpture from 1755.

According to Mariette, the choice of an adolescent model involved a deliberate and radical departure from the practice of antiquity, since ancient sculptors had chosen for their models fully formed adults. At this date, the superiority of the sculpture of Greek and Roman antiquity to the painting and sculpture of later ages was still universally acknowledged.[7] The most famous ancient statues were regarded as embodying ideal types of finished man- and womanhood. As such, the statues cited in Mariette's letter – the *Farnese Hercules* (fig.5, p.24), the *Apollo Belvedere* (fig.6, p.25), the *Medici Venus* (fig.7, p.26) and the *Belvedere Antinous* (fig.8, p.27) – provided eighteenth-century artists with their models of correct human proportion.

Regard for these masterpieces was reinforced in the minds of artists by the practices of basing both anatomical illustrations and the poses of models in academic life-classes on these and a handful of other ancient statues, notably the *Borghese gladiator* (fig.9, p.28) and the so-called *Dying Gaul* (fig.40, p.175).[8]

What the spectator was being invited to contemplate in the Bouchardon – the accurate representation of a body in transition from one state to another – was therefore something which fell outside the standards set by classical art. The sculptor's decision meant that he sacrificed the authority of the great statues of antiquity in his choice of proportions.[9] It also precluded others from judging his statue by the yardstick of ancient models. Bouchardon thereby distanced his enterprise both from classical tradition and from the practice of his contemporaries insofar as they followed that tradition. But that did not mean that they would have found the course he adopted mysterious. The study of anatomy and the live male model was central to the training of the academic artist, painter or sculptor in the eighteenth century. In practice it was always combined with study of antique models such as those cited by Mariette, but it was the practice of drawing from life which defined the Academy. Life drawing was something to which students had access only after training in drawing after engravings and then after the antique. The *Encyclopédie* described the *Académie de Peinture* as 'a public school where painters go to draw or paint, and sculptors to model, after a

7. See Francis Haskell and Nicholas Penny, *Taste and the antique: the lure of Classical sculpture 1500-1900* (New Haven, CT, and London, 1983). For Mariette's preference for the live model, see Guédron, *De Chair et de marbre*, p.124.
8. Haskell and Penny, *Taste and the antique*, p.5-94.
9. Mariette in Caylus, *Lettre*, p.125-27. In fact, there are ancient statues and gems which represent *Love* as an adolescent attempting to bend a bow and with which Bouchardon is likely to have been familiar. See above, n.6. Winckelmann considered the undeveloped and 'imperfect' forms of children's bodies could inspire only the third and humblest, 'comic' type of grace in ancient art (Winkelmann [J. J. Winckelmann], *Histoire de l'art chez les anciens*, 2 vols (the second in two parts) (Paris, H. J. Jansen, An II/1794-An XI/1803), vol.2, p.34, 36f.).

naked man who is called a *model*'. (The public exhibition of naked female models was of course prohibited on religious grounds.)[10] In spite of its classical subject and precedents, Bouchardon's statue was evidently intended to draw the spectator's attention to its dependence on the live model rather than the ideal figures exhibited by the sculptures of antiquity.

The reception of Bouchardon's statue at the court of Louis XV was not a disaster, but it was not a success, either. It was given two different positions in the state apartments at Versailles before being banished to a less prominent site at a secondary royal residence in 1754, a mere four years after it had been delivered to the Crown. This was an unexpected fate for an expensive and prestigious commission from the man regarded as France's greatest living sculptor. Hostile comment was muted – this was an official commission at a time when the Crown still possessed absolute authority, at least within the court, and those in a position to condemn the work outright may well have hesitated to do so, if only for political reasons. The critical reactions which were recorded were scattered and ambivalent. Unsurprisingly, many of them centred on the activity in which the god was engaged, together with the age at which Bouchardon had chosen to portray him.[11]

Diderot delivered his judgement on the statue in 1763, the year following the sculptor's death, in the *Correspondance littéraire*, an exclusive periodical which avoided official censorship by circulating in manuscript to a select international band of subscribers. It appeared in Diderot's highly critical review of the biography of Bouchardon written by one of the leading figures in French artistic life, the comte de Caylus. Diderot took the viewing of sculpture seriously ('I look at a painting, but I have to enter into dialogue [*m'entretenir*] with a sculpture').[12] The statue of *Love* was the only work by Bouchardon singled out for comment in the review. Although he did not say so, Diderot's observations picked up on the preoccupations of Mariette's 1750 letter to the *Mercure*, which was reprinted as an appendix to Caylus' life. This suggests that they were in part prompted by Mariette's account of the sculpture:

> It seems to me that it requires a lot of time for a child to turn into a bow the massive beam which armed the hand of Hercules. This idea shocks my imagination. I do not like Love employed so long at this manual work.

10. Jean Locquin, *La Peinture d'histoire en France de 1747 à 1785* (Paris, 1912; 1978), p.71-87; Guédron, *De Chair et de marbre*, and, on attitudes to the use of the female nude, p.25-33; on Mariette's views and their relation to the revival of academic interest in life drawing in the middle of the century, p.14f.
11. See Scott, 'Under the sign', p.84-87.
12. Grimm, Friedrich Melchior, *Correspondance littéraire, philosophique et critique, adressée à un souverain d'Allemagne, depuis 1753 jusqu'en 1769, par le baron Grimm et par Diderot. Première partie* (1813), vol.3, p.323.

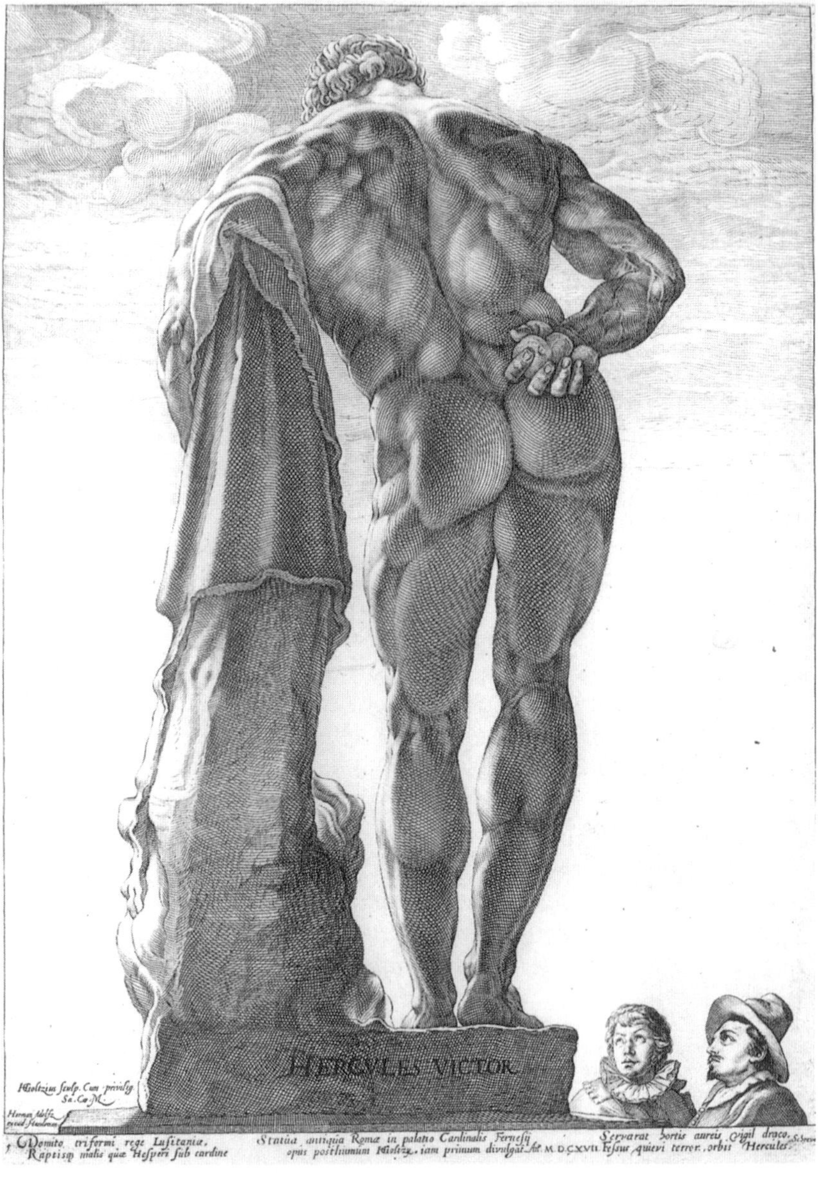
HERCVLES VICTOR
Domito triformi rege Lusitaniæ,
Statua antiqua Romæ in palatio Cardinalis Farnesij
Servarat sortis aureis vigil draco,

Figure 5: Hendrik Goltzius, *The Farnese Hercules*, engraving, *c.*1592, 41 × 30 cm.

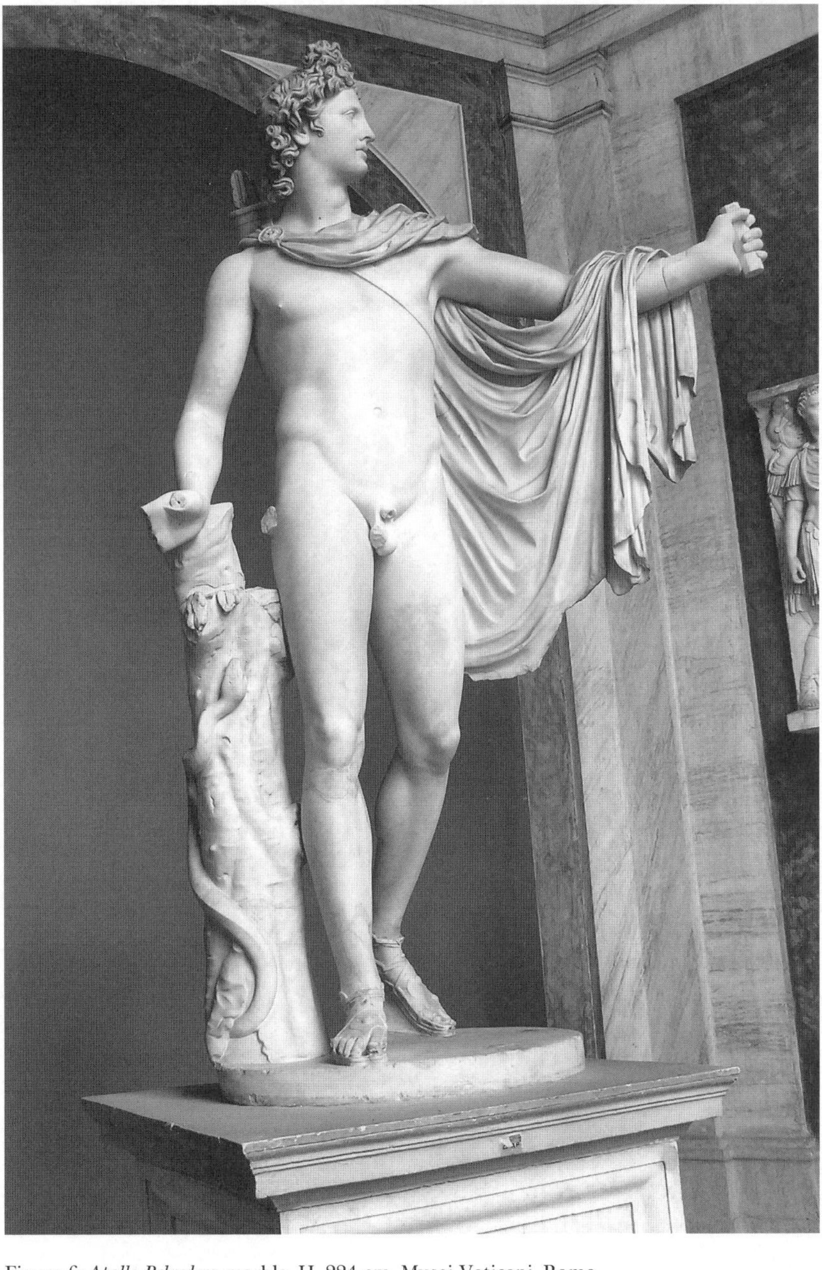

Figure 6: *Apollo Belvedere*, marble, H. 224 cm, Musei Vaticani, Rome.

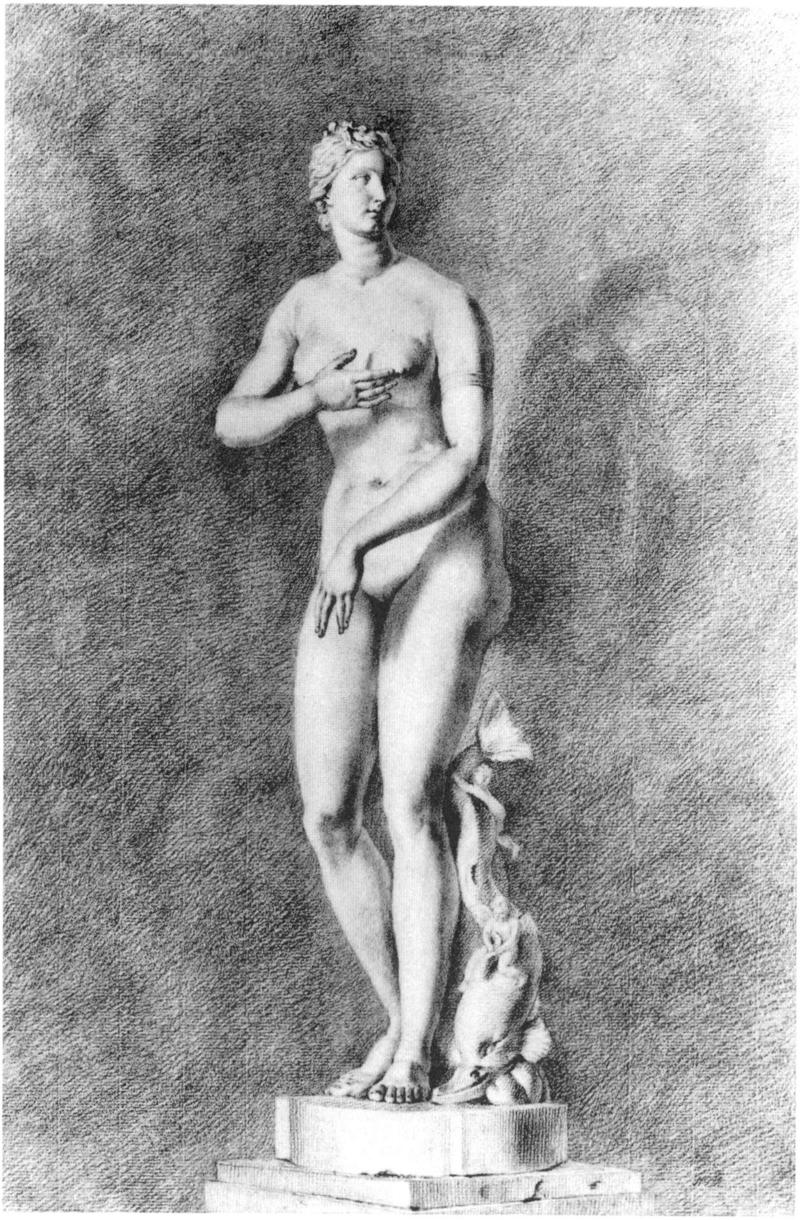

Figure 7: Giovanni Domenico Campiglia, *Statue of Venus with a dolphin, The Medici Venus*, drawing, red chalk, *c.* 1730, 53.7 × 37 cm, National Gallery of Scotland, Edinburgh.

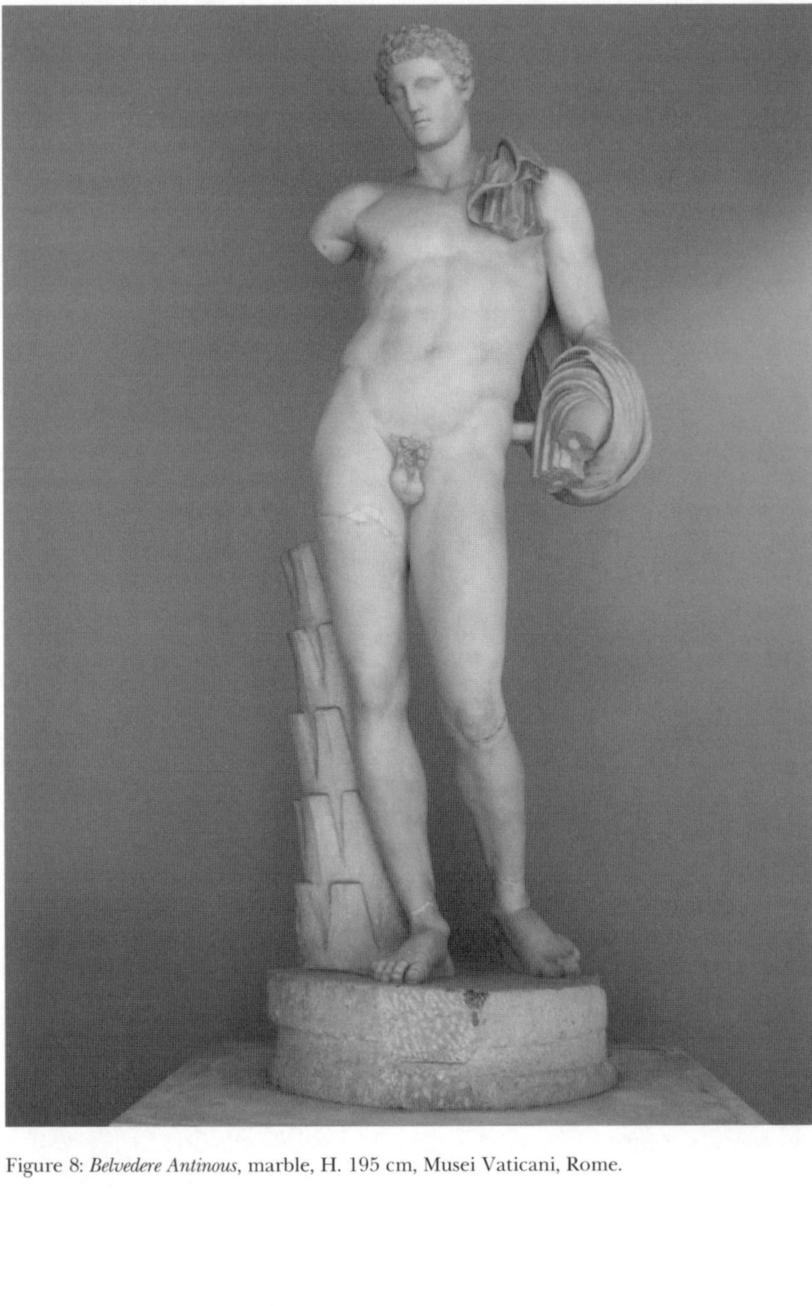

Figure 8: *Belvedere Antinous*, marble, H. 195 cm, Musei Vaticani, Rome.

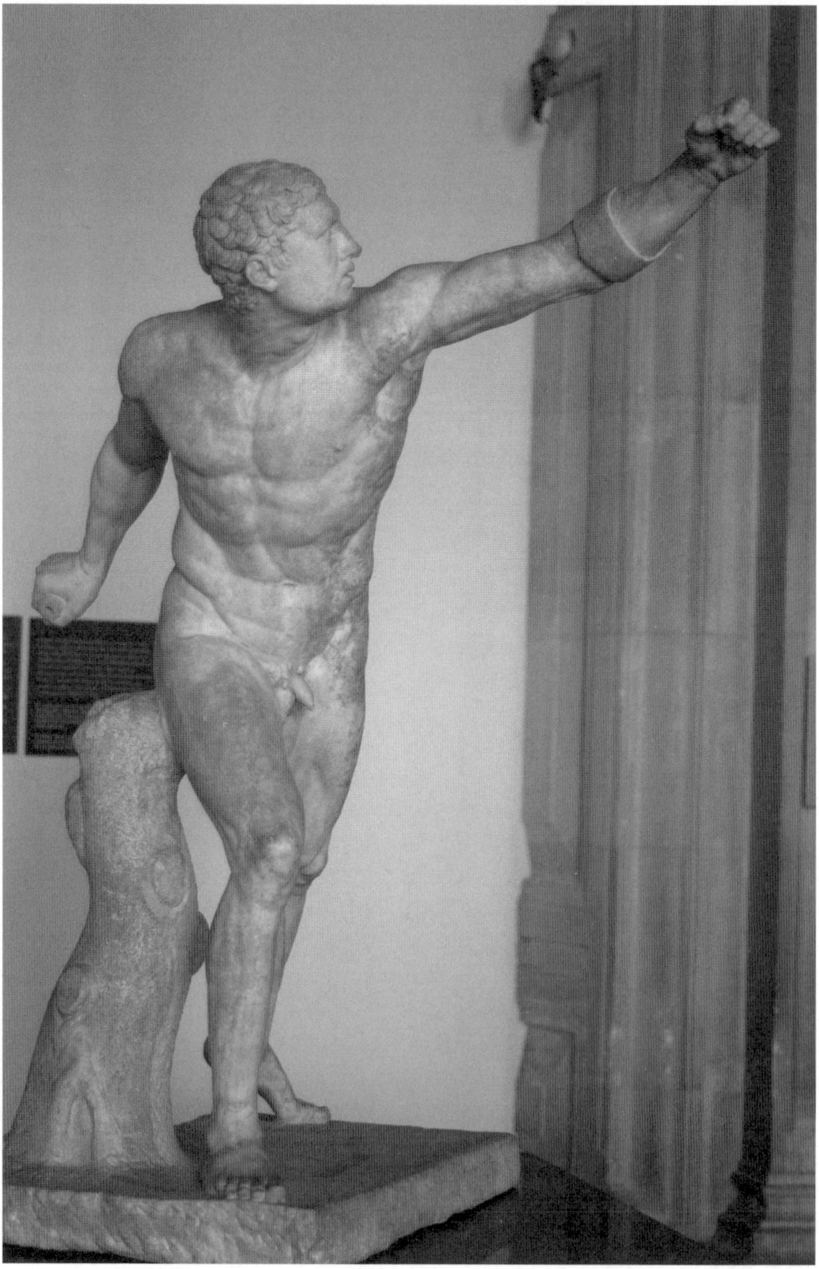

Figure 9: *Borghese gladiator*, marble, H. 199 cm, Musée du Louvre, Paris, Inv. 224.

There followed strictures on the statue's wings, inadequate for flight. Then, evidently affronted by what he regarded as the dismissive attitude exhibited by Mariette and Bouchardon to the authority of ancient sculpture, Diderot sketched a contrast between Bouchardon's approach and what some imaginary Greek or Roman artist might have made of the same subject:

> I think that an ancient, instead of bothering with this ingenious idea, would have tried to show me the tyrant of heaven and earth calm, lovable and frightening. These ancients, once you have got to know them well, become fearful judges of the moderns.

He went on to assert the superiority of classical sculpture to Renaissance painting – a commonplace of eighteenth-century critical opinion – before discussing Bouchardon's drawings.[13]

Diderot was not the only contemporary of Bouchardon to express indignation at the occupation which the sculptor gave to the god Love. The idea that physical labour was demeaning, a necessary but unmitigated ill, was still commonplace in early modern Europe, where it tended to be viewed by Christians as a consequence of the Fall. Critics expressed their distaste at the choice of such a subject accordingly.[14] But it was not the demeaning character of the god's occupation which upset Diderot. It was its duration. If he found it inappropriate that the god of love, the all-powerful 'tyrant of heaven and earth', should have been portrayed in an act of manual labour, he did not say so. Rather, it was the time required to accomplish the task which worried him. Diderot's reaction may well puzzle a modern reader. If there was nothing especially shameful about such activity in itself, how should its prolongation have made it so?

Diderot's position makes more sense if we compare it with a passage in his *Essais sur la peinture* written some three years later. In a chapter entitled 'What everyone knows about expression, and something everyone doesn't know', he set out to explain what he understood to be the effects of expression on appearance. He regarded expression as 'the image of feeling', registering all the 'shifts in his soul' in unequivocal terms on the subject's face and body. Taking as his example a famous ancient statue, the so-called *Belvedere Antinous* – one of those referred to in Mariette's letter to the *Mercure* (fig.8, p.27) – Diderot offered an account of the states of mind and body which were most attractive when registered in facial expression – health ('the cornerstone of

13. [Diderot], 'Fin de l'article sur Bouchardon', in *Correspondance littéraire*, vol.3, p.334.
14. See Scott, 'Under the sign' in *Manifestations of Venus*, ed. Arscott and Scott. For early modern views on labour, see the entry 'travail' in the *Encyclopédie*, and, for overviews, Lucien Febvre, 'Travail: évolution d'un mot et d'une idée', *Journal de psychologie* 21(1948), p.19-29, and Keith Thomas, 'Work and leisure in pre-industrial society', *Past and present* 29 (December 1964), p.50-62.

happiness'), serenity (the quality which he had imagined in an ancient statue of the god Love when he wrote his critique of Bouchardon), and an air of 'thoughtfulness and wisdom'. He explained how only slight alterations in the statue's expression would destroy the pleasure felt when looking at it. Although he acknowledged that people were attracted by different types of expression at different ages, according to their changing hopes and expectations of others, he maintained that they were generally drawn to those whose expression conformed with their idea of virtue, and repelled by those whose expression suggested vice. How could such readings be reliable or even possible? In large part because, according to Diderot, people acquired a habitual expression corresponding with the dominant passions and occupations of their lives. As an example of the effects of habit on the expression, not merely of the face, but of the body as a whole, Diderot described the expressions of Parisian street urchins and their transformation as they evolved into market traders:

> In the heart of the Saint-Marcel quarter, where I lived for a long time, I saw many children with charming faces. By the age of twelve or thirteen their eyes full of sweetness had turned calculating and intense, their pleasing little mouths had become oddly contorted, their rounded necks swollen with muscles, their ample cheeks marred by coarse bumps. They'd taken on the physiognomy of the market and the exchange. Driven to anger, insult, combat, cries, and humiliation in their pursuit of money, they'd acquired an air of sordid calculation, impudence, and wrath that would remain with them for the rest of their lives.[15]

This passage demonstrates the power of habit as Diderot and his contemporaries conceived it to transform both character and appearance. What changed angelic infants into aggressive and uncouth adults were the habits they contracted as street traders and porters. The changes which their way of life effected in their outward appearance were matched by corresponding transformations of character. Indeed, it is clear from Diderot's account that he saw the two types of change as part of the same process. That deformity of the spirit which resulted from a life dedicated to the mental and physical struggle for gain waged in competition with others was marked by the outward deformity of face and body – most obviously and unambiguously, by the undue muscular development which was the consequence of persistent physical exertion.

15. Denis Diderot, *Notes on painting* in *Diderot on art*, translated by John Goodman, 2 vols (New Haven, CT, and London, 1995), vol.1, p.210-12. The literature on expression is extensive. See, in particular, J. Montagu, *The Expression of the passions: the origin and influence of Charles Lebrun's conférence sur l'expression générale et particulière* (New Haven, CT, and London, 1994), R. Démoris, 'Les passions en peinture au dix-huitième siècle', in *Le Siècle de Voltaire. Hommage à René Pomeau*, ed. C. Mervaud and S. Menant, 2 vols (Oxford, 1987), vol.1, p.381-92.

In the case of the market trader, such deformity was registered in the muscles of the neck, swollen by carrying heavy weights, and the mouth and face, distorted by shouting. The effects of the habits of labour and self-interest on these human subjects are close to those which Buffon described in the case of the woodpecker – powerfully muscled necks, harsh looks, raucous voices and a lack of sociability or finer feeling. (According to David Garrioch, the street traders of eighteenth-century Paris tended to be unskilled and self-employed, 'lacking the centralised structure and official hierarchy of the corporate trades'.[16] It may therefore have been the case that such workers did to some extent lack the ties which Diderot might have interpreted as evidence of sociability.)

The views expressed in this passage on the ways in which habitual experience shaped identity depended essentially on the psychological theories of Locke and Condillac (a friend of Diderot). According to these two philosophers, the consciousness of the newborn child was a blank, devoid of innate ideas. What formed individual human consciousness was the succession of sensations which the individual received from outside – hence the label 'sensualist' which has been used, sometimes pejoratively, to describe their psychology.[17] Sensualist theory provided an essentially passive model of the formation of human identity. It also left little room, if any, for concepts of innate difference. The individual subject was formed by sensation, and was thus in principle at the mercy of any experiences which came its way. What transformed the marks of random experience into fixed character was habit. This was achieved by sheer dint of repetition. Habit could thus account for the link between expression and experience assumed by Diderot. It could also be seen as a determining cause, if not *the* determining cause, of difference between individuals. The habitual occupations and preoccupations of everyday life gave outward form to the muscles of the face and body as surely as

16. 'The master–journeyman relationship was absent, most street porters being self-employed. [...] They were not linked by common membership of a highly skilled occupation, by a city-wide corporate identity, or by a shared relationship with a master', David Garrioch, *Neighbourhood and community in Paris, 1740-1790* (Cambridge, 1986), p.115. On the poverty of the faubourg Saint-Marcel, see David Garrioch, *The Formation of the Parisian Bourgeoisie 1690-1830* (Cambridge, MA, 1996), p.10-12.

17. See K. M. Figlio, 'Theories of perception and the physiology of mind in the late eighteenth century', *History of science* 13 (1975), p.177-212, and the discussion in Tony Halliday, *Facing the public: portraiture in the aftermath of the French Revolution* (Manchester and New York, 2000), p.13-15, with further references. For the importance still accorded to habit by the *Institut*, see Martin S. Staum, *Minerva's message: stabilizing the French Revolution* (Montreal and Kingston, 1996), p.110-13. For an account of the mechanisms whereby habit was supposed to affect the appearance of the human body, see that in T. B. Eméric-David, *Recherches sur l'art statuaire considéré chez les anciens et chez les modernes* (1805; Paris, 1863), p.34. Eméric-David's memoir was originally a submission to an *Institut* competition crowned in the year IX/1800.

they shaped inner character. This applied to a market porter just as it did to a king or a priest.[18] The individual human consciousness had little or no means of resisting the effects of habit. The coarsening effect of their lifestyle on the inhabitants of the faubourg Saint-Marcel described by Diderot was thus a process which he could not but view as inevitable. Diderot's discussion stressed the affinity of native virtue for its counterpart in others, and flattered his readers by taking for granted their own virtuous inclinations. But his description of the street children makes it clear that they too once possessed such virtue, manifest in their originally angelic expression and comportment. We are left to conclude that Diderot himself, not to mention his readers, would have had no defence against a similar deformation of character had they been born into equally disadvantageous circumstances. Such was precisely the view expressed by Diderot's Scottish contemporary, Adam Smith, a few years later.[19] In practice, Diderot's endorsement of sensualist psychology was more qualified than Smith's and a good deal less complacent. As will be seen, he had important reservations about its sufficiency to explain every aspect of behaviour, and these increased towards the end of his life. But there is no question that it provided the overall framework within which he understood the formation of human character.

We are now in a position to appreciate why the question of duration bothered Diderot so much when he contemplated Bouchardon's *Love*. In one respect, that of strenuous physical labour, the experience of the children of the faubourg Saint-Marcel was matched by that which Diderot foresaw for the subject of Bouchardon's statue – the god, or possibly the model who posed as the god, since the statue was generally believed to have been based on a single individual.[20] Love might look blithe and innocent at this intermediary point in his labours, but so did the inhabitants of the faubourg Saint-Marcel at the outset of their own doomed careers. Armed with Diderot's foreknowledge, we cannot but

18. A view which Diderot expounded in greater detail in his *Salon of 1769*. See the discussion in Halliday, *Facing the public*, p.13. For a more detailed account of the process whereby habit was presumed to operate on expression, see ch.15 of Hogarth's *Analysis of beauty*, in William Hogarth, *Works* (London, 1838), vol.3, p.141, a text with which Diderot was familiar.

19. 'The difference between the most dissimilar characters, between a philosopher and a common street porter, for example, seems to arise not so much from nature as from habit, custom and education. When they came into the world, and for the first six or eight years of their existence, they were perhaps very much alike [...]. About that age, or soon after, they came to be employed in very different occupations. The difference of talents comes then to be taken notice of, and widens by degrees, till at last the vanity of the philosopher is willing to acknowledge scarce any resemblance', in Adam Smith, *The Wealth of nations* (1776), ed. Andrew Skinner (Oxford, 1978), p.120.

20. Etienne Falconet, *Œuvres*, 6 vols (Lausanne, 1781), vol.3, p.88. The surviving drawings bear this out (Scott, 'Under the sign', p.74).

foresee Love's transformation as a process of moral and physical degradation. The fact that Bouchardon's god is represented as a boy of a similar age to that of the children described by Diderot immediately prior to experiencing the corruption of the market place (twelve or thirteen years) only serves to reinforce the melancholy presentiment. When he contrasted Bouchardon's *Love* with the way a classical sculptor might have depicted the same god as 'the tyrant of heaven and earth calm, lovable and frightening', Diderot evidently envisaged a more secure and less effortful model. He may well have had in mind the terms in which Mariette had described the treatment of human physique by ancient sculptors. Following the indication given by Mariette, such a portrayal of the god would have given him the appearance either of a child or of a stable and fully-formed human being, proof against the degradations of habit.

Distasteful though he found it to contemplate in Bouchardon's statue, the effect of habitual activity and especially that of heavy labour on physical appearance and moral identity was something to which Diderot repeatedly returned. As Angelica Goodden has observed, 'Diderot's interest in the question of the body's adaptability became almost obsessive'.[21] This was surely because of the equivalence which he perceived between the effects of habit on the formation of the body and on that of the mind. He evidently believed that marks of adaptation in the body constituted a visible and inseparable component of the process which produced individual human identity as a whole. It was difficult for someone who subscribed to a sensualist psychology to picture the formation of character in any other way.

If the porters and market traders of the faubourg Saint-Marcel provided Diderot with a human equivalent to Buffon's woodpecker, where did he find his doves? Not, as one might expect, in one of the city's more affluent quarters, the faubourg Saint-Germain or the faubourg Saint-Honoré. Instead, the discussion in the *Essais sur la peinture* cited above transports us abruptly from urban Paris to the primal forest of Enlightenment myth:

> Each mode of living has its own character and expression.
> The savage has features that are solid, vigorous and pronounced, shaggy hair, a full beard, the most fully developed limbs: how could it have been otherwise? He's hunted, run, fought against wild beasts, exerted himself; he's managed to survive, and has engendered his like: the only two natural

21. *Diderot and the body* (Oxford, 2001), p.55. My reading of Diderot's critique differs from that of Jean Seznec, who did not relate Diderot's strictures to Mariette's comments, interpreting them rather in the light of Diderot's views on the use of allegory. See J. Seznec, *Essais sur Diderot et l'antiquité: the Mary Flexner lectures delivered at Bryn Mawr College, Pennsylvania* (Oxford, 1957), p.35-37.

> endeavours. There's nothing about him that's touched with impudence or shame. Rather an air of pride mixed with ferocity. His head is erect, held high. His gaze is penetrating. He's the master of his forest. The longer I consider him, the more he reminds me of the solitude and freedom of his domain. When he speaks, his gestures are imperious, his remarks energetic and brief. He is without law and without prejudice. His soul is quick to anger. He is in a state of perpetual war. He is flexible, he is agile; but he is strong.[22]

Unlike the inhabitant of the faubourg Saint-Marcel, the savage is endowed by Diderot with a mate – a female companion. Her manners are equally distant from those of her civilised counterpart. She is not ashamed of her nudity, and is ready to share the hardships of her husband's freely wandering life. Her looks are less fierce, however, and she is more easily frightened, thereby ensuring a measure of 'natural' dependency.

In their freedom to roam and their affectionate and harmonious love life, Diderot's savages resemble Bewick's doves, but the description of their habits is couched in different and broader terms. We are told that the male savage inhabits a forest, but not what sort of forest, that he lives by hunting, but not what or how he hunts, or how he asserts or maintains his mastery in the forest. This is not natural history. It is a rhetorical construction, fashioned to provide a contrast, not merely with the account of life in the faubourg Saint-Marcel which immediately precedes it, but with the life of civilised humanity in general. The savage woman's lack of interest in clothes, for example, is not the fruit of anthropological observation, but part of a standard discourse of denunciation directed against the appetite for fashionable and extravagant dress attributed to women by male writers in eighteenth-century society. On the other hand, this is scarcely a blueprint for practical reform. Diderot cannot have expected Parisian women completely to sacrifice clothes to an ideal of simple living. And if hunting and reproduction were the only two natural occupations, where did that leave those of the inhabitants of contemporary Paris – its philosophers, as well as its street traders? But if this diatribe was not intended to be taken seriously as natural history or as social prescription, it was nonetheless intended to be taken seriously. As a means of articulating criticism of contemporary institutions against which an author wished to protest, the appeal to a more or less fictional model of nature was a common enough device. It provided writers with a means of sanctifying as natural social institutions of which they approved (in this case, for example, the subordination of women to men in families) while damning as unnatural those which they disliked.[23] Unlike

22. *Diderot on art*, vol.1, p.210-12.

23. See, for example, Ludmilla Jordanova's observations in *Languages of nature: critical essays on science and literature*, ed. L. Jordanova (London, 1986), p.36-40, and, specifically on Diderot,

Bewick's accounts of the woodpecker and the dove, Diderot's descriptions of the street trader and the savage of the forest were juxtaposed, and he juxtaposed them with a clear polemical intention – that of making the reader uneasy about contemporary social organisation and what one aspect of that organisation – its reliance on the division of labour – did to people.

The contrast in physical appearance between man in society and man in nature is raised elsewhere in Diderot's writings, notably in the entry *Homme* (Man) in the *Encyclopédie,* the gigantic enterprise which he edited partly in conjunction with the mathematician d'Alembert. The *Encyclopédie* occupied most of Diderot's own working life and it was the project for which he became most famous. This article, an overview of the human condition, opens with a bitter-sweet paean to the dignity of Man [*sic*] and his achievements:

> a feeling, reflecting, thinking being who roams freely over the surface of the earth, who appears to be at the head of all the other animals which he dominates, who lives in society, who has discovered the sciences and the arts, who possesses a goodness and a malice peculiar to himself, who has given himself masters, who has made himself laws, etc.

Much of Diderot's description of man depends, like Bewick's account of the woodpecker, on Buffon. Diderot contented himself with occasional interjections of irony at those aspects of the human condition which he accepted with less equanimity than his Christian contemporaries, such as the brevity of life expectancy (according to Buffon, most human beings still died by the age of eight in eighteenth-century Europe). He also suppressed passages in Buffon which expressed views he did not agree with – notably Buffon's low opinion of physiognomics, the science of reading individual character through facial characteristics.[24] He also drew his readers' attention to the different proportions of the human body in the state of nature and in that of society:

> In the state of nature, the man who most easily performed all the animal functions would without contradiction be the best made, and conversely the best made would most easily perform all the animal functions, but it is not like this in the state of society. Each craft, each skill, each action demands peculiar arrangements of the limbs, given sometimes by Nature, or acquired by habit, but always at the expense of the most beautiful and the most regular proportions. Even the dancer, forced to support the weight of his body on the tip of his foot, will in time develop a disfigurement of this part

D. G. Charlton, *New images of the natural in France: a study in European cultural history 1750-1800. The Gifford lectures in the University of St Andrews 1982-1983* (Cambridge, 1984), p.127-29.

24. Jean Mayer, *Diderot, homme de science* (Rennes, 1959), p.329. Diderot's own faith in physiognomics is demonstrated in the chapter from the *Essais sur la peinture* discussed above.

> from the point of view of the sculptor who has set himself the goal of representing a well-made *man*, and not a dancer.
> It follows that the man of nature, he whom she had pleased to fashion in the most perfect manner, might perhaps excel at nothing; and that the artist who imitates nature would have to change all the proportions, according to the rôle in society into which he transfers him. If he wants to turn him into a docker [*crocheteur*], he will compress the thighs and thicken the legs; he will broaden the shoulders and bend the back; and so for the other occupations as well.[25]

Here once more the difference between man in nature and man in society was interpreted in terms of the effects of specialised labour and measured in terms of physical appearance. As in the *Essais sur la peinture*, Diderot presented those effects not merely as changing, but as deforming the body of man in society, and again he chose as one of his examples the effects wrought by a physically taxing and strenuous form of labour – that of the docker. The tone is more ironical, but the implied judgement on the effects of civilisation on human physique is nonetheless negative, even if the moral implication of those effects is not spelled out. But the note of condemnation was by no means always dominant in his treatment of this subject, particularly when he was offering guidance to artists whose job it was to represent humanity in a variety of situations. A recurrent theme in these and other discussions was the problems and challenges which the transformation of the body by occupation created for accurate artistic representation. In common with many of his contemporaries, Diderot believed that the character of the world and of human beings could be made sense of in terms of appearance. Beauty and deformity in the human form attested to the nature of an individual's formative experience. It was important from Diderot's point of view that the correspondence between experience and appearance should be legible and reliable. Artists, as specialists in the observation and interpretation of visible nature, had a special duty to realise that correspondence. If social experience transformed the body, then should not the successful work of art register such transformation? However unwelcome or even devastating the effects of social formation or deformation might be from a humanitarian point of view, they were what chiefly enabled artists and even writers to individuate character in representations of modern society. Failure to attend to them led to loss of verisimilitude. This is the argument of the first chapter of the *Essais sur la peinture*, 'My bizarre thoughts about drawing', which opens with reflections on how disabilities affect the comportment and appearance of the body as a whole. This leads into a critique of the way art

25. *Encyclopédie*, s.v. 'homme', 256b-259a.

students were taught to draw the body, and in particular a denunciation of practices in academic life classes, where the same model was made to assume a variety of poses, each of which was associated with a social role whose regular performance would have shaped the body differently in real life. Where did this emphasis on the deforming marks of experience leave the man of nature, the ideal man unmarked by specialised activity who was extolled elsewhere in the *Essais sur la peinture* and in the *Encyclopédie* article on Man? Nowhere, apparently:

> If I were initiated into art's mysteries, perhaps I'd know to what extent the artist should conform to accepted proportions, and I'd tell you; I do know, however, that they don't stand up against the despotism of nature, and that age and social condition dictate that they be sacrificed in a hundred different ways. I've never heard of a figure dismissed as badly drawn when its exterior organisation revealed its age and its capacity and custom of fulfilling its daily tasks. It is these tasks that determine both a figure's overall stature and the true proportions of its bodily members and their mutual consistency. It's from these that I see emerge the child, and the adult, and the old man; and the savage, and the civilised man; the magistrate, and the soldier, and the porter. If ever a figure would be difficult to capture, it would be that of a twenty-five-year-old suddenly formed out of clay, and who'd never done anything, but this man is a chimaera.[26]

'Accepted proportions' here refers to those ancient statues such as the *Belvedere Antinous* and the *Medici Venus* which artists were expected to take as models, while the impossible man formed fully grown from clay is none other than the Adam of biblical myth.[27] If the task of art was to represent credible human individuals formed in the real, postlapsarian world – individuals who appeared convincingly different from each other as a result of their different experiences of life – then the artist's starting point must be the rejection of such ideal stereotypes. That was the course Diderot had already proposed in his *Discours de la poésie dramatique* of 1758, where he had suggested that dramatists should study the way sculptors treated the effects of habitual occupation on physique and comportment in order to learn how to portray difference of character in the theatre.[28]

26. *Diderot on art*, vol.1, p.192.
27. As is evident from Diderot's 1760 review of Watelet's *Art de peindre* (*Correspondance littéraire*, vol.3, p.1-11) from which the text in the *Essais sur la peinture* in part derives.
28. 'Study bows the man of letters. Drill stiffens the soldier's step and raises his head. The habit of carrying burdens compresses the docker's midriff. The pregnant woman holds her head back. The hunchback holds his limbs differently to the upright man. These are the observations which, infinitely multiplied, educate the sculptor, teach him to change, strengthen, weaken, disfigure and reduce his ideal model from the state of nature to whatever state he pleases. It is the study of the passions, manners, characters and customs which teach the painter of man to change his model, and to reduce it from the state of

Similar concerns reappear in a *Question d'anatomie et de physiologie* addressed to a doctor, in which Diderot claimed to be gathering information for a lecture to be given to art students in St Petersburg. He asked the doctor to picture a lazybones [*fainéant*] of twenty-five years who had never done anything, and who had consequently preserved a body as beautiful as those drawn by the Renaissance painter Raphaël. What would happen, Diderot wanted to know, if such a man took up highway robbery in the manner of the demi-god Hercules. How would his new job affect his body, his expression, his mind? What would the effect then be if he gave up this new career, developed passions, incurred a disability?[29] This passage casts the man of nature in a new light – as unemployed man – although the terms used to describe the visible effects of physical exertion on his appearance (*altération, souffrir*) remain negative. It illustrates another paradox which Diderot's view of the effects of experience on the body necessarily entails: unlike the socially trained and socially useful man whose body and mind have been formed or deformed by his labours, the man who has never done anything, who is no more than an encumbrance on society, may have a body as beautiful as any imagined by a great artist – much like the dove, according to Bewick's account, among birds.

How is one to reconcile this Diderot with the one who was so disturbed by his encounter with Bouchardon's statue of Love, and who turned from it to the example set by ancient sculptors with such enthusiasm? This was a problem which evidently troubled Diderot himself. He returned to it more than once in his art criticism – in the reviews which he wrote for the *Correspondance littéraire* of the Salons, the exhibitions of paintings and sculpture by members of the French Academy held biennially at the Louvre. His reviews of the Salons of 1765 and 1767 both contain extended discussions of beauty with specific reference to the representation of the human form, although they reach somewhat different conclusions. In the *Salon of 1765*, Diderot's position is close to that set

---

man to that of good or bad, calm or angry man'. *Diderot, Œuvres esthétiques*, ed. P. Vernière (Paris, 1965), p.286. The sequel makes it clear that 'painter of man' describes the dramatist as well as the painter.

29. Diderot, 'Question d'anatomie et de physiologie', in Diderot, (ed.) J. Assézat and M. Tourneux, *Œuvres complètes* (1878-1879), vol.9, p.239-49. Diderot's editors print two responses from doctors; one, Diderot's friend, Petit, did not think that artists should bother very much with anatomy – detailed observation of people in everyday life should suffice. The other, anonymous respondent questioned whether mugging was a usual or an appropriate career choice for someone unaccustomed to physical exercise. He pointed out that important changes to the body resulting from exercise usually took place in the years preceding the age of twenty-five. He provided the sort of information Diderot asked for in some detail, both as regards the formation of muscles and the effect of habitual expression of the passions on the face.

forth in his earlier writings, though it is formulated in terms largely borrowed from the English artist and author William Hogarth.[30] Some observations on the *Farnese Hercules* (fig.5, p.24) inspire a digression on scale leading to a detailed examination of the proportions of that statue and the indications which they provide of relative muscular development. The strongly muscled neck is accorded particular significance as an index of strength – as it was in Diderot's description of the traders of the faubourg Saint-Marcel, or in Buffon's description of the woodpecker, for that matter. Diderot also observes that the head and feet of the statue are not increased in scale proportionately to the whole, an observation which he derived from Hogarth, who had added that this was 'contrary to all modern rule of enlarging every part in proportion'.[31] In a comparison which Diderot also owed to Hogarth, the proportions of this statue are contrasted with those of two others, the *Mercury* and the [*Belvedere*] *Antinous* (fig.8, p.27). Like Hogarth, Diderot saw the *Antinous* as occupying an intermediary position between the Hercules on the one hand and the more slightly built Mercury on the other. Unlike Hogarth, however, Diderot did not therefore regard the *Antinous* as the embodiment of the ideal, at least from a moral viewpoint. Instead, in language which recalls that which he applied to the hypothetical lazybones in the *Question d'anatomie et de physiologie*, he dismissed the statue as 'a man without a social function, a sluggard [*fainéant*] who's never accomplished anything, whose circumstances haven't altered his proportions at all. Hercules is the extreme of the working man, Antinous is the extreme of the lazy man'.[32] Diderot thus arrives at a similar paradox to that found in the *Question* – in terms of physique, the Antinous exemplified an ideal from which any variation could only represent a falling-off, yet at the same time the personal history to which that physique bore witness was morally unattractive because socially useless.

30. See the account in Seznec, *Essais sur Diderot*, p.23-42, to which the following discussion is indebted.

31. *Analysis of beauty* (ch.1) in Hogarth, *Works* (London, 1838), vol.3, p.35.

32. Diderot, *The Salon of 1765*, in *Diderot on art*, vol.1, p.66. Diderot replaced Hogarth's *Atlas* with the *Farnese Hercules*. The *Mercury* is probably the statue whose marble original is now in Florence (Haskell and Penny, *Taste and the antique*, no.61). There was a tradition in antiquity of placing statues of three male deities together in gymnasia – those of Eros (Love), Hermes (Mercury) and Hercules, since they excelled in friendship, eloquence and courage respectively; the unity of these three qualities being considered to produce harmony of character (Athenaeus, 13:56D). There is a precedent for Diderot's invidious comparison of the *Hercules*, this time with the *Apollo Belvedere*, in *De la poésie dramatique* (*Œuvres esthétiques*, p.217), although Diderot was more hesitant about condemning the Apollo when he made a similar comparison in a letter of 1762 to Sophie Volland – a letter which fleetingly confronted his two conceptions of the beautiful see Diderot, *Correspondance*, ed. Roth and Varloot (Paris, 1955-1970), vol.4 (1958), p.129 (no.277).

The discussion in the *Salon of 1767* is both more far reaching and more difficult to reconcile with Diderot's earlier views. Diderot presents a frankly idealist theory of beauty. He is critical of those who claimed that the beautiful is to be found in the real world (*la belle nature*). The notion of *la belle nature*, he asserts, is itself ideal. It belongs to the realm of the imagination, not reality. A portrait, even of a beautiful woman, could claim only a third-order relationship to ideal beauty. It is merely an artist's copy of an individual instance of beauty in the real world – itself for that reason secondary to the general idea, which is the highest form of beauty. Even the artist who painted the portrait of the beautiful woman would not be faithful to his model in all details, but would add or subtract something according to his own inner sense of what constituted beauty. Diderot cites a famous passage from Plato's *Republic* in support of his theory, but makes it clear that the form in which he uses it derived from 'the modern Plato', by which he means the contemporary German historian of classical art, J. J. Winckelmann.[33] To support his claim that the general idea could nowhere be found in nature, Diderot used his by now familiar argument about the deforming effects of habit and experience. Now, however, he included among the habits which vitiated natural beauty even those employments of the savage which he had described in the *Essais sur la peinture* as 'the only two natural endeavours', hunting and reproduction. Even Nature deforms. Where, then, was the artist to find a model of what was beautiful in the human form? From the antique – that is, from statues such as the *Antinous*, the *Apollo Belvedere* and the *Medici Venus*. But how had the sculptors who had created these masterpieces arrived at the general idea of beauty? As Diderot observes, they had no antiquity of their own to fall back on. He rejects the view that the embodiment of ideal human proportion for ancient artists – the canon or 'rule' of the ancient Greek sculptor Polyclitus – was based on a synthesis of beautiful parts derived from different existing bodies, the so-called selective *beau idéal*.[34] How, without a prior notion of what constituted beauty, Diderot wanted to know, could the ancients have

33. *Diderot on art*, 2:9-15. See also Annie Becq, *Genèse de l'esthétique française moderne 1680-1814* (1984; Paris, 1994), p.535-37. On Diderot and Winckelmann, see Jacques Chouillet, *La Formation des idées esthétiques de Diderot 1745-1763* (Paris, 1973), p.486-87; Else-Marie Bukdahl, *Diderot critique d'art. II. Diderot, les salonniers et les esthéticiens de son temps*, translated by Jacques Piloz (Copenhagen, 1982), p.50-54; Edouard Pommier, 'Winckelmann et la vision de l'antiquité classique dans la France des Lumières et de la Révolution', *Revue de l'art* 83 (1989), p.9-20.

34. Diderot, *Œuvres esthétiques*, p.2. For an account of Polyclitus' canon, see ch.4, below. Jaucourt, writing for the *Encyclopédie*, maintained that the canon was based on the selective *beau idéal* (vol.14, p.25 (s.v. 'règle')). The idea of a selective *beau idéal* was often linked to the story of the Greek painter Zeuxis, who was said to have composed a representation of Venus from the various beauties of individual women inhabitants of the southern Italian city of Crotona. See Régis Michel, *Le Beau idéal* (Paris, 1989), p.47.

made such a choice? According to him, they found ideal beauty, not by selective imitation, but by long observation, experiment, taste, instinct, 'a kind of inspiration vouchsafed only to rare geniuses, and perhaps a project, natural to idolaters, to elevate man above his condition and impress a divine character upon him, a character from which all that is contentious in our paltry, impoverished, shabby, and miserable lives had been excluded',[35] they had become aware of the most obvious deformities and had gradually extended that awareness to even the most minute details of the human body. They were thereby able to eliminate the defects of daily life – what Seznec called the stigmata of servitude[36] – in a process akin to that described in relation to the three statues in the *Salon of 1765*. This passage indicates that Diderot absorbed not merely Winckelmann's notion of ideal beauty, but his historicist explanation of the appearance of Greek art. According to Winckelmann, the superiority of Greek sculpture resulted from climate and from superior political, cultural and, as in Diderot's reference to the 'worshipper of idols', religious mores.[37] How then was the ideal to be attained in modern times, when these institutions were relatively decayed? Perhaps only, suggests Diderot, by a return to a state of barbarity – it would only be then that artists would become sufficiently aware of their ignorance to undertake the necessary research. Artists in more advanced eras 'remain mediocre simply because they are born knowing, so to speak'. They regard nature as though it were perfect rather than perfectible, so that they are content to copy nature for its own sake, and not in order to discover the ideal.[38]

The invocation of Greek cultural difference may have enabled Diderot to offer an historical explanation of his different views on the representation of the body, but there remains a fundamental contradiction between the two theories of imitation which underlie his prescriptions. The views set forth in earlier writings, such as the *Discours de la poésie dramatique*, the *Essais sur la peinture* and the *Question d'anatomie et de physiologie* can all be interpreted as expressing a more or less conscientious application to the question of the beauty of the human form – both its physical embodiment and its representation in art – of definitions of beauty which he had offered in the article *Beau* in the *Encyclopédie* (1751).

35. Diderot, *Œuvres esthétiques*, p.12.

36. Seznec, *Essais sur Diderot*, p.24.

37. See, for example, Winckelmann, *Histoire de l'art chez les anciens*, 2 vols (Paris, an II/1794-an XI/1803), vol.1, p.328 and, for religion, 368f. See also Diderot's own comments on Winckelmann in his *Salon de 1765*, in *Diderot on art*, vol.1, p.157.

38. Diderot, *Salon of 1767*, in *Diderot on art*, p.13-14. Later in the same *Salon* (p.26-28) there is an outburst against the representation of strenuous physical labour (in Hallé's *Scilurus ou la force de l'union*) whose vehemence recalls Diderot's reaction to Bouchardon's *Love*.

There he had suggested, among other things, that beauty consisted in justly proportioned relationships. If one part of a body was affected by particular circumstance, such as labour or injury, the whole body would change as a result. Such a body would be justly proportioned and thus in a measure beautiful because it obeyed the laws of natural necessity, which endowed it with inner coherence. As is clear from passages such as those in the first chapter of the *Essais sur la peinture* and the *Discours de la poésie dramatique*, this aesthetic also embraced the representation of deformity. Hence Diderot's repeated stress on the need to study the body as a whole, his strictures on life-classes in the *Essais sur la peinture* – they utilised models whose physique was inappropriate to the actions they were represented as performing – and his endorsement in the *Salon of 1765* of the non-canonical aspects of the Farnese Hercules identified by Hogarth – they were correct because they registered the actual effect of labour on the body. But the theory of ideal beauty according to Plato or Winckelmann which Diderot explicitly endorsed in the *Salon of 1767* presupposed a different basis for recognising beauty – a 'general idea' anterior to the marks which external experience would imprint on the body. It too accorded a place to deformity, but only as that which detracted from the beautiful – the negative which helped to define it, not its potential ingredient.[39]

These inconsistencies of position are usually interpreted in terms of aesthetic theory and, in particular, in relation to Diderot's own aesthetic preoccupations as critic and as original dramatist. What such interpretations leave out becomes evident if we take into account his earlier reaction to Bouchardon's statue and Mariette's account of it. At first glance, Bouchardon's minutely observed representation of an adolescent body at work appears to conform well enough with Diderot's repeated demands for minute attention to the conformation and modification of the human body. Yet Diderot rejected Bouchardon's approach in favour of the example set by the ancients in statues such as the *Antinous* – the idealised creations extolled by Winckelmann whose unblemished proportions Diderot elsewhere pilloried as those of a *fainéant*. He thus sketched out the issues to which he would return in greater detail in the *Salon of 1767*. It is evident that Diderot's misgivings about Bouchardon's statue did not originate in a concern with such aesthetic issues as realism, idealism or the sublime, even though they can be interpreted in terms of these labels. Had they done so, they might have been more easily resolved. The pain with which he reacted to Bouchardon's statue, and the uneasiness which impelled him to return

39. See Becq, *Genèse*, p.540.

to these issues in the *Salons* of 1765 and 1767, derived from elsewhere in his experience. It was Diderot's preoccupation with the moral and physical consequences of the division of labour which gave colour and weight to his aesthetic speculations. If we assume that his views on individual works of art originated in a preoccupation with art theory or that the concerns which drove them were primarily aesthetic, we risk falling into an error similar to that of which Diderot accused those academic painters and sculptors who ignored the study of real bodies in favour of unreflective devotion to theoretical models.

Why should Diderot have minded so much about the relationship of occupation to appearance and in particular its effects on the bodies and minds of those subjected, like the children of the faubourg Saint-Marcel, to harsh physical labour? His contemporaries by and large accepted the street urchin's lot with the same equanimity as that with which Buffon and Bewick regarded the fate of the woodpecker. It was God in his wisdom who had ordained that the woodpecker should toil its life away while the dove snacked and flirted, and equally it was He who had ordained that the children of the faubourg Saint-Marcel should lose their angelic innocence in the strenuous and competitive habits of the market place. The habits of the labouring and marketing poor insured that they would develop characteristic expressions and modes of behaviour as surely as the woodpecker developed its powerful beak and its raucous voice. The question of cause and effect – of why either the woodpecker or the children of the poor should be as they were – could safely be subsumed under that of the order of the universe. The lifestyle of the woodpecker was as it was because that was the will of God. The same could be said of the curse of work for humanity, or at least one portion of it – the so-called Third Estate, composed of commoners (the other two Estates, the clergy and the nobility were deemed to have their own responsibilities, but these did not include manual labour). The curse of work was a consequence of the Fall, a penalty decreed by God for Adam's disobedience (Genesis, 3.19).

Attitudes to the value of work were changing radically among Diderot's contemporaries. Buffon regarded work as a mark of the human domination over and power to transform nature. It was what distinguished the human from the non-human. No longer an immutable curse, it bore the seed, properly organised and divided, of perhaps unlimited future prosperity. For Adam Smith, the susceptibility of the human subject to the sort of mental and physical formation observed by Diderot in the inhabitants of the faubourg Saint Marcel was what made the division of labour, the source of future wealth, possible. These writers were evidently able to contemplate the brutalising effects of habitual labour without expressing Diderot's misgivings. Diderot's faith in progress was less robust. His model of history was if anything cyclical.[40] He chose to regard the effects of labour as a mark of what was contingent, arbitrary and unstable about the human condition – the transformative power of upbringing and habit on the most fundamental human characteristics. On one level, this position was fully consistent with his rejection of belief in a transcendent deity who shaped the universe – a view which, more forcibly expressed, had already led to his persecution and imprisonment at the hands of France's Christian establishment.[41] But his misgivings about the effect of specialised labour on individual character are more than the casual expression of a pessimist cosmology. They point to a more specific cause of uncertainty which surfaced repeatedly in his writings without ever being fully resolved. This is particularly evident in the *Encyclopédie*. The *Encyclopédie* set out to make available a compendium of hitherto scattered knowledge in one albeit voluminous publication. Most specifically – and it was for this that it became most famous – it presented for the first time a comprehensive picture of the productive forces of the kingdom of France. A key component of the project was therefore the dissemination of practical knowledge of methods of production, much of which had previously been the peculiar property of craftsmen and women, sometimes in the form of jealously guarded trade secrets, but often as skills transmitted orally from one generation to the next.[42] Many commentators have celebrated this aspect of the *Encyclopédie* as a pioneering attempt to cleanse manual skills of the stigma of baseness which attached to them by virtue of the curse of Adam, and to bestow on them the respect due to their social utility, thereby elevating the status of the artisan. On such a view, the artisan was the embodiment of a productive Third Estate at the expense of the clergy and the nobility – a prefigurement of arguments which would be made at the outset of the Revolution of 1789, most famously by Sieyès (see below). But as Cynthia Koepp has pointed out, the attitude of Diderot and d'Alembert was more complex than that. They valued the mechanical arts chiefly for their utility, but did not necessarily see that utility as conferring dignity on their practitioners as citizens. They argued for increased respect for artisans primarily as a means of enhancing productivity and the quality of production. When it came to individual trades, they tended to privilege more polite trades, such as carriage-

40. As witness his readiness to contemplate a return to barbarism as a possible solution to the decay of life drawing (*Salon of 1767*, p. 61.) See also Becq, *Genèse*, p.537. For Buffon, see Claude Blanckaert, 'La valeur de l'homme: l'idée de nature humaine chez Buffon', in *Buffon 88: actes du colloque international Paris-Montbard-Dijon* ed. J. Gayon et al. (Paris, 1992), p.583-600, and Adam Smith, *The Wealth of nations* (1776), ed. Andrew Skinner (1978), p.109-21.

41. See Diderot, *Lettre sur les aveugles*, ed. R. Niklaus (Geneva, 1951), p.44.

42. Jacques Proust, *Diderot et l'Encyclopédie* (Paris, 1962), p.203, 220.

making, and displayed anxiety about sharp practice among more lowly producers who catered to subsistence needs (including, presumably, the street traders of the faubourg Saint-Marcel). By codifying and disseminating craft secrets, they both undermined the authority of the individual practitioner and made possible the control and rationalisation of workshop practices from outside and above.

> To the extent that workers were perceived as marginal and disruptive, their private languages, their corporate groups, their rites and rituals served to insulate them somewhat from the dominant official culture, to render them culturally self-sufficient, and to provide some small defence against the kinds of economic movements transforming industry in the eighteenth century – in other words, to allow them a source of autonomous power. What we have in the *Encyclopédie* is a subtle and comprehensive expropriation of that nonliterate knowledge and hence power by the literate culture, an attempt, largely successful, to remove the inefficient and inarticulate world of work from the hands and mouths of the workers and to place it in printed form before the eyes of an enlightened 'management' whose ordered purposes it would serve.[43]

Viewed from this perspective, what Diderot saw as the brutalisation of heavy labour was part of a process to which his own writings contributed. The *Encyclopédistes*' approach was innovative but ambiguous. They proclaimed the social worth of artisans while putting into the hands of their masters a system of knowledge which could not but hasten their proletarianisation. An indication of Diderot's recognition of this process is attested by the vocabulary which he used to describe artisans collectively. Jaucourt, another contributor to the *Encyclopédie*, credited Diderot with restricting the meaning of the word *peuple* (people), formerly used to describe the nation as a whole, to workers and labourers alone. Diderot continued to use the word in its original sense as well, but he also used it as a term to describe the lower orders taken as a whole. Used in that sense, it was entirely pejorative. To 'depopularise' oneself meant, for

43. Cynthia J. Koepp, 'The alphabetical order: work in Diderot's *Encyclopédie*', in *Work in France: representation, meaning, organisation and practice*, ed. Stephen Kaplan and Cynthia Koepp (Ithaca, NY, and London, 1986), p.257. Georges Friedmann, 'L'*Encyclopédie* et le travail humain', *Annales ESC* 8 (1953), p.53-61. 'For Diderot, the wisdom of a mechanical art was embodied in its rules, not in the persons of its practitioners', in William H. Sewell Jr, *Work and Revolution in France: language and labor from the old regime to 1848* (Cambridge, MA, 1980), p.69. As Jacques Proust observed, the plates of the *Encyclopédie* exhibit no awareness of the deforming physical effects of manual labour with which Diderot was so concerned elsewhere. 'L'image du peuple au travail dans les planches de l'"*Encyclopédie*"', in Centre Aixois d'Etudes et de Recherches sur le dix-huitième siècle, *Images du peuple au dix-huitième siècle (Colloque d'Aix-en-Provence 25 et 26 octobre 1969)* (Paris, 1973), p.65-86 (67). On the charmed world of work evoked in the plates of the *Encyclopédie*, see Roland Barthes, 'Les planches de l'"Encyclopédie"', in *Le Degré zéro de l'écriture suivi de nouveaux essais critiques* (Paris, 1972), p.89-105.

Diderot, to make oneself better.[44] This attitude reveals an essentially urban perspective. It was only in an urban society that the social mobility implied in a notion of 'depopularisation' – like the division of labour on which it depended – was possible.[45] What was seen as improvement, whether personal or collective, depended on the same market mechanisms as the brutalisation which Diderot deplored.

The negative consequences of increased social specialisation were not restricted to the brutalising effects of hard labour, nor were its only victims the poor. Towards the end of his life, Diderot confronted and revised his views on this and related issues – the extent to which habit determined character, the moral justification of the division of labour and its place in society. The occasion was the posthumous publication of Helvétius' *De l'homme* in 1773. Helvétius' book presented a provocatively doctrinaire formulation of the sensualist position on character and experience. It provided an extreme statement of a view to which the younger Diderot would have subscribed without too much trouble, but at many of whose implications he now balked. Just as the views expressed by Diderot on the body and its representation have been interpreted by later commentators in relation to aesthetic theory, so there is a tendency to explain the opinions voiced in the *Réfutation suivie de l'ouvrage d'Helvétius intitulé l'homme* with reference to Diderot's discernment as a writer (he simply *knew* that everyone was different) or to his own presumed spiritual journey – was he, perhaps, rejecting materialism in favour of something more spiritual in his account of human development? In fact, Diderot found much to agree with in Helvétius' book and did not hesitate to recommend it to others. Nor, on the other hand, had his faith in sensualism ever been unqualified. Diderot had long been preoccupied with questions of physiology and psycho-physiology, and this was a preoccupation which increased in his later years. He had himself written extensively on these issues, most famously in *Le Rêve de d'Alembert*, but most ambitiously in his unfinished *Eléments de physiologie*. His views were heavily indebted to the *Elementa physiologiae* of the pioneering physiologist Albrecht von Haller, but he also drew on writings by Buffon and others, including Bordeu and Marat, the future revolutionary. Diderot saw in Haller's physiology of sensibility the basis for a holistic explanation of human psychology. He had already sketched theories which played off the relative strength of the component parts of

44. Roland Mortier, 'Diderot et la notion de peuple', *Europe* 1(1963), p.78-88 (84). For Jaucourt's more general comments on the changing use of the word *peuple*, see ch.5.

45. Smith, *Wealth of nations*, p.121-26. For the misgivings of the *Encyclopédistes* on the effects of urbanisation on artisans from rural backgrounds, see Friedmann, 'L'*Encyclopédie* et le travail humain', p.60f. Jean Fabre, 'L'article "Peuple" de l'"Encyclopédie" et le couple Coyer-Jaucourt', in *Images du peuple au dix-huitième siècle*, p.11-24 (22).

the nervous system, suggesting a greater role for innate difference than sensualist psychology in its pure form could easily accommodate. He was also interested in the role of possible interaction between the brain and the diaphragm in generating emotional reactions – an area in which speculation was largely unfettered by the existing state of knowledge, as he cheerfully admitted.[46] In his *Réfutation d'Helvétius* he set great store by this relationship and the possibilities which he saw it as offering for the differentiation of character in terms of the physical constitution of the subject anterior to sensation, attributing wisdom to the predominance of the brain; compassion and morality to that of the diaphragm. He also criticised Helvétius' failure to take into account medical differences such as those occasioned by the effects of different humours and the relative strength and weakness of the different fluids and fibres which composed the body.[47]

In an era which places as much faith in genes as ours, Diderot's scientific arguments against Helvétius appear crude and rudimentary. For us, they only confirm his ongoing acceptance of so much of the sensualist position. It was not in differences over physiological theory, however, that the chief grounds of Diderot's indignation lay. What overwhelmingly excited his ire was the complacency with which Helvétius regarded the disposition of society. This was a direct consequence of Helvétius' doctrinaire sensualism – if people were infinitely malleable, it did not really matter what they ended up doing individually. Adam Smith had drawn the same conclusion. When Smith contemplated the division of labour in society, he could admire the ingenuity of Providence. It is unlikely that Helvétius felt a similar impulse, but he could at least comfort himself with the knowledge that everyone would eventually adapt to the situation in which they found themselves. Diderot could not accept these views, even if this meant revising his earlier sensualist position. When he looked at the way that labour was divided in society he saw only a mess of broken dreams and wasted talent. He

46. 'Diaphragm, brain – little-known organs' (Diderot, ed. Jean Mayer, *Eléments de physiologie,* (Paris, 1964), p.290); Mayer, *Diderot, homme de science* (Rennes, 1959). On Diderot and Haller, see François Duchesneau, 'Diderot et la physiologie de la sensibilité', *Dix-huitième siècle* 31 (1999), p.195-216; Roselyne Rey, 'Diderot et les sciences de la vie dans l'Encyclopédie', *Recherches sur Diderot et sur l'Encyclopédie* 18-19 (1995), p.47-53, and T. Kaitaro, *Diderot's holism. Philosophical anti-reductionism and its medical background* (Frankfurt, 1997). According to Kaitaro: 'Diderot's philosophy is less related to the traditionally discussed philosophical sources [...] than to his medical and biological sources' (p.4). For the change in Diderot's attitude to sensualism in about 1773, see p.148. On the medical character of Diderot's criticism of Helvétius, see Anne C. Vila, *Enlightenment and pathology: sensibility in the literature and medicine of eighteenth-century France* (Baltimore, MD, and London, 1998), p.92f.

47. Diderot, *Réfutation suivie de l'ouvrage d'Helvétius intitulé l'homme* in *Œuvres*, vol.2, p.283, 336-38, 357, 366.

protested against what he saw as the haphazardness and inhumanity of this situation in the name of the conditions and aspirations of the individual human being:

> I agree that man reasons, as the fish swims or the bird flies; but each man is led by his organisation, his character, his temperament, his natural aptitude to combine one set of ideas rather than another. Chance and even more the necessities of life deal with us as they will; who knows that better than me? It is why for thirty years on end, against my inclination, I composed the *Encyclopédie* and composed only two plays. It is why talents are wasted and employments in society are occupied by men who are miserable or inadequate, and he who would have been a great artist is only a poor theology student or a boring lawyer. That is the true story of life, not all these sophisms [...] where the portrait of the author is served up to us as that of Man.[48]

Few would now agree with Diderot's self-assessment in this passage. The *Encyclopédie* is still regarded as the outstanding achievement of Enlightenment thought, while Diderot's plays are largely unperformed and unread. But that is not the point. Diderot's position was that there were innate differences which dictated the aptitudes and inclinations of individual human beings. If that is accepted, the division of labour according to the laws of the market (which is what 'chance and even more the necessities of life' amount to in this context) appears both wasteful of human resources in general and destructive of individual human happiness. Helvétius had accepted the worker's lot with philosophical complacency, as well he might – he himself had belonged to the wealthiest of France's élites, that of the farmers general or tax farmers. This was not lost on Diderot when he turned his attention to Helvétius' picture of life among the lower orders:

> I should be better persuaded of the delights of a joiner's day if it was a joiner who told me of them, and not a farmer general whose arms have never experienced how hard wood is or how heavy the axe. [...] So tiring is his labour, that the worker is more grateful for its cessation than for the benefit of his pay; it is not his reward, but the harshness and length of his task which occupy him throughout his day.

So exhausting was their work that 'nearly all the children of labouring folk are conceived on the mornings of Sundays or holidays'.[49] Diderot

48. Diderot, *Réfutation*, p.312f. On the financial constraints which dictated Diderot's contribution to the *Encyclopédie* and his relations with publishers and patrons in general, see Jacques Proust, *Diderot et l'Encyclopédie* (Paris, 1962), p.81-116. The discussion of beauty and imitation in the *Salon of 1767* was prefaced by a complaint about the low social status of artists and the difficulties which aspiring artists encountered, especially from the selfishness and stupidity of buyers, *Diderot on art*, vol.2, p.7-9.
49. Diderot, *Réfutation*, p.427.

upbraided Helvétius for declaring himself willing to saw stone – eight or ten hours of the saw would be enough to make the boredom of life in the court at Versailles appear attractive to anyone. As for Helvétius' claim that boredom was as bad as poverty, 'Behold the view of a rich man who has never been pushed to find a dinner'. Against Helvétius, Diderot regarded domestic service as even more demeaning than hard labour: 'If men who have strong shoulders and active legs prefer emptying a chamber pot to carrying a burden, that is because they have base spirits'. His diatribe against the conditions under which the poor were forced to work concluded with an allusion to Jean-Jacques Rousseau: 'Only the terrors of poverty and the effects of brutalisation can reduce man to such works. Ah! Jean-Jacques, how ill you argued the case for the savage as against the social state!'[50]

Here, Diderot expressed his feelings about the human consequences of the division of labour with unequivocal force. But they also interfered with his ability to take up consistent theoretical positions on a range of other issues. This is most evident in those passages in his aesthetic writings in which he turned for an ideal to those ancient statues whose perfect proportions he ridiculed elsewhere. Seznec was right to see in Diderot's fascination with the canonical statues of antiquity a reverence for classical culture, but the meaning which that culture had for him in this context needs to be defined more closely. Antiquity was a site of lost grandeur for Diderot, as it was for Winckelmann, but it was also a site of lost universals, a view which was gaining ground in the increasingly socially divided France of his later years.[51] He saw in antiquity a culture which had acknowledged and confronted the stigmata of inhuman social division and which had successfully risen above present deformity to an ideal of the human condition. The question of why Diderot's views on antiquity took this form, like that of why sculpture should have played so central a part in his discussion of individual human identity, will become clearer in the next chapter.

50. Diderot, *Réfutation*, p.429f.

51. See Régis Michel, 'Diderot et la modernité', in *Diderot et l'art de Boucher à David* (Paris, 1984), p.110-21 (119); J. Seznec, *Essais sur Diderot et l'antiquité: the Mary Flexner lectures delivered at Bryn Mawr College, Pennsylvania* (Oxford, 1957).

3. Temperament and the body

We now have some idea of the sort of connection which Diderot thought he saw between the appearance of the body and individual character, and how both were transformed by experience. But why did he take it for granted that there should be a connection between appearance and character in the first place? A clue to the answer is provided by the language in which he formulated his objections to Helvétius' assumptions about human sameness. There, he described natural character as the product of 'hardness or softness of fibre, soft or burning blood, thick or runny lymph, sharp or soapy bile, and the state of the hard or fluid parts of our machine'.[1] The choice of these substances – blood, lymph, bile, fibre and fluid – as the primary locations of difference between human beings may appear odd to us. Nowadays we explain difference in other ways – in terms of genes or psychological type. But Diderot's statement would have appeared relatively unremarkable to an eighteenth-century reader. Three of his categories – blood, lymph and bile – were what were known as humours. They had provided a staple ingredient of theories about the human body for over two thousand years.[2] The other categories relate to the theoretical replacements for the humoral classification offered by eighteenth-century medical theorists – in particular, by Albrecht von Haller, on whose writings Diderot's own physiological views were heavily dependent.

The fluids present in the human body were traditionally held to be composed of four humours, identified with what were thought of as four bodily juices – blood, bile, phlegm or lymph and black bile. By Diderot's time it was already recognised that there was no such thing as black bile, which is presumably why it does not appear on his list. The mixture of these humours was known as *krasis* or 'temperament'. At first, temperament was invoked primarily to explain a person's state of health, but in the course of antiquity the categories of temperament were increasingly linked to individual character type and outward appearance. Humoral theory was set forth in books attributed to the Greek physician Hippocrates, notably his *De Natura hominis* (*Of the nature of man* [*sic*]),

1. Diderot, *Réfutation suivie de l'ouvrage d'Helvétius intitulé l'homme*, in *Œuvres*, vol.2, p.283; see also vol.2, p.357.
2. On Diderot's use of humoral theory in his *Essais sur la peinture*, see Melissa Percival, *The Appearance of character: physiognomy and facial expression in eighteenth-century France* (Leeds, 1999), p.53.

which probably dates from the late fifth century BCE. In the second century of our own era another Greek medical writer, Galen, gave humoral theory the form in which it dominated Arab and Western medicine for the next fifteen hundred years. Galen's writings, translated into Arabic and then into Latin, were central not only to medicine, but to natural philosophy as a whole. What in part gave Galenism its authority and staying power was its integration of humoral theory within a doctrine of even broader scope – that of the elements. The union of matter with the four qualities of hot, cold, moist and dry was believed to form the elements of air (hot and moist), fire (hot and dry), earth (cold and dry) and water (cold and moist). These four elements made up the material world as a whole, according to the fifth-century BCE Sicilian philosopher Empedocles. The proportions of the elements within each individual human being determined individual characteristics. Sex, for example, was commonly related to difference in the relative heat of the individual body.[3] Each humour shared the constitutive qualities of one of the elements. Blood was hot and moist, like air; bile was hot and dry, like fire. Phlegm was cold and wet (water) and black bile was cold and dry (earth). The relationship between the elements in the outside world and humours in the human body was thus plausible (if not entirely straightforward). Air was ingested directly through the lungs and the elements in different amounts and combinations composed the food that people ate. Hippocrates and Galen were thus early and somewhat literally minded exponents of the doctrine that you are what you eat, though what might now be called metabolism also played its part. The humours were secreted by the organs (in the case of blood, the liver) and distributed throughout the body. All the humours were present in varying degrees in the body's blood.

Humoral theory was only one component of the complex and sophisticated medical model put forward by Galen – a model which drew on the writings of the Greek philosophers Plato and Aristotle as well as on those of Hippocrates – but it was a major component.[4] Temperament

3. Laurence Brockliss and Colin Jones, *The Medical world of early modern France* (Oxford, 1997), p.110. See also Thomas Laqueur, *Making sex: body and gender from the Greeks to Freud* (Cambridge, MA, 1990), p.25-28.

4. Galen's writings are voluminous. Arnulfe d'Aumont observed that 'writing cost him little' (*Encyclopédie*, s.v. 'Galénisme'). The standard edition is that by C. G. Kühn (20 vols. (Leipzig, 1821-1833)). For summaries of his doctrine, see Daniel Leclerc, *Histoire de la médecine, où l'on voit l'origine & les progrès de cet art, de siècle en siècle; les sectes, qui s'y sont formées; les noms des médecins, leurs découvertes, leurs opinions, & les circonstances les plus remarquables de leur vie* (Amsterdam, 1723), p.672-77; Laurence Brockliss and Colin Jones, *Medical world*, p.110-14; Vivian Nutton, 'Humoralism', in *Companion encyclopedia of the history of medicine*, ed. W. F. Bynum and Roy Porter, 2 vols (London, 1993), vol.1, p.281-91. For the history of Galenism, see O. Temkin, *Galenism: rise and decline of a medical philosophy* (Ithaca, NY, and London,

in its original sense meant the balance of humours. Galen recognised nine temperaments – the four mixed temperaments identified by Hippocrates, associated with the humours, four in which the single qualities – hot, cold, dry and moist – predominated, and an ideal temperament in which the properties of the other temperaments were equally balanced. The temperament of perfect balance (described by later commentators as the *temperamentum ad punctum*) could occur either in a whole individual (rarely) or in a particular organ or part of the body. The palm of the hand, for example, provided a good index to relative dryness/moisture and warmth/coldness of the humoral balance of the body as a whole.[5]

The identification of the theory of the temperaments with four distinct and stable character types rather than individual mixtures or 'idiosyncracies' was made at about the same time as that at which Galen wrote or shortly afterwards.[6] The theory positively invited application to everyday life and especially to other people. It provided a model which could account for both the diversity and the coherence of human identity. At the same time it enabled people to locate themselves and others in the spectrum of temperament identity on the basis of appearance. It provided an indication of what types of difference should necessarily go with each other and an explanation of why that was so. Identifying someone's temperament according to appearance was fairly straightforward – especially that aspect of appearance which is still called 'complexion' – a concept and a term which derive from temperament theory, where it was used to describe bodily make-up as a whole.[7] The colour of the outer surfaces of the body and particularly the skin was determined by the dominant humour or combination of humours in the blood. Complexion expressed temperament in part because the humours had distinctive hues indicative of their other qualities. It thus made possible a reading of character. A person of sanguine temperament – one in whose constitution blood predominated – would display both a ruddy complexion and a warm, impulsive disposition. The bilious or choleric, characterised by an abundance of yellow bile, were inclined to be sallow of skin, wiry of build and prone to anger, whereas the phlegmatic person was pale, flabby and – well, phlegmatic. Melancholics tended to be swarthy (thanks to the predominance of black bile). They were also introverted, sad and susceptible to mental derangement. There

1973). For the origins of humoral theory, see Raymond Klibansky, Erwin Panofsky and Fritz Saxl, *Saturn and melancholy. Studies in the history of natural philosophy, religion, and art* (London, 1964), p.1-15.

5. Galen, *De Temperamentis*, 1:8, 9; 2:1 (Kühn, vol.1, p.554-77).
6. Klibansky, Panofsky and Saxl, *Saturn*, p.55-66.
7. See Lynn Thorndike, 'De Complexionibus', *Isis* 49 (1958), p.398-408.

were more or less infinite possibilities for individual variations in temperament, known technically as 'idiosyncrasies', another term which we derive from humoral theory.

Temperament or combinations of temperament dictated a person's overall character, but variations also occurred in the same individual, particularly under the influence of age, disease or season. Different temperaments were believed to predominate at different stages in life. This again was something which simple observation verified, as babies – pale, snotty and generally phlegmatic – were transformed first into ruddy, sanguine children and then into sinewy, bilious adults before succumbing to withered and melancholic old age. Minor versions of the same cycle in bodily composition followed the times of the year, and even the quarters of the day (bile, for example, dominates from the third to the ninth hour of the day, when it is hot and dry; melancholy, from the ninth hour of the day until the third hour of the night, when it is cold and dry). Winter, the season of sniffles and sneezes, saw a peak in phlegm production, while the ruddier complexion brought on by a Greek spring – a change which might nowadays be attributed to suntan – had been explained by Hippocrates as a consequence of an increase in blood during the spring months. Melancholy increased with autumn. Each season brought with it risks from the characteristic diseases associated with the predominant humour.[8] Climate and prevalent winds also shared humoral qualities which helped determine temperament.

A knowledge of temperament became essential to the practice of medicine, since it enabled doctors to treat different conditions and diseases from one individual to another, depending both on temperament and on those external variables which influenced temperament – age, season and climate. It enabled them to predict the course of an illness and to prescribe appropriate curative or prophylactic action. It shed light on the otherwise mysterious and uncontrollable course of disease and enabled people to account for why one person survived an illness and another did not. Treatment was usually by means of diet and

8. Hippocrates, *De Natura hominis*, 7, 8, *Aphorism*, 3:18-31. A variant correlation of the humours with the four ages placed the phlegmatic last (Klibansky, Panofsky and Saxl, *Saturn*, p.10); an arrangement which came to predominate in later representations of the temperaments (*Saturn*, p.293 n.43). Both sequences are found in Galen (Elizabeth Sears, *The Ages of man: medieval interpretations of the life cycle* (Princeton, NJ, 1986), p.14). These associations survived the demise of Galenic medicine. Thus for Cabanis, writing at the end of the eighteenth century, 'the foetus is only organised mucus' (*Œuvres philosophiques de Cabanis*, ed. Claude Lehec and Jean Cazeneuve, 2 vols (Paris, 1956), vol.1, p.342; see also vol.1, p.332). For a particularly thorough characterisation of age by temperament, along with information on the diseases proper to each stage in life, see J. J. Virey, *Histoire naturelle du genre humain. Nouvelle édition* (Paris, 1824), vol.1, p.93-97. For the quarters of the day, see Thorndike, 'De complexionibus', p.408.

regime. It involved manipulation of what came to be known in the middle ages as the 'non-naturals' – so called to distinguish them from 'naturals' such as the humours. The non-naturals were things on which the body depended which were not, like the 'naturals', *of* the body – air, diet, movement and rest, sleep and waking, excretion and secretion, and the passions. The aim of regulating them was to establish a better balance between the humours in the body, whereby health would be restored. The variety in individual make-up which was built into the doctrine of the temperaments encouraged a broad perception of the state of health, disease being defined by loss of function.[9] From that point of view, Galenic medicine may have helped people live with their bodies in greater mental ease than we do. It encouraged more realistic expectations of what was and was not possible for the human body than its modern counterparts, whether alternative or mainstream. Galenism enabled people to make sense of what happened to them in life – changes in their bodies and personalities that came with age, the onset of a disease or medical condition – changes for which we are now offered very different explanations and remedies. Being able to explain changes over which they lacked total control doubtless helped people to come to terms with circumstances which it would otherwise have been hard to endure. Was temperament any less effective at doing that for ordinary people than genes are nowadays?

The enlightenment which temperament theory offered was not restricted to our immediate sphere. It also allowed people to connect the meanings of their lives to phenomena beyond the merely terrestrial – to the behaviour and 'influence' of heavenly bodies. At about the same time as Galen was setting his stamp on medicine, the Egyptian writer Ptolemy was fashioning models of astronomy and astrology which proved equally long-lived. Ptolemy's zodiac – the path through the heavens along which the seven wandering stars or planets appeared to travel as they circled the earth – provided a basis for the science of astrology. The planets, among which were reckoned the sun and the moon, were characterised by specific elements or combinations of elements. So were the particular fixed constellations associated with each of them along the path of the zodiac – hence the classification of 'star signs' retained in modern astrology – earth signs, water signs, etc. The conjunction of planets and constellations helped determine the influence of the stars on given events on earth.[10]

9. Temkin, *Galenism*, p.102; Leclerc, *Histoire de la médecine*, p.676.
10. See Lynn Thorndike, *The History of magic and experimental science*, 8 vols (New York, 1923-1958), vol.1 (1923), p.113; Tamsyn Barton, *Ancient astrology* (London and New York, 1994), p.60-62. In France, the connection of astrology with medicine as taught in universities was severed in the sixteenth century. See Brockliss and Jones, *Medical world*, p.111f.

The vocabulary of Galenism 'seemed able to respond in a differentiated way to the whole range of observable phenomena'.[11] From the second to the sixteenth century Galen's views provided the framework within which people viewed the workings of their bodies and minds and their relationship to the world around them. Self and world were experienced in fundamentally different ways to the selves and worlds that we inhabit. One reason that no-one will ever now know what it felt like to be Shakespeare or Michelangelo is that their perceptions and emotions were filtered and defined by a set of beliefs which has now largely vanished from human consciousness – Galenism. For centuries Galen's importance in Western thought rivalled that of Plato and Aristotle. The philosophies of Plato and Aristotle have survived their views on the science of nature, but Galen's has not. As Owsei Temkin explained, Galen's world view stood and fell with the natural model which underpinned it. 'Without medicine his philosophy was not viable'.[12] With its demise, a window closed on the past. But that is not to say that aspects of Galenism do not survive as part of the fabric of popular thought. Astrology, for example, appears to owe its survival to its Galenic rather than its Ptolemaic components. Few would now share Ptolemy's view that the sun and planets revolve around the earth, but the star signs of the zodiac command the faith of millions of horoscope readers. While more learned versions of astrology accord an important role to planetary influence in determining the events of people's lives, this is not what chiefly concerns most consumers of horoscopes. They are more attracted by that aspect of astrology which ties it most closely to temperament theory – the heuristic possibilities of attributing character type to star sign. Astrology thus embodies a survival of humoral theory into the twenty-first century. It testifies to our continuing appetite for conceptual tools which enable us to make sense of our own behaviour and that of the people around us. Nor is the survival of Galenism confined to horoscope readers. When it comes to talking about the physical and mental characteristics of others, people who ridicule faith in astrology as unscientific still employ the vocabulary of Galenism, sometimes echoing its overall concepts (temperament, idiosyncrasy, complexion, temperature), at others its individual categories (temperamental, bad- or good-tempered, ill- or good-humoured, sanguine, bilious, cholic, choleric, lymphatic, phlegmatic, melancholy) – not to mention the qualities on which those categories were held to be based (although when we call people cold, warm, dry or wet we are likely to be using these terms

11. J. Starobinski, 'Préface' in Galen, *L'Âme et ses passions*, translated by and ed. Victor Barras, Terpsichore Birchler and Anne-France Morand (Paris, 1995), p.xi.
12. Temkin, *Galenism*, p.1.

metaphorically). And that is when we are in good health. When sick, there are few who do not resort to the underlying assumptions of humorism as well as its language – as when we take warm drinks to combat the condition we still call a 'cold' (in spite of evidence from the thermometer that we are not exceptionally cold at all). Those who have continued to subscribe to versions of temperament theory regardless of scientific evidence (Rudolf Steiner, for example) have pointed to such persistence as evidence for the theory's underlying validity.[13]

Galenism went largely undisputed until the sixteenth century. It was a closed and a self-validating system. As long as its principles were unshaken, they were destined to receive 'nothing but their own echo' from the world. The multiplicity of possible explanations which they offered for specific phenomena made them impossible to falsify.[14] But once challenged with sufficient insistence, the precision and plausibility of Galen's explanations were revealed to be meaningless. The basis of Galen's humoral theory was attacked by the chemical theorists Paracelsus and Van Helmont, who replaced the traditional four elements with alternative sets. Blows also came from within. The thermometer, for example, was invented by Sanctorius in part as an aid to Galenic medicine. It supplanted subjective assessments of temperature of the sort prescribed in *De Temperamentis* with an objective scale of measurement. But the elevation of temperature to an independently verifiable phenomenon had the effect of demoting hot and cold, essential qualities in Galen's cosmos, to mere subjective human sensations (although modern thermometer scales still take their measure, like Galen's subjective model, from the boiling and freezing points of water).[15] It was the discovery of the circulation of the blood by Harvey which spelled the end for scientific Galenism as a total system. This was not merely because it played havoc with Galen's subtle and complex model of the dissemination of the humours through the body, but because it chimed in with another, plausible and deceptively straightforward model of the body

13. Rudolf Steiner, translated by D. S. Osmond, *The Four temperaments. A lecture given during the Winter of 1908-09* (London, 1929; 1949), p.7, 22; G. W. Allport, *Pattern and growth in personality* (New York, 1961), p.39; Dr Gilbert Childs, *Understanding your temperament* (London, 1995). For a fuller account of persistent humourism, see Cecil G. Helman, 'Feed a cold, starve a fever – folk models of infection in an English suburban community, and their relation to medical treatment', *Culture, medicine and psychiatry* 2 (1978), p.107-37. Vicky Rippere has demonstrated how lay views on how to cope with depressive behaviour perpetuate traditions of treatment by the non-naturals ('The survival of traditional medicine in lay medical views: an empirical approach to the history of medicine', *Medical history*, 25 (1981), p.411-14).
14. See Starobinski, 'Preface', in *L'Âme et ses passions*, p.xiif. D'Aumont made a similar criticism (*Encyclopédie*, s.v. 'Galénisme').
15. Temkin, *Galenism*, p.158. Cf. Galen, *De Temperamentis*, 1:9 (Kühn, vol.1, p.561).

itself – one which viewed living beings as complex machines. The seventeenth-century French philosopher René Descartes taught that human identity was composed of a material body and a spiritual soul which operated according to different principles, a view which did much to undermine Galenism. It was a model which Harvey's theory of circulation, with its central pump and its valves, fitted particularly well.[16]

If Galenism was dead by the end of the seventeenth century, why did Diderot still ground his view of human difference in the humours (three of them, at any rate)? This was no folkloric survival – Diderot was an attentive reader and translator of Haller's *Elementa physiologiae*, one of the most advanced medical texts of its day. Galenism may have been dead as a world philosophy, but its component parts lived on – particularly the doctrine of temperaments – in a broader context than that of medical theory. It was all very well for doctors to talk about the circulation of the blood – something that it was impossible for the lay person to observe directly – but the visible effects of temperament were part of everyone's experience. A medical expert might claim that the phlegmatic's blood circulated according to the same system as the sanguine's, but the difference between the two, whether in physical appearance or characteristic behaviour, remained as distinctive as ever. It could be verified by a walk down any crowded street. There was no need to resort to complex and arcane experiments or the writings of the learned.

Art shared with medicine the human body as its principal object of study.[17] Unsurprisingly, artists were encouraged to have regard to the temperaments when portraying human character and passion.[18] Representations of the temperaments and their characteristic appearance were common. Among the most famous in eighteenth-century Paris was the group of colossal figures which surrounded the base of a statue of Louis XIV erected in the Place des Victoires in 1685. These represented four captives and were the work, like the figure of the king above them, of the Dutch sculptor Martin van den Bogaert, known as Desjardins. They personified four nations whose defeat by Louis had been sealed by

16. Though Descartes himself, initially enthusiastic, rejected Harvey's arguments as too dependent on Galenic and Aristotelian models, supplying instead his own (mistaken) mechanistic model. See Richard Toellner, 'Logical and psychological aspects of the discovery of the circulation of the blood', in *On Scientific discovery: the Erice lectures 1977*, ed. Mirko Grmek, Robert S. Cohen and Guido Cimino (Dordrecht and London, 1981), p.239-59.

17. See Martial Guédron, *De Chair et de marbre: imiter et exprimer le nu en France, 1745-1815* (Paris, 2003), p.24f.

18. See Jennifer Montagu, *The Expression of the passions: the origin and influence of Charles Lebrun's conférence sur l'expression générale et particulière* (New Haven, CT, and London, 1994), p.19, and Melissa Percival, *The Appearance of character: physiognomy and facial expression in eighteenth-century France* (Leeds, 1999), p.44.

the peace of Nijmegen. Following the example provided by Pietro Francavilla on the pedestal of an earlier royal statue, that of Henri IV formerly on the Pont Neuf, Desjardins personified each nation by a man of different age and corresponding temperament. The statue of the king was destroyed at the Revolution, but those of the captives were saved as masterpieces on the grounds of their outstanding quality as works of art, in spite of what was judged their ideologically offensive content.[19] They are now in the Louvre. In each case, it is temperament which conditions the captive's reaction to adversity. The youthful and sanguine figure of *Spain* looks up hopefully towards his conqueror (fig.10, p.60), whereas the more mature and bilious personification of *Holland* (fig.11, p.60) strains furiously against his (now vanished) shackles as he meditates rebellion. The older *Brandenburg* (fig.12, p.61) appears to be identified as phlegmatic, acknowledging the humiliation of his position but nonetheless submitting to a superior power. Finally, the *Holy Roman Empire*, apparently personified as the bowed and aged embodiment of melancholy (fig.13, p.61), is lost in despair, insensible to the victor who once posed haughtily above his head. Complexion, of course, could not be evoked in monochromatic bronze sculpture, but gesture, physique, skin and even hair quality – smooth and bouncy in the case of sanguine *Spain*, dry and listless in that of the *Empire* – contribute along with age to the establishment of temperament identity.[20] The figures were also intended to represent national characters in line with temperament, although their original national identities were utterly forgotten by the end of the eighteenth century.[21] It was only their forcefully differentiated responses to the humiliation of defeat which continued to speak meaningfully to

19. See E. Pommier, *L'Art de la liberté: doctrines et débats de la Révolution française* (Paris, 1991), p.29-37. Francavilla's captives had already been removed from the base of the statue of Henri IV on the Pont Neuf (see Jeffrey Merrick, 'Politics on pedestals: royal monuments in eighteenth-century France', *French history* 5 (1991), p.234-65 (253)). On the monument itself, see Lorenz Seelig, *Studien zu Martin van den Bogaert gen. Desjardins* (Munich, 1980), p.27-204; Gérard Sabatier, *Versailles ou la figure du roi* (Paris, 1999), p.481-91; Thomas W. Gaehtgens, 'La statue de Louis XIV et son programme iconographique', in *Place des Victoires: histoire, architecture, société*, ed. Isabelle Dubois, Alexandre Gady and Hendrik Ziegler (Paris, 2003), p.9-35.
20. It is by no means clear which of the older pair, *Brandenburg* and the *Empire*, is intended to personify phlegm, and which melancholy. See Seelig, who appears to favour the latter identification (*Studien*, p.60), but compare the personification of *phlegma* in the engraving by Jacob I de Gheyn illustrated by Klibansky, Panofsky and Saxl, *Saturn*, pl.142. The place of the phlegmatic in the cycle of the temperaments was in any case subject to variation (see n.6 above) and, even in arrangements where both were represented as old, the order of the two was sometimes inverted (Klibansky, Panofsky and Saxl, *Saturn*, p.296 n.53, p.370). In terms of affective response, both figures on Desjardins' monument are necessarily self-absorbed in comparison with the two younger captives.
21. See the debates reported by Pommier, *L'Art de la liberté*, p.29-37.

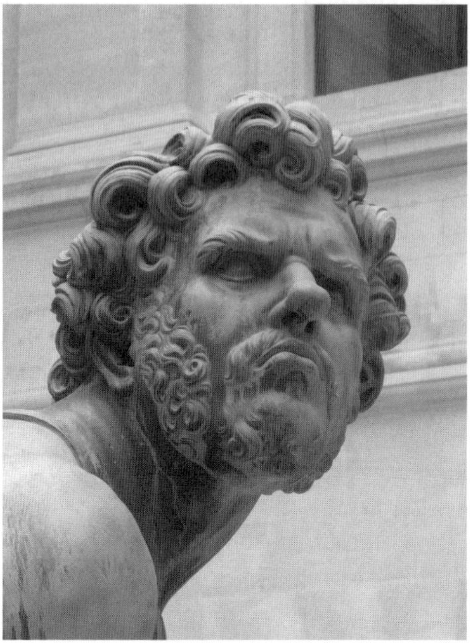

Figure 10: Desjardins (Martin van den Bogaert), *Spain* (sanguine), bronze, H. 220 cm, Musée du Louvre, Paris, RF 4407.

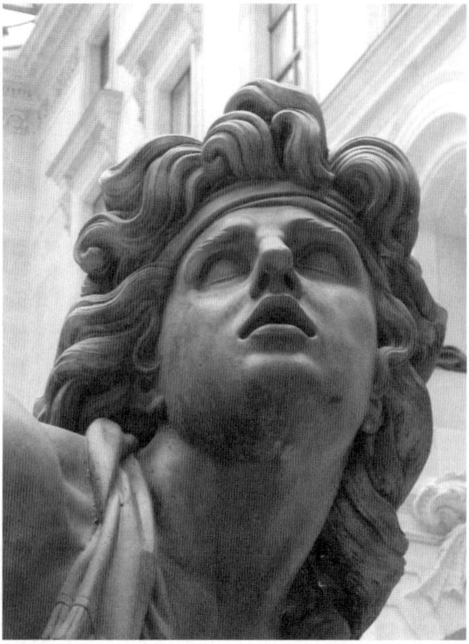

Figure 11: Desjardins (Martin van den Bogaert), *Holland* (bilious temperament), bronze, H. 220 cm, Musée du Louvre, Paris, RF 4410.

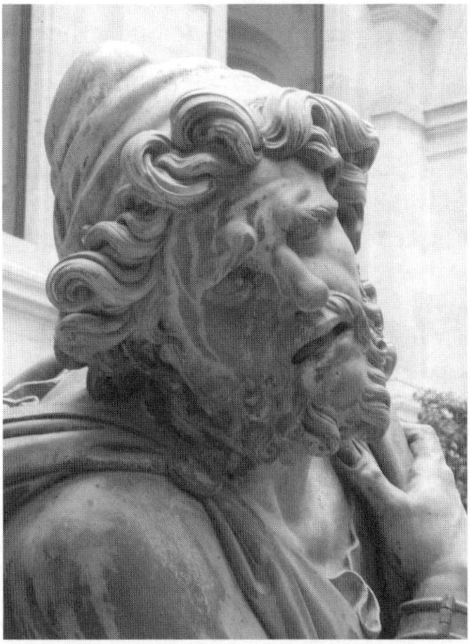

Figure 12: Desjardins (Martin van den Bogaert), *Brandenburg* (phlegmatic), bronze, H. 220 cm, Musée du Louvre, Paris, RF 4409.

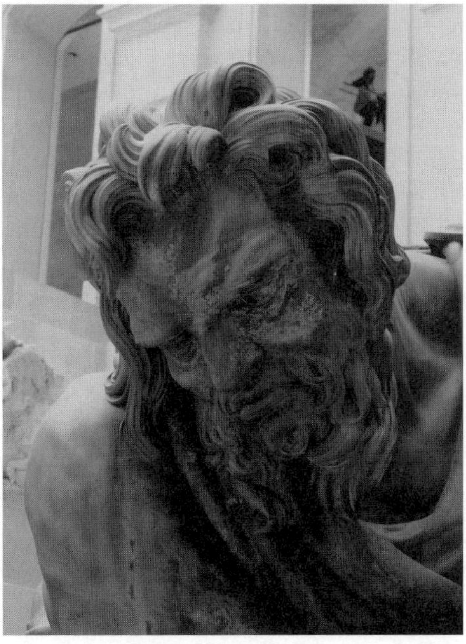

Figure 13: Desjardins (Martin van den Bogaert), *Holy Roman Empire* (melancholy), bronze, H. 220 cm, Musée du Louvre, Paris, RF 4408.

passers-by. Such mute witnesses could only reinforce what spectators felt that they already knew about the way that temperament and age affected behaviour.

But it was not merely common sense that revolted at the denial of temperament theory. Medical diagnosis and treatment had for centuries been based on the existence of the humours and variations of temperament. The model for the interaction of the body and its environment on which medical treatment continued to depend – that of the naturals and the non-naturals – was itself part of the Galenic world view. It was accepted not merely by doctors but by all those who endeavoured to regulate their own health in accordance with a conception of hygiene grounded in the healing power of nature. Medical specialists did not command even among the educated elite the respect accorded them today. The daily practice of medicine was not yet the province of health professionals. It remained an issue of self-administration and self-regulation, as demonstrated by the medical entries in the *Encyclopédie*.[22] The prescription of a patient's relationship to the non-naturals presupposed the presence of the naturals, including the humours. Even writers who were vehemently opposed to the humoral theory of Galen, such as Boerhaave, ended up accepting substitute classifications which look to a modern reader very similar to the system they were intended to replace. Boerhaave, who accepted a mechanistic model of the workings of the body, rejected humorism. He described how observations of the blood conducted with the help of the microscope had demonstrated that bile was not a component of the blood and that black bile had been misidentified. But he held on to the notion of four elements, and two of the elements which he recognised were the same as Galen's. Not only were body fluids largely composed of water, but the solid parts of the body consisted ultimately of earth. The other elements in the composition of the body were oil and salt. Like the traditional humours, these could be found in balanced or unbalanced mixtures (*temperies*, *intemperies*), producing disorders in the latter case. This yielded a system remarkably similar to the original model of four temperaments, with four distinctive types of character associated with the preponderance of one or another of the individual elements. Unsurprisingly, the description of the 'earth' temperament corresponds with the traditional characterisation of the melancholic in salient respects (dryness, dark complexion, sadness, leanness). Apart from the emphasis given, predictably enough, to thirst, the characterisation of the salty tempera-

22. See William Coleman, 'Health and hygiene in the *Encyclopédie*: a medical doctrine for the Bourgeoisie', *Journal of the history of medicine and allied sciences* 29 (1974), p.399-421. For the survival of Galenic theory in popular medical textbooks even in the nineteenth century, see Laqueur, *Making sex*, p.150f.

ment reads remarkably like that of the bilious in the old scheme of things. The preponderance (or *intemperies*) of water and especially oil yielded characteristics similar to those associated with the phlegmatic temperament of the ancients. Only the sanguine temperament is difficult to identify with any of Boerhaave's replacements.[23] To a patient being treated by one of Boerhaave's followers the difference between his model and that of the Galenists would not have been easy to discern.[24]

Temperament helped people to live their lives and to make sense of their feelings. It enabled them to come to terms with behaviour and inclinations which attracted censure or even legal penalties when judged by the moral standards of church, state and society at large. In this respect it functioned very differently from the dualism of Descartes, as well as from the sensualist psychology of the followers of Locke and Condillac.[25] At the end of the eighteenth century, it helped the aged Casanova to make sense of his own notorious earlier career as he looked back on a life during which his character had been successively phlegmatic, sanguine and bilious, and to accept the melancholy which he recognised as inevitably the final stage of that progression through the temperaments which had constituted his life.[26] An artist's attraction to one body type rather than another – something which might nowadays be explained in terms of sexual preference or gender orientation – was construed as a consequence of the artist's temperament.[27] What would nowadays be seen as the consequences of sexual attraction could be explained as the effect of temperament, especially in situations where moral opprobrium might have been incurred. An instance of this is provided by Casanova's younger contemporary, Jean-Claude Delamétherie. Delamétherie was editor of the influential *Journal de physique* and a force to be reckoned with in the scientific world of pre-

23. Hermannus Boerhaave, *Praelectiones academicae in proprias institutiones rei medicae, edidit et notas addidit Albertus Haller* (Turin, 1742-1745), vol.1, p.510-13.
24. The same was true of procedures adopted by followers of the rival, iatrochemical school, who also rejected the humours (and to whose theories Boerhaave's in this instance appear to have been indebted, despite his vigorous disclaimer (*Praelectiones*, p.512)): 'All that had really happened with the acceptance of iatrochemical ideas was that a new explanatory stage had been introduced between the facultative and temperamental levels. As a result, it remained usual to deploy Galenic temperamental accounts of health and disease alongside iatrochemical ones' (Brockliss and Jones, *Medical world*, p.148).
25. See above, ch.2. Their view of the innate sameness of human character was in accordance with conventional Christian teaching. Thus the eighteenth-century physiognomist Bougeant held that 'because the soul is the same in every human being, it cannot be the cause of the great variety in human characters, a fact which is more readily explained by subtle differences in the temperaments' (Percival, *Appearance of character*, p.23).
26. Klibansky, Panofsky and Saxl, *Saturn*, p.122 n.163.
27. Girard Audran, *Les Proportions du corps humain mesurées sur les plus belles figures de l'antiquité* (Paris, 1683), n.p.

and post-revolutionary Paris. Under the Consulate he published a book blending natural history with human psychology which made considerable use of temperament theory to explain the varieties of human behaviour and belief. Differences in outlook between Islam and Christianity, for example, were attributed to the temperaments of their founders – sanguine and melancholic/misanthropic respectively.[28] Delamétherie's book covered similar ground to other popular texts of the day, designed to exploit the vogue for natural history brought about by the success of Buffon's *Histoire naturelle de l'homme*. But his approach to some topics was highly unorthodox, particularly when it came to family values. The eulogies of matrimony and exhortations to marry and multiply which are practically inescapable in the moral literature of this period are surprisingly absent from Delamétherie's text, concerned though it is with the morality of everyday life. Delamétherie asserted that, far from being the havens of affective pleasure they were cracked up to be, most marriages degenerated quickly into mere business partnerships. On the other hand, he was unstinting in his praise for the lot of the spinster and the bachelor – a eulogy reinforced by warnings of the consequences of reckless breeding for the welfare of the matrimonially inclined.[29] Elsewhere, Delamétherie drew attention to aspects of human behaviour over which his contemporaries preferred to cast a veil of silence, particularly in literature aimed at a wide readership. Most unusually, he included a section on deficiency of attraction to the opposite sex, which he linked explicitly to same-sex attraction. While condemning what he stigmatised, conventionally enough, as a 'criminal inclination' towards members of one's own sex, he was remarkably indulgent towards the defect which inspired it, informing his readers that it involved 'a need which is not, in truth, of the first necessity'. Nor was his condemnation of 'criminal inclination' always so harsh. His citation of an accusation about the sexual habits of Julius Caesar reported by the historian Suetonius – that he was a husband to every woman and a wife to every man – is not accompanied by any expression of disapprobation. The anecdote appears in a discussion of the loose morals of great men, which it was used to illustrate and, by implication, to justify ('One might even say', Delamétherie added, 'that most men of energy are much given to the pleasures of love' – which is not at all how

28. J. C. Delamétherie, *De l'homme considéré moralement; de ses moeurs, et de celles des animaux*, 2 vols (Paris, An IX/1802), vol.1, p.xix. There was already a tradition whereby depictions of the four apostles (Dürer) and the four evangelists (Rubens) were associated with the four temperaments (Klibansky, Panofsky and Saxl, *Saturn*, p.366-72). To express his own theory of temperament, which appears to incorporate elements from those of Stahl and Haller, Delamétherie created a language of pseudo-algebraic formulae (*De l'homme*, p.xxv-xxviii).

29. *De l'homme*, vol.2, p.262f.

most of his contemporaries described behaviour such as that attributed to Caesar by Suetonius). He repeated the anecdote later on, in the course of attempting to demonstrate that fidelity in marriage was neither 'natural' nor particularly prevalent in civilised societies (this passage immediately succeeds that in which Delamétherie addresses a paean to celibacy).[30] What makes Delamétherie's interest in same-sex attraction relevant to the present context is the chapter devoted to 'caresses'. According to Delamétherie the habit of caressing one's fellow beings was eminently natural, part of our animal inheritance (he was an early advocate of the view that human beings were descended from monkeys), but also an indicator of civilisation:

> Social man is even more *caressant* than the man of nature and the animals. His sensibility is more delicate; his feelings, more lively.
> He has two ways of expressing his feelings; he employs gestures, like the animals. A mother takes her child in her arms, plays with it, covers it with kisses [...] The lover caresses his mistress in the same way; the friend, his friend [...]
> Words supply man in society with a second way of expressing his feelings [...] The expression of these caresses will always be modified by temperament. The caresses of he who has a phlegmatic temperament will be cold; those of the bilious man will be full of heat and physical expression [*démonstrations extérieures*].[31]

No reader of Cuvier's somewhat sour obituary of his friend could doubt the essentially bilious nature of Delamétherie's own temperament.[32]

Identities based on gender and gender orientation are social constructs. There was no space for the public affirmation of an identity based on same-sex attraction in eighteenth-century European culture. In spite of the enlightened views of Helvétius (to whom Delamétherie's may to some extent be indebted) and Diderot, a more or less universal stigma was still attached to men suspected of having or desiring sexual relations with other men. Acts of sodomy had been punishable by death until the Revolution. They were decriminalised by the Jacobins, but by 1802 courts were once again handing out prison sentences for same-sex acts.[33] It would be anachronistic to describe Delamétherie as gay or even homosexual, nor do his relationships appear to have been any more

30. *De l'homme*, vol.1, p.81f., vol.1, p.215, vol.2, p.269. See also Suetonius, *Caesar*, 52.
31. *De l'homme*, vol.2, p.162f.
32. Michaud, *Biographie universelle*, s.v. 'Métherie'.
33. See Jeffrey Merrick and Bryant T. Ragan, Jr, ed., *Homosexuality in early modern France: a documentary collection* (Oxford, 2001), p.171-228. For the views of Helvétius and Diderot, see Bryant T. Ragan Jr, 'The Enlightenment confronts homosexuality', in *Homosexuality in modern France*, ed. Jeffrey Merrick and Bryant T. Ragan Jr (New York and Oxford, 1996), p.8-29.

homosocial (or less heterosocial) than those of his contemporaries. Details of his biography might suggest a homosexual identity to a modern reader, if only in negative terms. It was evidently his failure to marry and father offspring which marginalised his position in the provincial property-owning bourgeois family from which he sprang.[34] The alternative which he offered to marriage was celibacy, not same-sex cohabitation. As has been seen, he condemned some varieties of same-sex love as 'criminal inclination'. It is clearly impossible to determine where Delamétherie or his friends drew the line between a bilious caress and a criminal inclination, although an obvious interpretation of the latter might be relations involving acts of sodomy, subject to the death penalty under the Old Regime. At the same time, it is difficult not to read evidence of personal inclination into his observations on caresses between friends and on the propensity of the bilious to such behaviour. It is no longer possible to say what Delamétherie got up to in his private life, though it is easy enough to imagine circumstances under which biliousness of temperament might have been invoked to explain a caress too far. More importantly, perhaps, in Delamétherie's long life, a sense of temperamental identity may have provided the naturalist himself with an explanation or a consolation for feelings and behaviour which, defined in other terms, would have aroused near universal hostility in society at large. Temperament theory appears to have done for Delamétherie what a sense of gay identity accomplishes for us in a twenty-first-century culture where identity is centred on gender and gender orientation. In a discussion of Foucault's views and the construction of sexual identities, David Halperin has invited us to 'inquire into the construction of sexual identities before the emergence of sexual orientations'.[35] The way Delamétherie deployed temperament theory suggests that such identities may not always have been constructed in primarily sexual or even gender terms. It was not there that Delamétherie saw the essence of his own (or presumably other people's) individuality, but in the idiosyncrasy of his temperament.

As its endorsement by Delamétherie indicates, the doctrine of the

34. Born in 1743 at La Clayette, a village in the Mâconnais, Delamétherie initially trained for the priesthood, a career which he abandoned when his elder brother died, presumably without issue. In spite of pressure from his family, he failed to marry, explicitly recognising another brother, Antoine (elected a deputy in 1789), as head of the family and making over all but an annuity from his inheritance. He later made over more money to Antoine when the latter was in difficulties and died in straightened circumstances, apparently as a result (information from Cuvier's biography in Michaud, *Biographie universelle*, s.v. 'Métherie' and from www.galichon.com/genealogie/html/celebre/delametherie (copyright Jérôme Galichon)).

35. 'Forgetting Foucault: acts, identities and the history of sexuality', *Representations* 63 (1998), p.93-120 (109).

temperaments proved resilient on the theoretical level, too. Not all that we now classify as Galenic was seen as such by our early modern precursors, and the doctrine of the temperaments was firmly rooted in the pre-Galenic writings of Hippocrates and in those of other, later figures. It would be easy for a reader of modern medical history to imagine that a rejection of Galen represented a rejection of ancient Greek medical authority in general. This was far from being the case. Medicine remained firmly attached to its ancient roots throughout the period covered in this book. Its languages were Latin and Greek, not yet those of modern Europe. All important medical texts continued to be written and published in Latin. Haller's most influential publication, the *Elementa physiologiae corporis humanae*, exerted Europe-wide influence during the second half of the eighteenth century without ever being translated into French or English.[36] The chief beneficiary of Galen's loss of credit in the eighteenth century was no modern doctor, but the even more venerable Hippocrates. Hippocrates' stock rose astronomically during the later seventeenth and eighteenth century in what has been called a 'Hippocratic renaissance'.[37] Humoral theory had been formulated by Hippocrates seven hundred years before Galen. Hippocrates had lived in the age of the Greek city-states. Although a Greek, Galen had served the Roman overlord, as physician to the emperor, Marcus Aurelius. Hippocrates was now cast as the heroically independent ancient doctor – the earlier and the wiser – whose modest productions could be effectively contrasted with the brilliant and more sophisticated but less profound writings of his more worldly successor.[38] This re-evaluation of two great ancient medical authorities was in line with a more general transformation of the Enlightenment's relationship to antiquity. It was not dissimilar to a revised view of the relationship of

36. The work translated by Bordenave and published in 1769 as *Elémens de physiologie* was a translation of Haller's earlier *Primae lineae physiologiae.*

37. By Jackie Pigeaud ('Cabanis et les rapports du physique et du moral' in *Revue médicale de la Suisse Romande* 106 (1986), p.47-59 (52)). Neo-Hippocratism was associated with the influence of the seventeenth-century English physician Thomas Sydenham, and with a concern for what would now be regarded as environmental considerations. See Sergio Moravia, *Filosofia e scienze umane nell'età dei lumi* (1982; Florence, 2000), p.164-71.

38. See for example d'Aumont (*Encyclopédie*, s.v. 'Galénisme'); P.-J.-G. Cabanis, 'Coup d'œil sur les révolutions et sur la réforme de la médecine', in Cabanis, ed. J. Lehec and C. Cazeneuve, *Œuvres philosophiques* (1956), vol.2, p.98-108 (Hippocrates) and vol.2, p.115f (Galen). By contrast with Galen, Hippocrates was characterised as a disinterested patriot, impervious to the seductions of foreign wealth and power, as in the painting by Girodet of *Hippocrate refusant d'aller donner les secours de son art aux ennemis des Grecs* [*Hippocrates refusing the Gifts of Artaxerxes*] (Salon of 1795, Paris, Faculté de Médecine), an anecdote reported by d'Aumont in the *Encyclopédie.* For this and other aspects of the cult of Hippocrates during the Revolution, see Nina R. Gelbart, 'The French Revolution as medical event: the journalistic gaze' in *History of European ideas* 10 (1989), p.417-27.

the two great epic poets of Greece and Rome, Homer and Virgil, which pitted the authentic and 'original' genius of Homer against his later, more polished but less forceful Roman imitator, Virgil. Nor was it unlike the periodisation of ancient art introduced by Winckelmann, who taught his readers to prefer the severely classical style of sculpture deriving from fifth-century BCE originals (the age of Hippocrates) to later, more elegant ancient art.[39] The eighteenth century came to prefer its antiquity on the rough side. Since the humours were central to Hippocratic medicine, they remained central to the preoccupations of eighteenth-century medical writers and practitioners. But the humoral theory presented in the writings attributed to Hippocrates was vague and sometimes contradictory. In practical terms, the elevation of Hippocrates ensured that what was effectively the Galenic version of temperament theory would continue to provide doctors and others with a point of reference, but with increased latitude for modification.[40]

Diderot's citation of the humours, then, was no isolated throwback to a pre-mechanist and pre-modern view of medicine prompted by a layman's lack of specialised knowledge. By the mid-eighteenth century, there was renewed interest in the idea of temperament among medical writers as well.[41] The capacity of the mechanistic model of the body to explain phenomena of health and disease proved limited – a severe limitation in what purported to be a medical doctrine.[42] The various schools of medical thought which proliferated during the early eighteenth century in Europe investigated the possibilities of more theoretically acceptable replacements for humoral theory. The two writers most often credited by later eighteenth- and nineteenth-century medical writers with rewriting temperament theory in modern, scientific

39. See Kirsti Simonsuuri, *Homer's original genius: eighteenth-century notions of the early Greek epic (1688-1798)*, (Cambridge, 1979); Winckelmann, *Histoire de l'art chez les anciens*, 2 vols (the second in two parts) (Paris: H. J. Jansen, an II/1794-an XI/1803), vol.2, p.28-33; Alex Potts, *Flesh and the ideal: Winckelmann and the origins of art history* (New Haven, CT, and London, 1994), p.18-46.

40. Thus, for example, H. A. Wrisberg opined that 'the theory the temperaments of the human body, in the sense commonly received by physicians, and taught in the schools [...] savours too much of the ancient and particularly of the Galenical doctrine', but immediately went on to expound a version of temperament theory which relied substantially on that very doctrine, though with modifications' (Baron Albertus Haller, M.D., translated by William Cullen, M. D., *First lines of physiology, printed under the inspection of William Cullen, to which are added* [...] *all the notes and illustrations of Prof. Wrisberg*, 2 vols (Edinburgh, 1786), vol.1, p.85-89). See below for Lavater.

41. See Harvey Mitchell, 'Rationality and control in French eighteenth-century medical views of the peasantry' in *Comparative studies in society and history* 21 (1979), p.81-112 (85).

42. See for example Roger, 'The Living world', p.271, Keith Thomas, *Religion and the decline of magic: studies in popular beliefs in sixteenth- and seventeenth-century England* (1971, Oxford 1991), p.787f.

form were Stahl and Haller, both of whom struck blows at the mechanistic model offered by Descartes, though from rather different directions. Both also produced versions of temperament theory which owed much to mechanistic views of how bodies worked. They sought to explain temperament in terms of the solid parts of the body, not just the humours. Stahl is more famous nowadays as a chemist than as a doctor – he thought he found the principle of combustion in a substance which he called 'phlogiston', and which he considered to be one of the elements. He also supposed the existence of 'soul' as a principle which informed all living matter. Nonetheless, his version of temperament theory appears to have assumed a substantially mechanical model of the body. Stahl's writings are notoriously difficult to understand and interpret, but a perhaps rationalised and almost certainly simplified picture of his views on temperament was disseminated by later eighteenth-century writers on the subject. According to them, a combination of factors – differences in the composition and consistency of the blood and the diameter of the principal blood vessels – was supposed to yield an easier or a more obstructed blood flow in different individuals. It was this which produced the effects, physical and mental, which had previously been attributed to the humours alone. Differences in moral character – the cheerfulness of the sanguine, or the indolence and timidity of the phlegmatic – were thus related to the relative ease with which the fluids circulated. Healthy, corpulent blood pulsed vigorously through the body of the man of sanguine soul, whereas the blood of the phlegmatic was watery and moved through narrow vessels and swollen solids, resulting in low body heat, weakness and habitual paleness. The soul of the phlegmatic was in a state of malaise. The vessels of the melancholic body were broad enough, but the composition of the blood was thick and its progress therefore sluggish.[43]

Haller's position was somewhat different. He pioneered an essentially physiological model of the body which stressed the two properties of sensibility and irritability, present in nerves and muscles respectively. He demonstrated that the fibres of muscles displayed what he called irritability – a property peculiar to living matter which could not be explained in mechanistic terms. His emphasis on the solid parts of the body rather

43. This account is based on Charles-Louis Dumas, *Principes de physiologie, ou introduction à la science expérimentale, philosophique et médicale de l'homme vivant* (Paris, An VIII/1800), p.422 (citing Stahl's Theoria medica vera of 1708); Henri-Marie Husson, *Essai sur une nouvelle doctrine des tempéramens* (Paris, 1799), p.11; Jacques Lordat, *Exposition de la doctrine médicale de P.-J. Barthez, et mémoires sur la vie de ce médecin* (Paris, 1818), p.234f.; P. M. Marion de Procé, *Quelques vues générales sur les doctrines des tempéraments, et sur le tempérament lymphatique en particulier; thèse présentée et soutenue à la Faculté de Médecine de Paris; le 11 août 1812* (Paris, 1812), p.6.

than the soul or the humours has attracted the label 'solidist' to his views, to distinguish them from 'animists' (followers of Stahl) and humorists (in this sense only, followers of Galen). Haller's solidism provided the basis both for a new approach to human psychology and for a regenerated theory of temperaments as well. The latter is expounded in his most substantial and best-known work, the *Elementa physiologiae corporis humani.* Haller grounded temperament in the relative strength and weakness of the solid parts and the degree of irritability present. Thus, for example, a bilious temperament could be explained in terms of the combination of high levels of irritability with strong, resistant fibres. A melancholy person combined high levels of irritability with weak fibres; a phlegmatic, weak fibres with low irritability. There was little room left for the humours, which had still haunted the composition of the blood in Stahl's model. Haller thought that the ancients had been wrong in identifying the components into which blood could be broken down with the humours and thereby with the elements – misled, he implies, by an appetite for teleological explanations. Thus, for example, they had identified blood serum as bile because of its yellow colour (although it was neither bitter nor inflammable, like bile) and water as phlegm. Haller believed, like Galen, that the constitution of the blood depended on diet (poor people, for example, had yellowish blood as a result of their enforced vegetarian diet), but he denied that this was a determining factor in temperament.[44] Temperament derived, not from the fluid and changeable parts of the body, such as the humours, but from its stable solid parts. Temperament depended on the inherent warp [*congenitum stamen*] of the individual body's fibres.[45] If temperament depended on the balance of humours in the blood, Haller argued, it would change with changes in our diet. In order to prove that this was not the case, Haller conducted experiments on himself, abstaining both from meat and from wine over different periods. He registered no change in his temperament as a result. Conversely, he observed that children nourished on the same

44. Albrecht von Haller, *Elementa physiologiae corporis humanae*, 8 vols (Lausanne and Berne, 1757-1766), vol.2, p.140-48 (Book 5). Haller's account depends in part on that of his master, Hermannus Boerhaave, whose *Praelectiones academicae in proprias institutiones rei medicae, edidit et notas addidit Albertus Haller* (Turin, 1742-1745), he edited. On Haller, see Anne C. Vila, *Enlightenment and pathology: sensibility in the literature and medicine of eighteenth-century France* (Baltimore, MD, and London, 1998), p.13-28. On the significance of Haller's approach, see also Gerhard Rudolph, 'La méthode Hallérienne en physiologie', *Dix-huitième siècle* 23 (1991), p.75-84. For Diderot and Haller, see François Duchesneau, 'Diderot et la physiologie de la sensibilité', *Dix-huitième siècle* 31 (1999), p.195-216, who notes that, although Diderot's views were heavily indebted to Haller's, he tended to assimilate irritability to sensibility, like other French writers (p.209). See also ch.7.

45. 'Non adeo a fluidis partibus, aut a victu, quam a congenito stamine temperamenta pendere multa demonstrant' (*Elementa physiologiae*, vol.2, p.147).

milk and the same diet exhibited different characters – restless and angry or gentle and sleepy – before exposure to external factors had had an opportunity to influence the balance of humours. Similarly, different plants, grown in the same soil and nurtured with the same water, produced very different sap. This was evidently a consequence of differences in the original constitution of their solid parts, not their nutrition. The brains of animals and of humans were revealed on analysis to contain similar elements without producing similarity of temperament.[46] This was thus a more determinist version of temperament theory than that offered by the ancients.

Haller questioned the identification of the humours with the components of the blood, but he still believed in temperament. Not being bound by the traditional quadripartite classification, he was in a position to identify new temperaments. This he duly did, adding a fifth temperament to the usual four. He called this the *temperamentum baeoticum, quadratum, rusticum* – a temperament little noticed, he added, by earlier doctors. According to Haller, people endowed with this temperament exhibited the low levels of irritability and sensibility encountered in phlegmatics, but whereas the fibres of the phlegmatic were weak, those associated with the muscular temperament, as it came to be known, were strong. Ever laconic, Haller provided little information on his new temperament, but the three adjectives which he chose would have given his readers a fair indication of what he was talking about. *Baeoticus* (more properly, *Boeoticus*) refers to a region of ancient Greece, Boeotia, associated etymologically and culturally with the rearing of cattle. *Boeoticus* is used to describe those with the same occupation and the same presumed character as the inhabitants of Boeotia – rustic, backward and above all slow-witted. *Rusticus* means 'country-dwelling' and thus 'peasant'. It too is generally used in a pejorative sense. *Quadratus* describes build and is a more neutral term. It was the word used by the ancient Roman medical writer Celsus to describe bodies which are neither slim nor fat but the mean between the two ('corpus autem habilissimum quadratum est, neque gracile neque obesum' (*De Medicina*, II, 1, 5)). It may have been a medical term. It means literally 'four-square' and was used in that sense to describe stockily built individuals, for example by the historian Suetonius in his account of the emperor Vespasian.[47] Cabanis later described Haller's *temperamentum baeoticum, quadratum, rusticum* as the *temperamentum musculosum torosum*, the 'knotty muscular temperament', and more simply as the muscular

46. *Elementa physiologiae*, vol.2, p.147f.

47. Suetonius, *Vespasian*, 20. Suetonius also described him as firm-muscled ('compactis firmisque membris'). See Jackie Pigeaud, 'Homo quadratus. Variations sur la beauté et la santé dans la médecine antique', *Gesnerus* 42 (1985), p.337-52.

temperament. Though mentioned only briefly in Haller's text, the muscular temperament was to attract considerable attention by the end of the century.

With Haller's revision, temperament theory was definitively severed from the humoral explanations offered by the ancients. Paradoxically, this operation secured it a new lease of life. To the young Marion de Procé, writing over sixty years later, Haller's identification of the muscular temperament in particular appeared a momentous event in the progress of human knowledge – the sort of event which a writer of a later generation might have described as a 'paradigm shift'. It had made possible the opening up of this branch of medicine to the true principles of philosophy:

> In effect, the moderns, knowing how to appreciate the value of the results which the ancients obtained from exact observation of natural phenomena, soon recognised what was hypothetical, vague or too narrow in their [humoral] theory: they rejected it, and realised that the temperaments should be made to depend on the modifications which anatomy and physiology revealed in the principal organs of the body, rather than in varied nuances offered by humours and qualities, most of which were imaginary.[48]

Marion de Procé was neither alone nor even unusual in according such significance to Haller's achievement. Another writer saw in Haller's theory of temperament a decisive reorientation of perceptions of cause and effect in the natural world and a turning away from teleological explanations. Whereas the ancients had believed that when they named the temperaments they were classifying them by their causes, modern doctors, thanks to Haller, realised that they were naming them from observation of their effects.[49] This enabled them to think up new sets of causes, more attractive to a modern world view.

But what had Haller actually done, and what had been the result of his conceptual leap? By identifying the temperaments with physiological characteristics, he had distanced himself, not merely from the humours, but from the Galenic medical philosophy with which they had been bound up. Temperament remained the basic framework for classifying

48. P. M. Marion de Procé, *Quelques vues générales sur les doctrines des tempéraments, et sur le tempérament lymphatique en particulier; thèse présentée et soutenue à la Faculté de Médecine de Paris; le 11 août 1812* (Paris, 1812), p.8. Marion de Procé is nowadays best remembered for his discoveries as a marine biologist. See his 'Sur plusieurs espèces nouvelles de poissons et de crustacés observées dans un voyage de France à Manille', *Bulletin de la Société philomathique de Paris*, 1822, sér. 3, vol.9, p.129-34.

49. 'ils croyaient les nommer par leurs causes, tandis que nous ne pensons tirer leurs noms que de leurs effets évidens' (Henri-Marie Husson, *Essai sur une nouvelle doctrine des tempéramens* (Paris, 1799), p.9). Marion's and Husson's estimate of the importance of Haller's temperament theory was shared by Cabanis and J. N. Hallé (see below).

human types, but the model it now provided was descriptive rather than prescriptive. It no longer offered the possibility of treatment by correcting the humours one with another to arrive at a more satisfactory temperamental balance – Haller's experiments and observation of the effects of diet on himself and others demonstrated the unfeasibility of that. It no longer offered the possibility of treatment at all. Haller's metaphor for the fibre wherein temperament was now held to reside – the 'inherent warp' of the body's fabric – was well chosen. Temperament based on the quality of the fibres – the *stamen* or warp on which cloth was woven on a hand-operated loom – depended on qualities of relative strength, weakness and irritability which were innate, built into the fabric of the body itself and thus immutable. Temperaments based on the humours were subject to the influence of external factors such as age, season and diet. Since every body was made up of the same humours in different proportions, the same basic ingredients were common to all. This meant that even the most phlegmatic person would have bilious moments if pushed too far, just as the most perfectly sanguine individual might experience feelings of melancholy under appropriate circumstances. There was a common substratum to what it meant to be human. But this was no longer entirely the case with Haller's temperaments. Difference was now inscribed in the very constitution of the individual's fibres. The over-bilious or melancholic subject could no longer hope to attain relative equilibrium through judicious manipulation of the non-naturals. By the same token, the slow wits and physical strength which Haller and his readers attributed to peasants were not the result of upbringing or a life of physical toil. They were innate. They marked their possessors off as qualitatively different – as people whom nature had destined to feel and think differently from others. The temperament you were born with was what you were stuck with. Galen's philosophy of 'you are what you eat' was replaced with the 'you are what you inherit' of geneticism to come.

That was what Haller was at last able to observe, what the humoral basis of temperament theory had prevented his predecessors from noticing before – that there was one category of people who were constitutionally different from the rest of the human race – the *boeotii*, the *rustici*, those on whom the biblical curse of Adam fell most directly and who were condemned to work the land with the sweat of their brows. Their muscles and their sensibilities operated differently from those of other people. They were, as his choice of adjectives indicated, both different and inferior. This was something which Haller's colleague, Heinrich August Wrisberg, spelled out in the long note on temperaments which he added to his edition of Haller's earlier *Primae lineae* (which had taken a more conservative line on temperament theory):

> The body [of a person endowed with the 'boeotic or rustic' temperament] is lusty, full of juices, a small irritability in its strong muscles, and some stupour in its small nerves. Persons of this sort are capable of no education; and whatever they undertake savours of a low turn of mind.[50]

They were country yokels (as an experienced alpinist – he was the first poet of mountain scenery to gain international fame – Haller had doubtless been able to observe the rural peasantry at close quarters). In Haller's revision, temperament no longer gave out its reassuring message that we were all the same, all different – that each temperament carried with it its own advantages and disadvantages, but that in the final analysis no one temperament was better or worse than the others in any absolute sense. Freed from the constraints of humoral theory to look for the evidence for temperamental difference in the people around him, Haller identified an indicator of social difference which he promptly recast as genetic. He had discovered a physiological justification for class difference.

Where Haller showed the way, others followed. It was not until the 1790s that the muscular temperament attracted much attention, but the idea that, liberated from its humoral basis, the doctrine of the temperaments could provide an index of identity linked to distinctions of social behaviour was one which bore immediate fruit. The philosopher Immanuel Kant used temperament theory as a way of exploring social difference in his *Observations on the feeling of the beautiful and sublime*, published in 1764, a mere four years after the publication of the second volume of Haller's *Elementa physiologiae*. As its title suggests, Kant's treatise is about aesthetics. More specifically, it lays the ground for a theory of aesthetic responses and their moral equivalents. The nature of the high or sublime style in poetry had been discussed in an ancient Greek treatise, *On the sublime*, attributed to Longinus. The question of what constituted the sublime, and of what distinguished it from the merely beautiful had been taken up more recently by Edmund Burke in his *Philosophical inquiry into our ideas of the sublime and beautiful*, which had appeared in 1756. According to Burke, the sublime in art as in nature suggested feelings of awe and fear akin to those experienced in conditions of actual danger. The sublime was characterised by vagueness, vastness and the impression of power. The beautiful, on the other hand, inspired sensations like those of sexual pleasure and was described in terms of harmony and grace. As Kant put it, 'the sublime *moves*, the

50. In Haller, *First lines*, vol.1, p.89. For the concern of eighteenth-century medical theorists with the health of peasants, as well as their low opinion of peasants' moral and intellectual capacity, see Harvey Mitchell, 'Rationality and control', especially p.91, 108.

beautiful *charms*'.[51] The sublime was identified by Burke with masculinity; the beautiful, with the feminine. What was unusual about Burke's categorisation was the extent to which it emphasised the psychological response of the spectator rather than qualities of the object itself. Kant followed Burke in that respect. After a brief introductory discussion of terms, the second and longest section of the *Observations* analyses responses to the beautiful and the sublime in terms of the four temperaments. There is no reference to Haller's *Elementa physiologiae*, although Kant was an earnest admirer of Haller (the first section of the *Observations* closes with the citation of Haller's poetry as an example of the sublime).[52] Whether or not he was aware of Haller's revision of temperament theory, his discussion of temperament is at one with Haller's approach insofar as he omits any direct reference to the humours. Kant's interest in relating temperament to issues of social distinction also accords with Haller's views. He uses the temperaments as indicators of aesthetic response and moral character rather than physical type. Kant used only the four Hippocratic temperaments (not the muscular), but these, together with the aesthetic judgements which he attributed to them, provided him with a hierarchy of moral worth related to distinction of taste which are ultimately based on social distinctions.

At the top of Kant's scale of temperaments came the melancholic – he [*sic*] who 'has above all the feeling for the sublime' and prefers it to 'the deceiving charms of the beautiful'. Kant's analysis of the melancholic character is couched in terms which anticipate the language used by newspaper astrologers of our own day to describe those born under different star signs:

> He looks upon the change of fashions with indifference and their glitter with disdain. Friendship is sublime, and therefore belongs to his feeling. [...] Affability is beautiful, thoughtful silence, sublime. He is a good guardian of his own and others' secrets. Truthfulness is sublime, and he hates lies or dissimulation. He has a high feeling of the dignity of human nature. [...] He is a strict judge of himself and others, and not infrequently is weary of himself as of the world. [...] Insult and injustice kindle vengeance in him. He is then much to be feared. He defies peril, and disdains death. [...] He is in danger of becoming a visionary or a crank.[53]

The sanguine, on the other hand, 'has a predominating feeling for the beautiful'. He is warm and sympathetic, but impressionable and impul-

51. Immanuel Kant, translated by John T. Goldthwait, *Observations on the feeling of the beautiful and sublime* (1959; Berkeley, CA, Los Angeles, CA, and London, 2003), p.47. On Kant and temperament theory, see Raymond Klibansky, Erwin Panofsky and Fritz Saxl, *Saturn*, p.122.
52. Kant, *Observations*, p.50.
53. *Observations*, p.64-66.

sive ('he must never be a judge', warns Kant). The bilious appears to have a feeling for the sublime, but it is only:

> That sort of the sublime which one may call the splendid. It is actually only the gloss of sublimity and a strongly conspicuous colour which conceals the inner content of a thing or person who perhaps is only evil and common, and deludes and moves by appearance. [...] His benevolence is politeness, his respect ceremony, his love concocted flattery. [...] He has no feeling for the beauty or the worth of actions, but for the judgement that the world might pass on them.[54]

The unfortunate phlegmatic is devoid of appreciation for either the sublime or the beautiful, however debased, so that 'this disposition does not belong in the context of our deliberations'. So utterly devoid of aesthetic or moral grace is the character of the phlegmatic that he would rather read Defoe's *Robinson Crusoe* than Richardson's novel *Sir Charles Grandison* (a yardstick and a judgement which might surprise or pain twenty-first-century arbiters of literary taste, but which would have been readily endorsed by Diderot).[55] The varieties of literary appreciation evidently replaced the humours as the basis for Kant's classification of the temperaments.

Sections three and four of Kant's *Observations* analysed response to the sublime and the beautiful in terms of gender and race respectively. In the light of Burke's views, it is unsurprising that the ideal male response should have been identified with that of the melancholic, whereas the typical female subject displayed the sanguine's preference for the beautiful.[56] Since the sanguine is the temperament associated pre-eminently with youth, Kant's characterisation of women amounts tacitly to the infantilisation of their judgement. It is little wonder that he should view 'the epoch of growing old, so terrible to every woman' as almost an anomaly in the case of what he predictably enough describes as 'the fair sex'.[57]

The characterisation of racial stereotypes according to temperament followed a standard pattern which usually related temperament to

54. *Observations*, p.67f.
55. *Observations*, p.70-72. *Sir Charles Grandison* is a novel by Samuel Richardson. In his *Eloge de Richardson*, Diderot took the ability to appreciate Richardson's novels, including *Grandison*, as the mark of a superior sensibility which he related to a melancholy temperament. See the analysis in Vila, *Enlightenment and pathology*, p.155-62.
56. *Observations*, p.81 (with Kant's note), 61.
57. *Observations*, p.92f. For a fuller discussion of Kant's characterisation of women in the *Observations*, see Ludmilla Jordanova, 'Sex and gender', in *Inventing human science: eighteenth-century domains*, ed. Christopher Fox, Roy Porter and Robert Wokler (Berkley, CA, and London, 1995), p.166-69. Women were also classified as sanguine by Roussel in his *Système physique et moral de la femme* (Paris, Chez Vincent, 1775). See the discussion in Vila, *Enlightenment and pathology*, p.252f.

climate on the basis of presumed hot/cold and moist/dry qualities. Given the moral and aesthetic hierarchy which Kant imposed on the temperaments, English readers might have been more flattered to learn that their national character was melancholic, than the Dutch when told that they were phlegmatic (though the latter might at least console themselves with the knowledge that their fellow-countryman, Desjardins, had represented Holland as bilious – the polar opposite of phlegmatic – on the monument to Louis XIV in the Place des Victoires). Gender-oriented readings of the *Observations* see the third section as the most significant for an interpretation of the book as a whole. That was not Kant's own approach, however, even though this text is significant for the ways in which gender came to be conceptualised in the nineteenth and twentieth centuries.[58] Like Delamétherie, he interpreted characteristics which relate to gender in terms of temperament, not the other way round.

Those familiar with Kant's later writings will recognise in the responses of the melancholic and the sanguine the distinction of disinterested aesthetic response from mere sensory pleasure which would later inform his critical theory. The mature Kant would present aesthetic judgement in terms of universals, rejecting the empirical approach adopted in the *Observations*.[59] In the earlier work, however, it is used chiefly as a tool of social discrimination. This is nowhere more evident than in Kant's account of the aesthetic responses of the bilious man. His description of the latter's self-consciousness – his concern for effect and for outward show – are very much how one might have expected an eighteenth-century bourgeois to have judged the comportment of the courtier as characterised in a famous passage by Norbert Elias – the person for whom affective life was experienced in public and designed for public consumption.[60] Kant's very emphasis on innate taste itself expresses the critical position of a new social caste for whom aesthetic response was experienced in private and probably alone – the readers of English novels, for example. But innate taste is very much a matter of temperament. You either have it or – as in the case of the unfortunate phlegmatic – you don't. This is implicit in Kant's assertion that it is wrong to dismiss those who do not share our own values as deficient in understanding – what they lack is our capacity to feel.[61] It is at this point

58. See the discussion in Paul Mattick, *Art in its time: theories and practices of modern aesthetics* (London and New York, 2003), p.55.
59. Immanuel Kant, translated by Werner S. Pluhar, *Critique of pure judgement* (Indianapolis, IN, 1987), p.163-65.
60. Norbert Elias, translated by Edmund Jephcott, *The Court society* (Oxford, 1983), p.110-16.
61. Kant, *Observations*, p.2. In this respect, though not in others, the phlegmatic was close to the muscular temperament according to Haller (*Elementa physiologiae*, vol.2, p.147).

that Kant's view of temperament joins hands, as it were, with Haller's – for both men, it is a question of *congenitum stamen*. Casanova passed from sanguine priapism to melancholic old age in a single lifetime, but it is difficult to imagine Kant's bilious extrovert or Haller's stolid *Boeoticus quadratus rusticus* accomplishing a similar voyage. If at times the Kant of the *Observations on the feeling of the beautiful and sublime* sounds more like Russell Grant than the future author of the *Critique of pure reason*, this is not because, like Russell Grant, he subscribed to a modified version of humoral theory such as that embedded in modern astrology. There is no mention in the *Observations* of the traditional basis of temperament in humoral theory. But there is an assumption of immutable difference among temperament types which accords with Haller's version of temperament theory. There is, for example, no advice on how to make the taste of the bilious less superficial and worldly. No crash course in the sentimental novel is likely to wean the phlegmatic from his appetite for *Robinson Crusoe*. Like the hebetude of Haller's peasant, the characters of the temperaments as described by Kant are innate. Underlying social intention is of course more crudely evident in Kant's *Observations* than it is in Haller, but that is in part because the project of social distinction lies closer to the surface in Kant.

Another commentator who used temperament theory as a means of classifying aesthetic response made explicit reference to Haller's *Elementa physiologiae*. This was Haller's compatriot, the Swiss pastor and physiognomist, J. C. Lavater. Physiognomics – the science of reading individual character from appearance – was almost as old as humoral theory, with whose history its own was bound up. Haller also believed in aspects of physiognomic theory – especially in what was known as pathognomy, or the effects of habitual expression on the muscles of the face, a belief shared, as has been seen, by his French disciple Diderot.[62] The *Elementa physiologiae* was in fact one of Lavater's sources for his observations on the physiognomies of the mentally deranged.[63] But Lavater's faith in physiognomics went further than mere pathognomy. He held that there was a strict conformity of outer, physical appearance with inner, moral character: 'a beautiful appearance was precisely indicative of a beautiful soul and vice versa'.[64] He shared Haller's determinist views of the capacity of

62. See ch.2. See also Haller, *First lines of physiology, printed under the inspection of William Cullen, M. D.* (Edinburgh, 1786), vol.2, p.43f.

63. Sander L. Gilman, *Seeing the insane* (1982; Lincoln and London, 1996), p.62. Cf. Haller, *Elementa physiologiae corpus humani*, 8 vols (Lausanne, 1760-1769), vol.5 (1769), p.570-74.

64. David Bindman, *Ape to Apollo: aesthetics and the idea of race in the eighteenth century* (London, 2003), p.95. This book contains a good general introduction to Lavater (p.92-123). On French attitudes to physiognomists, see Melissa Percival, *The Appearance of character: physiognomy and facial expression in eighteenth-century France* (Leeds, 1999). Percival has already

individual character for change.[65] He was therefore well-disposed to a theoretical position which stressed the immutability of temperamental difference. There are three passages on the physiognomy of temperament in the *Essay on physiognomy*. In the first Lavater stressed the role of the 'solid' parts of the face as indicators of temperament as against the more usual criteria derived from complexion and movement (expression). To support his argument he accompanied this text with an engraving of four profile heads illustrative of the temperaments. These are executed in an austerely linear manner, thereby eschewing the means then available to engravers of indicating variations in colour or complexion (hatching, stipple).[66]

His most extended discussion of temperament embraced with enthusiasm the revised version of temperament theory set forth in Haller's *Elementa physiologiae*. Like Diderot, however, and like Haller's colleague Wrisberg, he was reluctant to dispense with traditional temperament doctrine entirely. For Lavater, temperament was only one visible index of character, but it was a privileged one, given its venerable history in medical science. In particular, Lavater remained attached to the Galenic notion of the idiosyncrasy – his belief, to use his characteristic metaphor, that within the 'grand Magasin de Dieu' there existed an 'individual prescription' for each of us. At the same time, following Haller and Haller's own master Boerhaave, he rejected the traditional identification of four elements, pointing out that scientific progress had by now identified many more than that – what about mercury, for example, or ether? Not to mention more recently discovered elements, such as electrical matter, magnetic fluid and phlogiston?[67] But he attempted to argue, confusingly, that the presence of new elements should be measured in terms of irritability and elasticity. He even went so far as to predict the invention of new machines for the 'barometric and thermometrical evaluation' of degrees of irritability which would lead to vastly improved accuracy in the diagnosis of temperament. This was followed by exercises which may appear far-fetched to later readers. These include an attempt to characterise the temperaments by analogy with the qualities of the elements traditionally believed to compose them – the lightness, for example, of the bilious temperament, always ready, fire-like, to rise upwards, or the tendency of the melancholic to sink in the direction of

suggested a link between 'the reawakening of interest in the temperaments' in the 1780s and the spread of Lavater's writings on physiognomy (p.53).

65. 'Man is as free as a bird in a cage' (J. G. [*sic*] Lavater, *Essai sur la physiognomie, destiné à faire connoître l'homme et à le faire aimer*, 4 vols (The Hague, 1781-1803), vol.2, p.19). References are to this, the first French edition of Lavater's *Essai*, unless otherwise stated.

66. Lavater, *Essai*, vol.1, p.262.

67. Lavater, *Essai*, vol.3, p.85f.

its prime constituent element, earth. He went on to speculate on the qualities of irritability demonstrated in lines, such as those which describe profiles (profile reading was one of Lavater's preoccupations). This is followed by a series of illustrations demonstrating not merely the traditional temperaments but instances of mixed temperament as well.[68] There is no mention of the muscular temperament.

Lavater's reading of Haller's account of the temperaments was very confused, thanks largely to his determination to entangle it in a web of lore related to traditional temperament doctrine from which he was prepared to discard little or nothing. The procedure adopted in his other principal discussion of the temperaments is not unlike that of Kant. Like Kant, Lavater provided his readers with a measure of their own temperaments and those of others based on the differentiation of aesthetic response. In Lavater's case, this took a visual form.[69] An engraving depicts a group of four men confronted with a famous picture of the day, Chodowiecki's *Les Adieux de Calas*, widely known as an engraving (fig.14, p.82).

As in Kant's *Observations*, their aesthetic response is determined by and explained in terms of temperament. Each man typifies one of the four temperaments – providing an illustration, as it were, of the mid-points of four sliding scales.

The choice of Chodowiecki's image is significant. It suggests further affinities between Kant and Lavater, culturally and ideologically. The Calas affair had shocked enlightened Europe in the 1760s. Jean Calas, a French protestant, had been tried and executed by the Catholic authorities in Toulouse in 1762 for the presumed murder of his son. It was alleged that he had killed his son (who had probably committed suicide) in order to prevent him from converting to Catholicism. Calas' death was public and protracted (he remained conscious for the two hours during which his limbs were broken on the wheel – a torture extended in the hope that he would 'confess' his crime, which he stubbornly failed to do). His family was persecuted (his daughters were imprisoned in convents in order to force their conversion to Catholicism) but one of his sons escaped to Switzerland, where he succeeded in persuading Voltaire to take up the case. There followed a vigorous campaign, as a result of which the judgement of the Toulouse court was overturned by the Council of State in 1764. Calas was declared innocent a year later.[70]

68. Lavater, *Essai*, vol.3, p.85-116. Lavater's highly eclectic vision resembles and in some respects presumably derives from the characterisations provided by medieval commentators, such as those discussed in Thorndike, 'De Complexionibus'.

69. Lavater, *Essai*, vol.2, p.68f; see also vol.3, p.89.

70. Lavater, *Essai*, vol.2, p.69. For the significance of the Calas affair, see Sarah Maza, *Private lives and public affairs: the causes célèbres of pre-revolutionary France* (Berkeley, CA, Los Angeles, CA, and London, 1993), p.27-33.

The campaign helped initially to fashion a new public sphere by articulating a collective public sense of outrage. For a time the campaign centred on the first and most notorious engraving of the Calas family. In April 1765 Grimm described to readers of the *Correspondance littéraire* how surviving members of the Calas family had been brought to Paris and presented to the king, Louis XV. Apart from a modest indemnity accorded them by the king, they were now destitute, as a result of their persecution. Grimm proposed to raise money by means of a public subscription for an engraving of survivors based on portraits taken of them by the artist and writer Carmontelle in the Concierge prison in Paris (fig.15, p.83).

The subscription aroused so enthusiastic a response that the legal authorities in Toulouse attempted, at first successfully, to block its publication – an acknowledgement of the potential power of such modes of mobilising and articulating public opinion. This only increased the public's enthusiasm. Diderot described the subscription as 'the most authentic evidence of the contempt in which are now held those religious opinions which have so often stifled humanity in the breast of man'.[71] The final subscription list read like a roll call of enlightened Europe, from the philosopher Helvétius to the ten-year-old composer Mozart. The widow Calas presented her own copy of the engraving to Voltaire, who hung it over his bed. Chodowiecki's engraving after his own painting was designed as a pendant to Carmontelle's (or a reduced version of it by a German engraver). It purported to depict an earlier moment in the drama – Calas taking leave of his family before his execution. The portrait-like restraint of Carmontelle's engraving has been replaced by the expressive and compositional language of history painting, but the moral contrast – between the cruel and unjust state machine symbolised by the prison setting on the one hand and the unassuming family virtue of its victims on the other – remains the same. This aspect was reinforced by Lavater, who included on the previous page of the *Essay on physiognomy* an engraved detail from Chodowiecki's plate showing only the heads of the father and the daughter who embraces his head.

The use of Chodowiecki's *Les Adieux de Calas* as a thermometer of aesthetic response is thus fraught with ideological assumptions about the sort of moral judgement and emotional reaction to be expected from a spectator. The engraving had been designed implicitly to polarise the

71. In a letter to Sophie Volland of 18 August 1765, cited in Bernard Gagnebin, 'La gravure de la malheureuse famille Calas' in *Gazette des Beaux-Arts* 1319 (1978), p.197-202 (n.9), whose account I have followed here. On the Chodowiecki, see Peter H. Feist, 'Chodowieckis Calas', in *Ars auro prior, studia Joanni Bialostocki sexa genario dicata*, ed. Alijca Dyczek-Gwizdz (Warsaw, 1981), p.575-83.

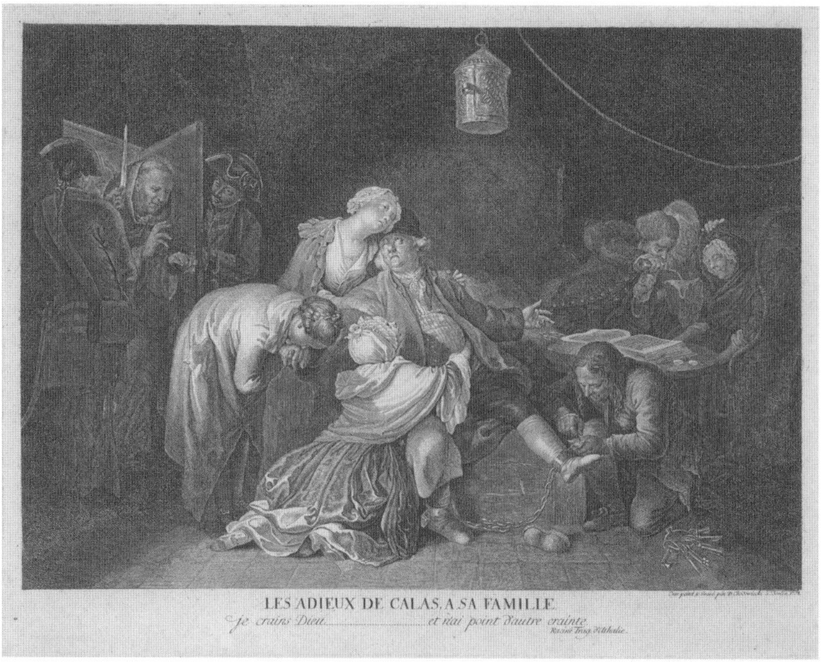
LES ADIEUX DE CALAS, A SA FAMILLE
Je crains Dieu .... et n'ai point d'autre crainte

Figure 14: Daniel Chodowiecki, *Les Adieux de Calas à sa famille*, etching, 1768, 34.2 × 44.5 cm, British Museum, London.

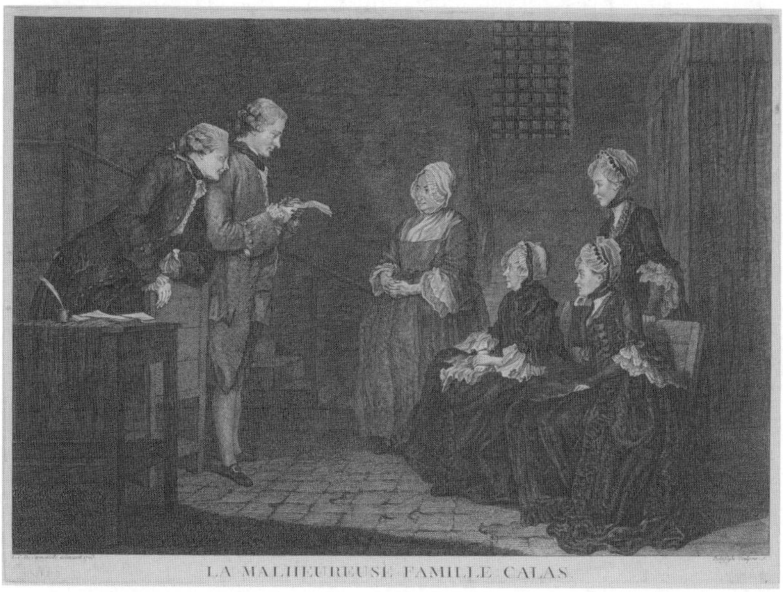

Figure 15: Jean-Baptiste Delafosse after Louis Carmontelle, *La Malheureuse famille Calas*, etching and engraving, 31.1 × 43.3 cm, British Museum, London.

'natural' virtue of the Calas family against the bigotry and superstition of the Catholic hierarchy. Its use in Lavater, in another engraving also by Chodowiecki, is designed to illustrate and define the temperaments according to differences of response to an image where the edifying spectacle of family affection is combined with the pathos of the immediate situation. As in Kant's account of the temperaments, the most 'feeling' responses come from the sanguine (third from left, shedding tears) and the melancholic (second from left, head bowed in contemplation). The bilious or choleric man (far right) is indignant rather than sorrowful, more concerned to arouse the sympathy of others than to experience or express his own. The unfortunate phlegmatic again comes off worst, being too lazy and unresponsive even to rise from his chair. The four temperament types preserve their traditional 'complexions', insofar as these can be reproduced in a monochrome engraving – thus, for example, the phlegmatic man is fat and snub-nosed; the bilious, angular, with a lined and boney face. Lavater's and Chodowiecki's characterisation of the individual temperaments may be less overtly judgemental than Kant's, but it is only marginally so. It constructs a similar hierarchy. The more authentic responses are again attributed to the melancholic and the sanguine, to whom the representatives of the other two temperaments are subordinated in the composition of the group. It also preaches the same overall message – that aesthetic response to cultural artefacts provides an index to moral character.

There is one noticeable consequence of the new characterisations of the four temperaments provided by Kant and Lavater which is especially apparent in Chodowiecki's engraving. This differs from traditional representations of the temperaments, particularly those which link the temperaments to the four ages of man, as in the case of Desjardins' *Captives*. If the phlegmatic temperament was assigned to old age rather than infancy, there was relatively little real difference in the characterisations of the two older and colder temperaments – the phlegmatic and the melancholic.[72] For Kant and Lavater, however, they stand at opposite poles.

Why did both Kant and Lavater take aesthetic response as the measure of temperamental difference? And why were they both so keen not merely to differentiate the responses appropriate to different temperaments, but to judge them as well, arranging them hierarchically? The subject of Chodowiecki's engraving provides a clue. What was surprising about the Calas affair was not the inhumanity of the punishment inflicted on the old man – Christian Europe had experienced far worse excesses of sectarian cruelty during the previous thousand years and

72. See above, n.15.

more – so much as the speed with which the authorities were forced to renounce the earlier verdict. It was an indication of the new-found power of public opinion. The emergence of an articulate and independent public sphere in a world where systems of democratic representation were as yet unknown was the great event of mid-eighteenth-century political culture.[73] But it was not just the outcome of the Calas affair which was decisive for the development of the public sphere. It was the nature of the case itself – the 'demonstration that the ordeals of an obscure family could become a matter for public concern and educate those unused to thinking of public matters as a concern to each and every citizen of the nation'.[74] It established the image of the bourgeois family at the heart of the new public sphere, thereby indicating that the authentic public sphere was constituted by private people, not the aristocratic world of courtly display which still monopolised state power in early modern Europe.[75]

It is not merely the subject of Chodowiecki's engraving which is significant in this context. It is the fact that it is an engraving – a multiple produced in significant quantities to be disseminated, to be discussed and above all to generate feeling throughout enlightened Europe. It was not in what we now think of as political life that that the public sphere made its first appearance – it was only with its advent that what we now call political life became thinkable. It was above all in the sphere of cultural production and consumption that the change most visibly took place. It was symptomatic of the cultural habits and geographical distribution of those who composed the new public sphere that during the later stages of the Calas affair attention and controversy should have centred on an engraving. The mode of production and circulation of engravings also enabled private individuals to demonstrate a collective public voice. Engravings like Chodowiecki's *Adieux de Calas* and English novels such as those referred to by Kant were distributed internationally. They were available to middle-class consumers on a grander scale than any earlier comparable type of luxury goods – through subscription libraries in the case of books, and through display in printshop windows in the case of engravings. Both engravings and books helped give a sense of collective identity to the new, scattered and far-flung public of private citizens on the basis of shared cultural habits and moral and political assumptions. For producers who knew how to supply what the market wanted – people like Samuel Richardson, whose novel *Sir Charles*

73. See Jürgen Habermas, translated by Thomas Burger with the assistance of Frederick Lawrence, *The Structural transformation of the public sphere* (Cambridge, 1989; 1992).
74. Maza, *Private lives*, p.65.
75. Habermas, *Structural transformation*, p.30.

Grandison so impressed Kant – the rewards were spectacular.[76] But this was an audience among whom patterns and habits of cultural consumption were sharply distinguished from those of the older court audiences who consumed their entertainment gregariously and against whom members of the new public sphere increasingly defined themselves, as in Kant's contemptuous description of the taste of the bilious man.[77] Consumers such as Kant, Lavater and their readers were part of a new, anonymous republic of readers and spectators who encountered each other only through their common culture of consumption. Through the dissemination of cultural artefacts, they shared intimate feelings and responses to novels or engravings with people of whose names, faces and identities they remained utterly ignorant. They shared a culture where emotional transparence was matched only by anonymity. A new critical literature was created which responded to the needs of the new public. It helped make the new public aware of its own identity, in part by making it aware of right and wrong ways of enjoying art, encouraging attitudes of self-consciousness and criticism of the habits of others. Chodowiecki's plate of the temperaments may well have suggested to Lavater's French and English readers the regular public exhibition of painting and sculpture which had recently become an established feature of cultural life in Paris and London – an environment in which a mixed and anonymous public were able to scrutinise both the art and each other's responses to it.[78]

Interpreted from this perspective, the responses of Kant's melancholic transform possible weaknesses in the position of the new type of cultural consumer into strengths. The serial isolation of the bourgeois scholar and novel reader, denied the promiscuous sociability of court life, creates favourable conditions for the sort of independent, reflective judgements which Kant attributes to his melancholic.[79] His emphasis on the deficiencies rather than the strengths of the sanguine sensibility effectively demoted the critical status of the one group who stood to gain most from the new privatised patterns of cultural consumption – women, who now found themselves potentially on a par with men, freed from the restrictions imposed on their consumption of public culture. Kant's characterisation of women as sanguine implied that, though women may have had

76. See John Brewer, *Pleasures of the imagination*, p.125-29.

77. Cf. Habermas, *Structural transformation*, p.36f.; Norbert Elias, translated by Edmund Jephcott, *The Court society* (Oxford, 1983), p.110-16.

78. See Thomas E. Crow, *Painters and public life in eighteenth-century Paris* (New Haven, CT, and London, 1985); David Solkin, ed., *Art on the line: The Royal Academy at Somerset House 1780-1836* (New Haven, CT, and London, 2001); Richard Wrigley, *The Origins of French art criticism: from the ancien régime to the Restoration* (Oxford, 1993).

79. The best-known anecdote of Kant's own life concerns his appetite for novels.

an appetite for good literature – after all, their hearts were in the right place – they lacked judgement. It is easy to see in the inauthentic responses of Kant's bilious subject the representative of the style of cultural consumption which was on the way out or at least under threat as a result of new fashions – that of the courtier. The courtier witnessed court entertainments staged under highly controlled and ritualised conditions where the appropriate response depended on larger issues than individual subjectivity. Phlegmatics simply belong to another world, aesthetically, morally and, by implication, socially. In this context, the justice of Pierre Bourdieu's description of Kant's aesthetic position as that of a member of the dominated fraction of the dominant class – the class, as it were, of the professional melancholic – becomes apparent:

> This pure aesthetic is indeed the rationalisation of an ethos: pure pleasure, pleasure totally purified of all sensuous or sensible interest, perfectly free of all social or fashionable interest, as remote from concupiscence as it is from conspicuous consumption, is opposed as much to the refined, altruistic enjoyment of the courtier as it is to the crude, animal enjoyment of the people.[80]

From one perspective, the shift described in this chapter from a humoral to a solidist model of the temperaments – from Galen to Haller – can be comprehended as part of a larger movement in the intellectual history of the West. It is explicable in terms of the change in outlook described by Michel Foucault in his book *Les Mots et les choses* (*The Order of things*) – the shift from a world perceived in terms of resemblances and affinities, analogy and sympathy (or antipathy) to one ordered in terms of identities and differences.[81] Henri Gouhier had already singled out the replacement of a system of signs by a system of laws as characteristic of the development of a mechanistic model of the human body associated with Descartes.[82] Richard Sennett has plausibly linked the acceptance of the theory of the circulation of the blood to the advent of mercantile capitalism, citing among other evidence the prevalence of medical metaphors relating to circulation in the writings of early economists such as Adam Smith.[83] But what these analyses do not account for is the

80. Pierre Bourdieu, translated by Richard Nice, *Distinction: a social critique of the judgement of taste* (Cambridge, MA, 1984), p.493. Bourdieu's comments relate to the Kant of *The Critique of pure judgement*.
81. Michel Foucault, *Les Mots et les choses. Une archéologie des sciences humaines* (Paris, 1966), p.64 and *passim*. Keith Thomas, *Religion and the decline of magic* provides a social context for these developments.
82. Henri Gouhier, 'Le refus du symbolisme dans l'humanisme cartésien', in *Umanesimo e symbolism*, ed. E. Castelli (Padua, 1958), p.65-74.
83. Richard Sennett, *Flesh and stone: the body and the city in western civilization* (London, 1994), p.271 and *passim*.

concern with establishing terms of *social* discrimination betrayed by Haller's characterisation of the muscular temperament – a concern even more evident in Kant's and Lavater's discussions of the temperaments. As will be seen, this concern played an equally decisive role in the attitudes of eighteenth-century commentators to the question of how or whether ideal human beauty could be embodied in sculpture.

4. Temperament and the ideal: ancient and modern

Identification of temperament depended a great deal on the ability to interpret the visual evidence offered by complexion, build or individual comportment. The tradition of linking temperament to individual human appearance and its representation stretches back to Galen himself. Galen set great store by the appearance of the human body in ways which went far beyond the characterisation of temperament by complexion. To an extent unthinkable to a modern consciousness his philosophy of medicine was bound up with what might nowadays be regarded as questions of aesthetics. In his reflections on the configuration of the human body he looked for the purpose underlying form – the purpose of appearance.

At the heart of Galen's views was a notion of justice – it was just, for example, that the muscles of the upper arm should be bigger than those of the lower arm, since the size of the muscles should be equivalent to that of the parts which were to be moved. Scattered through his writings but especially in his treatise *De Usu partium* (*Of the use of the parts* [*of the body*]) are attempts to provide a rationale for the appearance of the human form related to models of function (*dynamis*) and utility.[1] In some cases, where functional utility was not evident (at least to Galen), he was prepared to attribute an aesthetic will to Nature. He pictured Nature as a sculptor or skilled artisan fashioning form. Nature had finished off details with which she was particularly pleased with decorative flourishes, such as the ear, the foreskin, lips or nostrils. The artistically rounded human buttock (contrast those of the ape), was also largely decorative in purpose. Nature added such details as a craftsman of quality might add vine or ivy leaf decoration to a bowl or the hilt of a sword.[2] But Nature, unlike the craftsman, created the whole being, not merely its outward form. The idea of justice was also relevant in the case of temperament, where the just balance of the basic elements was to be aimed at as much as possible. There are two significant passages in Galen's writings in which he related

1. This is a brief and partial treatment of complex issues. For a fuller discussion, to which the present account is indebted, see Jackie Pigeaud, 'L'esthétique de Galien' in *Métis* 6 (1991), p.7-42. See also his *L'Art et le vivant* (Paris, 1995), p.127-53.
2. Pigeaud, 'L'esthétique de Galien', p.18. Cf. *De Usu partium*, 11:13 in *Galen on the usefulness of the parts of the body Peri chreias moríon De Usu partium* ed. and translated by Margaret Tallmadge May (Ithaca, NY, 1968), vol.2, p.529.

the idea of beauty as justice of proportion both to the proportion of the constituent parts of the body and to the balance of the elements in temperament. In both cases, he cited a treatise and a statue by the famous Greek sculptor of the fifth century BCE, Polyclitus – a circumstance which has given rise to considerable speculation about Galen's views on the embodiment of perfection in physical appearance. The more baffling of these passages is in his treatise on the temperaments, *De Temperamentis*. There, Galen stated that an artist who sought to represent the most beautiful (*eumorphotatos* or 'best formed') man or horse, ox or lion, would seek out the mean (*to meson* or the 'middle term') within each species. He added that a statue known as the *Canon of Polyclitus* had acquired its name (*canon* means 'rule' or 'yardstick' in Greek) from having the commensurability or proportion (*symmetria*) of all parts accurately related to each other. He went on to describe the perfect canon of the temperaments. The man who had all the elements in balance would be *eusarkos* (literally, 'well-fleshed').[3] Galen's other mention of the *Canon of Polyclitus* occurs in a passage which criticises the views of the Stoic philosopher Chrysippus. Galen accused Chrysippus of confusing beauty with health when dealing with the soul, even though, when dealing with the body, he had managed to distinguish *symmetria* (proportion) in the elements which compose the body from *symmetria* of the body's parts – a distinction which Galen clarified with a reference to the *Canon of Polyclitus*, since that did indeed deal with the *symmetria* of the parts. He gave the additional information that the sculptor had first written his treatise on the canon and then produced his statue to exemplify it.[4]

These passages are difficult to interpret, in large part because, unlike the readers Galen was writing for, we do not possess the *Canon of Polyclitus*, at least in its written form. We do have more or less damaged and more or less faithful copies of two statues by Polyclitus which later writers associated with the *Canon*, the *Doryphorus* (fig.16, p.92) and the *Diadumenos* (fig.17, p.93). (Polyclitus' originals have long since disappeared.) 'Doryphorus' means 'spear carrier' and the figure would originally have carried a spear in its left hand. The *Diadumenos* is represented as a victorious athlete tying the winner's ribbon (or diadem) around his head – hence the name by which the statue is known. It seems likely that the *Canon* should be identified with one of these (the Roman author Quintilian appears to have identified it with the *Doryphorus* (5.12.21) and this has become the favourite candidate of modern art historians). Without Polyclitus' text it is difficult to know what was so special about the proportions of these figures, how we should set about measuring

3. *De Temperamentis*, 1:9 (Kühn, vol.1, p.566).
4. Galen, *De Placitis Hippocratis et Platonis*, 5:3.

them or even how accurately the surviving copies reflect the proportions of the originals. Polyclitus' text appears to have been well known in antiquity, at least in name, to judge by the number of surviving authors who refer to it, but none of these sheds much more light on its content than Galen.[5]

Difficulties of another order are raised by Galen's argument in the first passage mentioned above, that in *De Temperamentis* 1:9. He appears to have compared one sort of proportion – the balance between the humours – with another, that expressed by the internal relationships. The use of *to meson* or 'the mean' is clear enough in the first instance. The balance between the humours could quite properly be described as a mean or combination of means. This is corroborated by the procedure which Galen himself recommended earlier in the same chapter for arriving at a just measure of the elements of hot and cold or dry and moist – mixing equal quantities of ice with boiling water and of dry earth with water respectively. Relative degrees of heat, cold, dryness and moisture could then be measured as deviations from the mean measures arrived at by this procedure.[6] But it is by no means clear how ideal bodily proportion could be arrived at by following a similar procedure. It is unlikely, for example, that taking an average of everyone's measurements would yield a measure of perfect beauty, even though a casual reading of this passage in *De Temperamentis* appears to suggest that this might have been what Galen was recommending. It would appear that Galen was attempting to bring together two essentially dissimilar types of mean – one relating to external proportion, the other to internal constitution – and two types of rule or canon – that of beauty (which depended on commensurability) and that of the perfect balance of temperament, which would have involved a balance of the elements and, as a secondary effect, that effect on overall corporeal appearance suggested by the term *eusarkos* (well-fleshed). This was a project peculiar to Galen himself, not something which his fifth-century BCE predecessors, either Hippocrates or Polyclitus, could have envisaged.[7]

5. The evidence is set forth and evaluated in Andrew Stewart, 'The canon of Polykleitos: a question of evidence' in *Journal of Hellenic studies* 98 (1978), p.122-31. See also his *Greek sculpture: an exploration* (New Haven, CT, and London, 1990), vol.1, p.160-63, 264-66. For an overall account of Polyclitus and the question of the Canon see Paolo Enrico Arias, *Policleto* (Florence, 1964). English texts of these and other relevant passages in Galen are given in Gregory V. Leftwich, 'Polykleitos and hippocratic medicine', in *Polykleitos, the Doryphorus and tradition*, ed. Warren G. Moon (Madison, WI, 1995), p.38-51. For the context which linked medicine to sculpture in the classical period, see Guy P. R. Métraux, *Sculptors and physicians in fifth-century Greece. A preliminary study* (Montreal and Kingston, 1995).
6. Galen, *Medicorum Graecorum opera quæ extant. Editionem curavit C. G. K. Gr. and Lat.*, ed. C. G. Kühn, 26 vols (Leipzig, 1821-1833), vol.1, p.561.
7. Jackie Pigeaud, 'L'esthétique', p.26, and 'Homo quadratus'. See also Métraux, *Sculptors*, p.65-67.

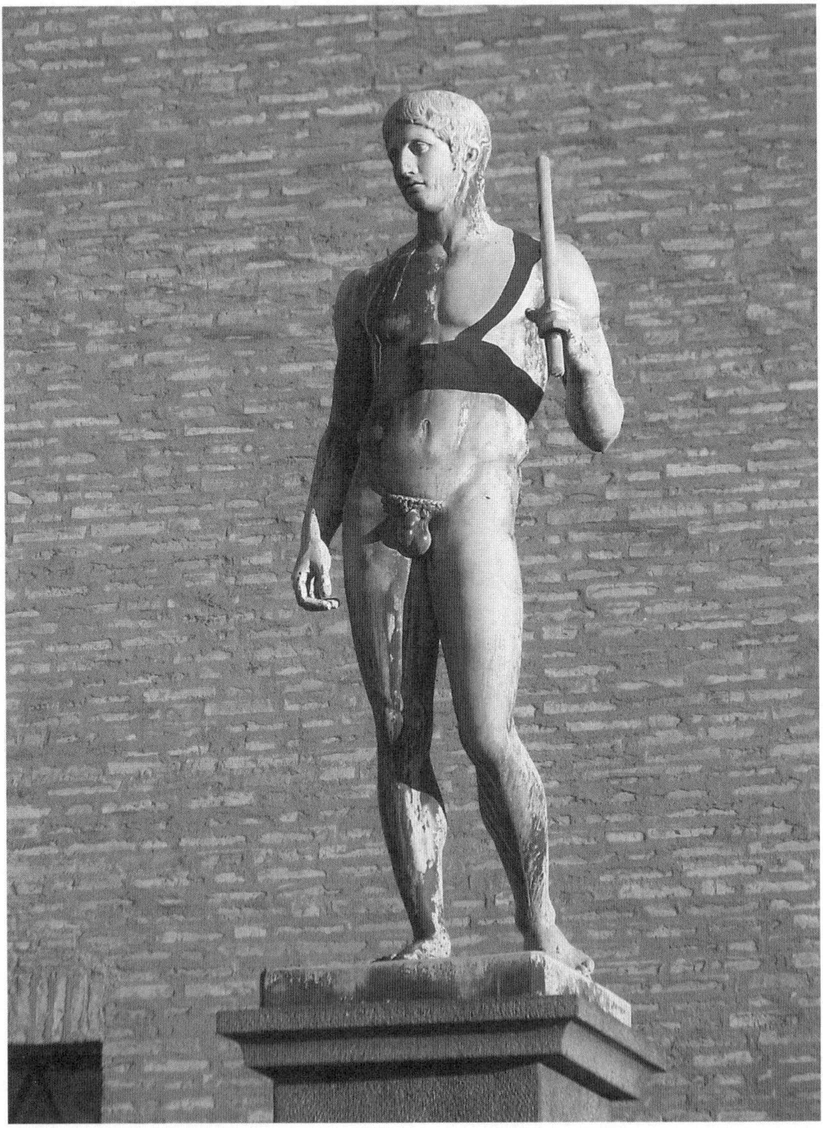

Figure 16: Polyclitus, *Doryphoros*, bronze copy, *c.* 450-40 B.C., Götaplatsen, Göteborg, Sweden.

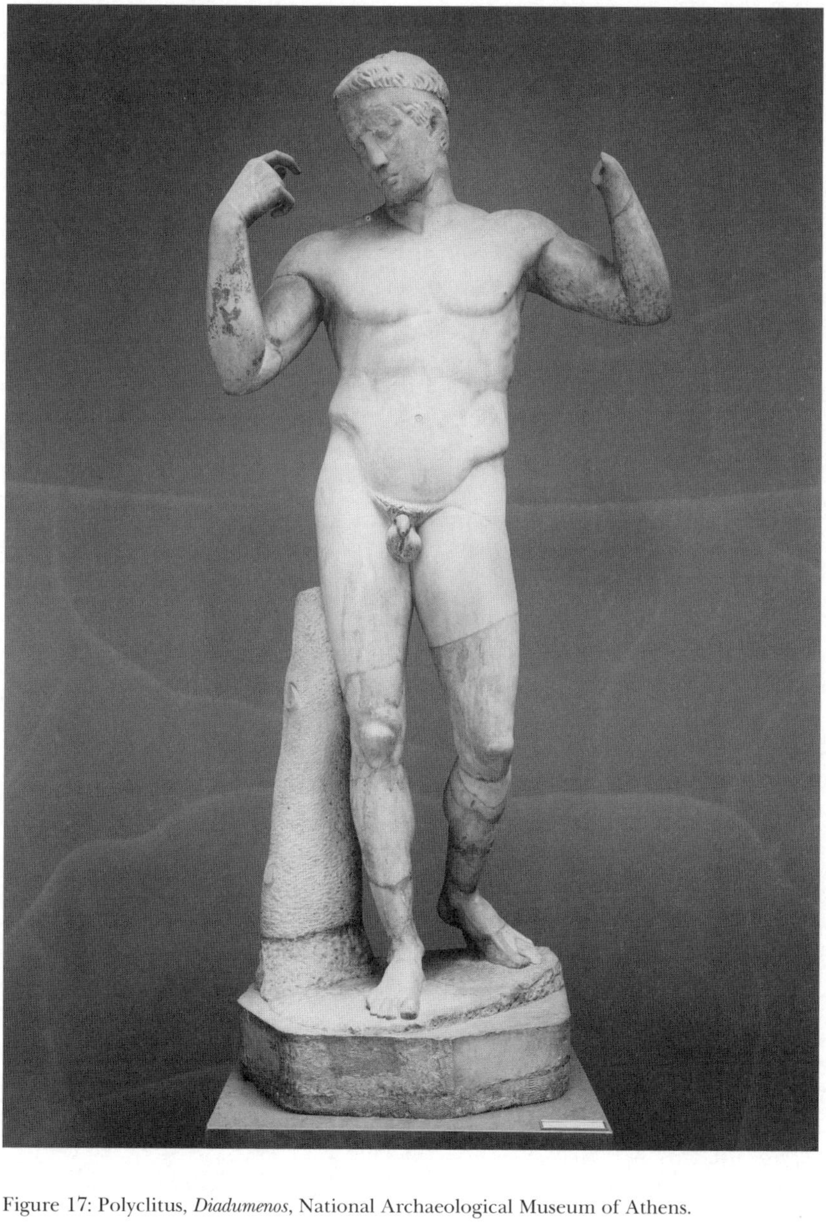

Figure 17: Polyclitus, *Diadumenos*, National Archaeological Museum of Athens.

This was not a problem for Galen's successors. They accepted what he said – however they interpreted it – as part of that heritage of antiquity by whose authority modern culture regulated its own perceptions and expectations of the world. Obscure though the passage in *De Temperamentis* may have appeared, an overall message – that the healthy body was the body beautiful – seemed clear. Its appearance in one of the most authoritative textbooks in Western medicine constituted an invitation to medical writers of later generations to find a correlation of perfect health with perfect beauty, of the healthy body with its representation in art. They concluded that the *beau idéal* was to be identified with the canon, a view which survived throughout the eighteenth and early nineteenth centuries.[8] Galen's account of Polyclitus and his *Canon* appeared to be corroborated by passages in other ancient writers who dealt with Polyclitus in the context of the history of art, notably Pliny the Elder. Galen's procedure in equating perfection of proportion with perfect balance of the humours may have acquired plausibility from the writings of other ancient authors who linked the question of human proportion to cosmic considerations, notably that which opens the third book of Vitruvius' *De Architectura* (see below). Speculation about the precise nature of the connection was as yet untrammelled by the need to square it with the appearance of any specific work of art. It was not until 1863 that the canon of Polyclitus were identified with surviving ancient sculptures. Then it emerged that versions of what turned out to be the *Doryphorus* had been discovered during the previous century, but that they had not been connected with the descriptions of the statue in the surviving literary accounts. A bust with the features of the *Doryphorus* published in 1767 was identified as a portrait of Lucius Caesar, a grandson of Augustus who died in childhood. This was on the basis of likenesses on medals but also because of the bust's facial expression, which an over-imaginative interpretation assimilated to that found in representations of Lucius' father, the consul Agrippa. Nor was a version of the whole figure discovered in 1797 identified as such.[9] No-one, it

8. See *Encyclopédie méthodique (Médecine)*, s.v. 'tempérament' (article by Gibert), vol.13, 1830, p.221-24; H. M. Husson, *Essai sur une nouvelle doctrine des tempéramens; présenté et soutenu à l'École de Médecine de Paris, le 18 nivôse, An VII de la République* (An VII), p.5; J. J. Virey, 'De l'emploi des caractères d'histoire naturelle et de physiologie humaine dans la peinture; par J. J. Virey du Val-de Grâce', in *Magasin encyclopédique, ou Journal des sciences, des lettres et des arts*, rédigé par A. L. Millin. VIe année, (An VIII/1800), p.159.

9. Haskell and Penny, *Taste and the antique*, p.118. Engravings of the bust were published in 1767 (Reale Accademia Ercolanese di Archeologia, *Le Antichità di Ercolano esposte* (Naples, 1757-1792) (1767), vol.5, p.181-5). For the discovery of the statue, see Adolf Michaelis, 'Tre statue Policletee', *Annali dell'Istituto di correspondenza archeologica* 50 (1878), p.7 n.1. Guédron's statement in his otherwise excellent discussion of the fortunes of the canon in eighteenth-century France that the Doryphorus was well known through Roman

appeared, had recognised perfection when they saw it – merely (in the case of the bust) good breeding. But the lack of surviving statues identifiable with those of Polyclitus had not prevented artists and scholars from searching out alternative models of perfection from the same stock of classical Greek sculpture (in Roman copies) which had produced the *Doryphorus* and the *Diadumenos*. The favourite candidate, overwhelmingly, was the *Apollo Belvedere* (fig.6, p.25) (the *Antinous*, Diderot's preference, was also cited, but less frequently). When the Dutch anatomist Petrus Camper presented his theory of the facial angle, whereby humans of different races and animals were arranged in what purported to be an ascending scale of perfection which depended on the angle formed by two lines of the face, he discovered that the most intelligent and morally endowed human head of all was that of the *Apollo Belvedere*.[10] The man usually hailed as the inventor of modern psychiatry, Philippe Pinel, took the head of the same statue as the ideal measure against which to set those of maniacs and idiots, evidently undeterred by the possible obtuseness of people with marble heads.[11]

Galen was by no means the only ancient author to deal with Polyclitus and his *Canon*, nor were his the texts to which artists and those interested specifically in the history of art most readily turned for such information. They were more likely to consult the potted history of ancient sculpture given in the thirty-fourth book of the elder Pliny's *Natural history*. Pliny's discussions of Polyclitus and another sculptor, Lysippus, attracted considerable interest in the eighteenth century, not least because they appeared to imply that ancient art had changed and in some respects even improved in the era of Lysippus – that is, at a period later than that of Phidias and Polyclitus, commonly reputed to have been the greatest

copies is incorrect (*De Chair et de marbre: imiter et exprimer le nu en France 1745-1815* (Paris, 2003), p.39). As indicated by a passage which Guédron himself quotes from Émeric-David, the Canon was still regarded as irrecoverable in 1805 (p.52).

10. Pierre Camper, *Dissertation sur les variétés naturelles qui caractérisent la physionomie des hommes des divers climats et des différens ages* (Utrecht, 1792), p.41, 44 (cf. pl. 2, fig.4). For an extended consideration of this phenomenon, see Jackie Pigeaud, 'De la beauté physique à la beauté morale: les anciens et les modernes', in *L'Art et le vivant*, p.297-343.
11. Sander Gilman, *Seeing the insane* (1982; Lincoln and London, 1996), p.73. For other instances see Henri-Marie Husson, *Essai sur une nouvelle doctrine des tempéramens* (Paris, 1799), p.28; Montesquieu (Charles-Louis de Secondat, baron de La Brède et de Montesquieu), 'Mes pensées', *Œuvres complètes* (Paris, 1949), vol.1, p.1261; J.-L. Moreau (de la Sarthe), *Histoire naturelle de la femme, suivie d'un traité d'hygiène appliqué à son régime physique et moral aux différentes époques de la vie* (1803), p.253 (where the Apollo is, as often, cited in conjunction with his presumed female equivalent, the Venus de' Medici). On Husson and Winckelmann, see Roselyne Rey, 'La transmission du savoir médical', in François Azouvi, *L'Institution de la raison: la révolution culturelle des idéologues* (Paris, 1992), p.29-49 (143).

artists of antiquity.[12] Eighteenth-century reactions to these passages – and especially to Pliny's vocabulary – are particularly relevant in the present context because of what they reveal about changing attitudes to the project of identifying a universal ideal of male beauty as exemplified by the *Canon of Polyclitus*.

Pliny reported several facts about Polyclitus, some of them demonstrably wrong – for example, the identity of Polyclitus' master. He described the *Diadumenos* as having the appearance of 'a man, yet a boy' and the *Doryphorus* as having that of 'a boy, yet a man'. He also listed the *Canon* (the statue) separately from both the *Diadumenos* and the *Doryphorus* (probably mistakenly). He added that Polyclitus was:

> The only man who is said to have embodied the principles of his art in a single work [...] He is considered to have brought the scientific knowledge of statuary to perfection, and to have systematized the art of which Pheidias had revealed the possibilities. It was his peculiar characteristic to represent his figures resting their weight on one leg; Varro however says that they are square [*quadrata*] and almost exactly after the same type.[13]

This passage was subjected to an extended critique by the French sculptor Etienne Falconet, who published his own, French commentary on Pliny's text in 1772. On the scope of the canon, he accused Pliny of having misunderstood his sources (which in this instance he had not). Falconet argued that a figure sufficiently correct to serve as a rule could do so only for figures of its own sex, character and age. He doubted whether a canon of universal proportion was even possible. Jaucourt, a contributor to the *Encyclopédie*, had suggested that Polyclitus made use of the selective *beau idéal* to arrive at his *Canon*.[14] Falconet rejected this explanation too. To prove his point he cited Bouchardon's practice in the case of his 'très-bel Amour' (i.e., *Love making himself a bow from the club of Hercules* (fig.4, p.19)). Falconet claimed that Bouchardon had used a single model, thereby implying that it was only by the use of a single live model that the highest beauty in art could be realised. This had also been true of the horse used by Bouchardon as a model for that in his equestrian statue of Louis XV.[15] Thus Falconet, like Mariette, though from a different perspective, singled out Bouchardon's statue of *Love* as an example of a

12. See Alex Potts, *Flesh and the ideal*, p.73.
13. *The Elder Pliny's chapters on the history of art, translated by K. Jex-Blake with commentary and historical introduction by E. Sellers* (Oxford, 1896), p.43-45 (Pliny, *N. H.*, xxxiv, 2); and p.xv-xix for the role of Varro.
14. *Encyclopédie*, vol.14, p.25 [s.v. 'règle']. For Diderot's rejection of this view, see above, ch.2.
15. Etienne Falconet, 'Notes sur trois livres de Pline l'ancien, où il traite de la peinture et de la sculpture', in *Œuvres d'Etienne Falconet, statuaire, contenant plusieurs écrits relatifs aux beaux-arts* (Lausanne, 1781), vol.3, p.84-88. For a vigorous expression of Falconet's esteem for Bouchardon, see his undated letter (*c.*1766) to Diderot in Diderot, *Correspondance*, vol.6, p.123.

practice – the minute imitation of a single model – which implied a rejection of the classical ideal of universal types. Commenting on a later passage in the same chapter of Pliny, Falconet understood a statement by Varro to the effect that Polyclitus' statues were 'almost exactly after the same type' as a hostile criticism (although this is by no means obvious from the tone of Pliny's report).[16] Falconet's position accords with an increasing concern for particularity of body type among artists and critics who expressed their dissatisfaction with the use of a single, 'universal' model in academic life classes. Such a model was the legendary Deschamps, famous for having posed for 'more than forty years' at the Academy of Painting in Paris, where he was said to have provided the model for 'almost all the figures in paintings of the French school' produced during that period:

> There is a legitimate complaint that, in large schools, there was only one model, or two at most. This gives students the impression that there is only one nature, it hides from them the countless differences, and familiarises them with mannerism, even as they are made to work from nature.[17]

But Falconet reserved his most extended and trenchant criticism for another characteristic of Polyclitus' figures recorded by Varro and reported by Pliny – that they were 'square'. The adjective used by Pliny, *quadratus*, is one which we have already encountered. It was used by Haller in his description of the Boeotian or muscular temperament. It was also the word used by Renaissance editors to translate *eusarkos* (well-fleshed) in the passage in Galen's *De Temperamentis* which discusses Polyclitus'.[18] This was perhaps because it had been used by the classical medical writer Celsus to describe another mean – that between thin and fat. The meaning attached to *quadratus* by Pliny is unclear. It may have been intended to translate a Greek word, *tetragonos*, which has a specific signification in an aesthetic context, or it may simply record the personal reaction of the two Roman writers, Varro and Pliny, to the figures of Polyclitus. If the latter is true, it is possible that it is used in the same sense as in the passages in Celsus and Suetonius already referred to in the discussion of Haller.[19] That is how it was understood by Pliny's eight-

16. 'Cette petite phrase n'est point un éloge', Falconet, *Œuvres*, vol.3, p.90.
17. Claude-Henri Levesque in Watelet and Levesque, *Dictionnaire des arts de peinture, sculpture et gravure*, 5 vols (Paris, 1792), vol.3, p.471f., s.v. 'modèle'. Deschamps was employed for forty six years, from 1725 to 1771 (Locquin, *La Peinture d'histoire*, p.79). Also see Locquin for similar expressions of dissatisfaction by Cochin, Diderot and others, and ch.2. Women were, of course, not allowed to pose at the Academy under the *ancien régime*.
18. Kühn 1:567.
19. See the discussion in J. J. Pollitt, *The Ancient view of Greek art: criticism, history and terminology* (New Haven, CT, and London, 1974), p.263-69. For the Pythagoreans, the word *tetragonos* also had connotations of perfection, including moral perfection, and justice, notably in a

eenth-century French editor, Gabriel Brotier, and that is how it was understood by Falconet as well. Brotier and Falconet took it for granted that the adjective referred to the type of body represented rather than the mode of representation.[20] Falconet evidently considered that the use of this adjective jeopardised the status of the *Canon*:

> If Polyclitus' figures were square [*quarrés*] (according the testimony of Varro which Pliny does not contradict, and which he seems even to agree with, they were of average proportion, a bit heavy, fleshy and lacking elegance) what then was that beautiful proportion, that *rule* of art which he had made, and which the other artists studied so much? Polyclitus could evidently not have made the Apollo [Belvedere].[21]

Falconet apparently regarded the *Apollo Belvedere* as the embodiment of the non-*quadratus*. The social assumptions underlying Falconet's attitude become explicit in his commentary on a later passage in Pliny's text. There the word *quadratus* reappears in what is apparently a reference to the *Canon* of Polyclitus included in an account of the work of the later sculptor, Lysippus:

> [Lysippus'] chief contributions to the art of sculpture are said to consist in his vivid rendering of the hair, in making the heads smaller than older artists had done, and the bodies slimmer and with less flesh, thus increasing the apparent height of his figures. There is no word in Latin for the canon of symmetry [*symmetria*] which he was so careful to preserve, bringing innovations which had never been thought of before into the square canon of the older artists [*quadratas veterum staturas permutando*], and he often said that the difference between himself and them was that they represented men as they were, and he as they appeared to be.[22]

---

famous fragment of the lyric poet Simonides (543) where it is used to describe the perfect citizen. These are dismissed by Pollitt in this context, but are discussed by Deborah Tarn Steiner, who also proposes that the *Doryphorus* was intended to incarnate the perfect citizen as hoplite: 'Confronting the viewer with an idealised image of his own body and role within the state, the statue offers a paradigm of both physical and civic excellence, of a self-regulation that enables a man to fulfil his part in a public enterprise' (*Images in mind: statues in archaic and classical Greek literature and thought* (Princeton, NJ, and Oxford, 2001), p.39-44 (44)). If so, the view that *quadratus* translates *tetragonos* might be relevant to the interpretation of *De Temperamentis* I, 9, since *tetragonos* could also be linked to the Pythagorean doctrine of the four virtues appropriate to the four ages (Pindar, *Nem.* 3:74 f.) and thus perhaps of the four elements (Steiner, *Images*, p.43).

20. See Brotier's note *ad loc.* (*Caii Plinii Secuni Historiae Naturalis libri XXXVII*, 1779 edition, 6:350). See below for the views of Winckelmann, whom Falconet took to task for what he regarded as a misinterpretation of Pliny's use of *quadratus* (*Œuvres*, vol.3, p.117).
21. Falconet, *Œuvres*, vol.3, p.90. Following Brotier, Falconet also quoted Celsus, whose approval for the *corpus quadratum* – the square-built body as mean between the fat and the slim – he somewhat grudgingly acknowledged but did not share. The Apollo was also singled out by Falconet in his contribution to the *sculpture* article in the *Encyclopédie* (vol.14, p.834, s.v. 'Sculpture').
22. *The Elder Pliny's chapters on the history of art*, p.51-53 (Pliny, *N. H.*, xxxiv, 2).

Evidently recalling Suetonius' use of the word *quadratus* to describe the build of the emperor Vespasian (see above), Falconet argued, reasonably enough, that if Lysippus' predecessors really had represented men both 'as they were' and 'square', most Greek men must have looked like Vespasian. This he refused to believe. Instead he suggested that:

> He must have thought and said that his predecessors copied common nature without principle or selection, just as they found it in the first comer; that as for him, he made men of the most elegant and noble form and proportion, such as nature offered at her best.[23]

Here, *quadratus* is aligned with 'common'; the beautiful, with what is 'elegant and noble'. These are socially rather than aesthetically defined terms. The unfortunate Vespasian, evoked by Falconet to provide the middle term in the equation of *quadratus* with 'common', had been characterised in similar terms by Suetonius himself – familiar with his inferiors, particularly at mealtimes, coarse and forthright in his speech and especially his jokes.[24] Falconet may have had little time for the embodiment of universal beauty as exemplified in the *Canon* of Polyclitus, but the embodiment of gentility was something he evidently took seriously – sufficiently so to foist it onto Lysippus, regardless of lack of evidence. The continuation of Falconet's account makes it clear that his readiness to interpret Pliny's account of Lysippus in this way was driven by considerations nearer home – the practice, as he understood it, of Lebrun, Louis XIV's first painter and first director of France's Royal Academy of Painting and Sculpture, and that of his successors. According to Falconet, Lebrun and his followers had said to their students: 'When you copy nature, do not make what you see; remember the *Hercules* [Farnese] and the *Laocoön*; make the arms with big muscles, the legs with big square [*quarrés*] calves, sharply delineated nipples and prominent, rounded six-packs.'

But then Bouchardon had appeared, together with the painters François Le Moine and Carle Vanloo. They had taught how to see accurately and record gracefully the beauties of nature, and how to correct faults by referring to the great masters and the sublime principles of the best antiquity. Clearly Falconet was concerned to make a point about changing taste and practice in the mid-eighteenth century. But he was also proscribing a certain type of model, that exemplified by

23. Falconet, *Œuvres*, vol.3, p.113f. Some critics expressed similar misgivings over the robust build of statues of Polyclitan types once these had been plausibly identified in the nineteenth century. See Adolf Michaelis, 'Tre Statue Policletee', *Annali dell'Instituto di Correspondenza Archeologica* 50 (1878), p.10.

24. *Vespasian*, 21-23.

the – to his mind – over-muscled bodies of the *Farnese Hercules* (fig.5, p.24) and the father in the *Laocoön* group (fig.18, p.101). He was right to claim that these two figures had been accorded pre-eminence in the previous century. They had been given pride of place in the collection of engravings which Girard Audran had published in 1683 to illustrate the proportions of the finest ancient statues.[25] Falconet recognised that the hallmarks of Lysippus' figures – the smaller heads, the lighter, less fleshy bodies and more elongated figures – were not precisely the opposite of 'square muscles', but they were the opposite of 'square and common builds [*tailles quarrées et communes*]':

> The principal merit of Lysippus was to have known how to go beyond the servile imitation of common nature; to have developed in his statues what particularly pleases; what moves the soul without violating the truths of nature; what appears to distance itself from scrupulous exactitude while in reality approaching all the more to truth and beauty of the first order.[26]

Lysippus, then, had encouraged his students to modify what they saw, at least according to Falconet – much as Lebrun had done. But the values underlying what Falconet presumed to have been the advice of these two artists were surely different. The respect accorded to the *Laocoön* and the *Farnese Hercules* in the seventeenth century had accorded with beliefs about the social and natural order. In his compilation of engravings designed to illustrate the proportions of ancient statues, Audran had arranged the figures in a hierarchy of physical prowess. First came the *Laocoön* and the *Farnese Hercules*, followed by the *Antinous* and the *Apollo Belvedere*, two Venuses (the Callipygian and the Medici) and more ephebic male figures. The sequence ended with adolescence and infancy, embodied in the two sons of Laocoön and a Cupid respectively. Such a hierarchy echoed that of the patriarchal society in which Audran lived, but it also obeyed what he might have identified as the 'order of nature', arranged on a sliding scale from the physically strongest to the weakest members of society. The preference for certain physical types which Falconet attributed to Lysippus was also governed by a sense of social distinction, but one which attached to the spectator, not to the body represented – the ability (or otherwise) to distinguish the elegant and the

25. Girard Audran, *Les Proportions du corps humain mesurées sur les plus belles gigures de l'antiquité* (Paris, 1683). Audran's publication continued in use by students until the early nineteenth century (Guédron, *De Chair et de marbre*, p.43).

26. Falconet, *Œuvres*, vol.3, p.114-16. The judgement that such body types are apt to 'move the soul' may have been prompted by Falconet's reading of Winckelmann (see below). For other critiques of what were now perceived as the excessively muscular figures of earlier artists including Michelangelo, see Guédron, *De Chair et de marbre*, p.65f.

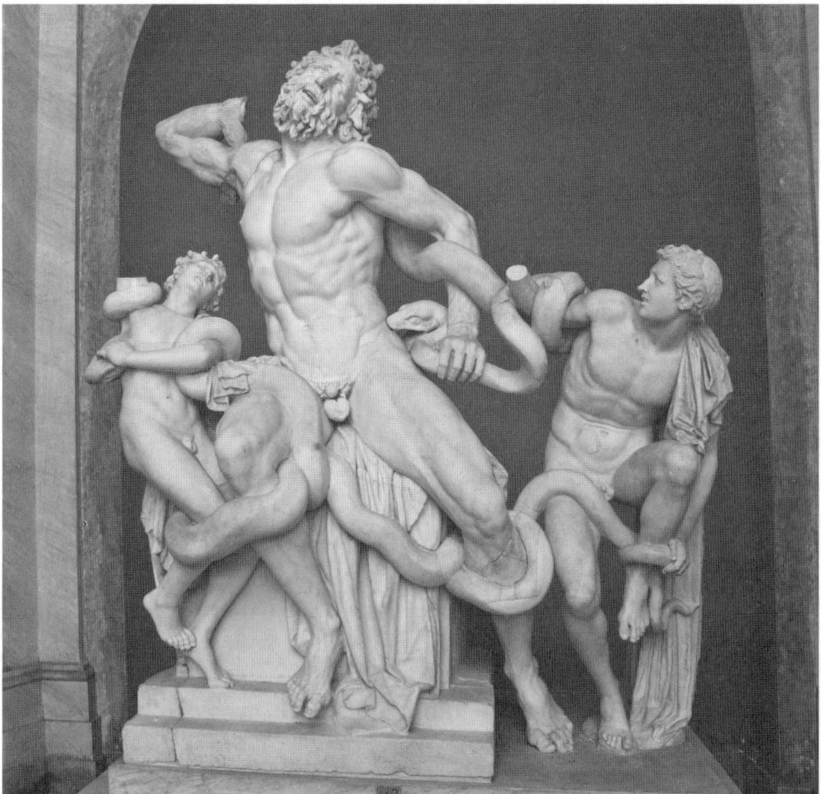

Figure 18: *Laocoön*, marble, H. 242 cm, Musei Vaticani, Rome.

noble from the common and the *quarré*. In this his approach resembled those of Kant (see above) and Winckelmann, whom he had read.[27]

Underlying Falconet's necessarily hypothetical reading of Pliny's account of Lysippus and earlier sculptors is the unfavourable interpretation he gives of the word *quadratus* as applied to bodies. This interpretation accords with Haller's use of the same adjective to describe the build typical of the muscular temperament. It appears to have been only from the middle of the eighteenth century that the adjective *quadratus* acquired this pejorative meaning, and this occurred, strikingly, in fields – medicine, aesthetics – where it had hitherto been used to describe a bodily build which was acceptable or even desirable. The word had carried a positive sense for Celsus and for the Latin translators of Galen. Suetonius had used it as a neutral descriptive term – so, apparently, had Pliny, whatever precisely he had meant by it. It had also been used in relation to the ideal human body by the Roman architectural writer Vitruvius. In a discussion of how to work out proportion in the plan of temples, Vitruvius offered a set of ideal proportions for the body which may be indebted to Polyclitus' lost *Canon*. He then explained how the ideal human body, laid flat on its back with its limbs extended, could be inscribed in a circle, with its centre at the navel: 'And just as the human body yields a circular outline, so too a square figure may be found from [*lit.*, in/on] it' (Non minus quemadmodum schema rotundationis in corpore efficitur, item quadrata designatio in eo invenitur).

This was to be achieved by measuring the figure from the bottom of the feet to the top of the head, and from one outstretched hand to the other.[28] The idea that the ideal human body contained proportions which could thus be related to the design of a square does not appear to have offended either Vitruvius' Roman readers or those later artists and theorists who took up his vision in fifteenth- and sixteenth-century Europe. It appeared to justify the use of the proportions of the ideal human body as a yardstick which could be applied to other forms. The very fact that Vitruvius claimed universal applicability for the measurements which he offered was fundamental to his message as an architect and to the attraction which his system exerted on later generations. The perfect figures within which the ideal body could be inscribed appeared to confirm the divine nature of the plan on which that body was based. But the ideal body also related to actual human bodies, with all their

27. As Alex Potts observed in relation to Winckelmann, 'while the ideally beautiful figure is not in itself the symbol of an enlightened middle class, the proper understanding of it is' (*Flesh and the ideal*, p.159; see also p.205).
28. Vitruvius, translated by Morris Hickey Morgan, *The Ten books of architecture* (New York, 1960; 1914), p.73 (*De Architectura*, III, 1:3).

individual imperfections. It was the norm which connected them with each other. Like the *meson* (mean) evoked by Galen in his discussion of Polyclitus' *Canon*, Vitruvian man offered the ideal as an embodiment of the norm, an embodiment which emphasised the common identity of the human race (or, at least, the 50 per cent of it who were male). It was only the existence of all the innumerable individual men in the world which could hold in place the common value of the ideal created by the theoretical intersection of their measurements. Later, this passage fascinated artists who included Dürer and Leonardo da Vinci. Leonardo's graphic demonstration of Vitruvius' idea in a drawing now in Venice has itself become an icon for later generations, the embodiment of an emphatically humanist vision of the universe, with man [*sic*] as the measure of all things but also with a single man as the measure of all men (fig.19, p.104).[29] The would-be universality of the four square Vitruvian canon was losing its appeal by the mid-eighteenth century, at least for artists. The ideal proportions of the body on which Vitruvius based his calculations (*De Architectura*, III,1:2) were accepted by Buffon, though with reservations about their universal applicability.[30] But Watelet was not concerned with the 'one canon fits all' stance implied by the traditions surrounding Polyclitus and Vitruvius. Instead, like Girard Audran before him, he emphasised the need to distinguish the various proportions appropriate to differences of age and sex. He did not discuss the *Canon* of Polyclitus specifically, but he used the adjective *quarré*, by which Falconet translated *quadratus*, to describe the figure appropriate to the older male, and he cited the *Laocoön* (fig.18, p.101) as an example of this build, as Falconet himself would do.[31] In aesthetic as well as medical vocabulary the idea of the *quadratus* or 'four-square' figure was now associated with a specific type of physique, one whose appearance was to be explained in terms of age and experience, rather than with a norm or universal ideal.

Haller and Falconet, moreover, both associated the term *quadratus* with the appearance of people in specific social categories – categories to which they clearly did not expect their readers to belong. Each used pejorative terms to 'place' the type of the *quadratus* body socially –

29. See Erwin Panofsky, 'The history of the theory of human proportions as a reflection of the history of styles', in *Meaning in the visual arts* (New York, 1955), especially p.67-70 and 88-100, and, on the role of theories of human proportion in aesthetic theory, Panofsky, *Idea: a concept in art theory* (New York and London, 1968), p.52-55.

30. Georges-Louis LeClerc, comte de Buffon, *The Natural history of birds. From the French of the Count de Buffon*, translated by W. Smellie, 9 vols (London, 1793), vol.4, p.135-141.

31. Watelet and Levesque, *Dictionnaire des arts de peinture, sculpture et gravure*, 5 vols (Paris, 1792), vol.3, p.471f.; p.75-86 (80). See also the *Encylopédie*, 13:469, s.v. 'Proportion' (article signed D. J. (i.e., Jaucourt) but with text from Watelet). See the discussion in Guédron, *De Chair et de marbre*, p.48f.

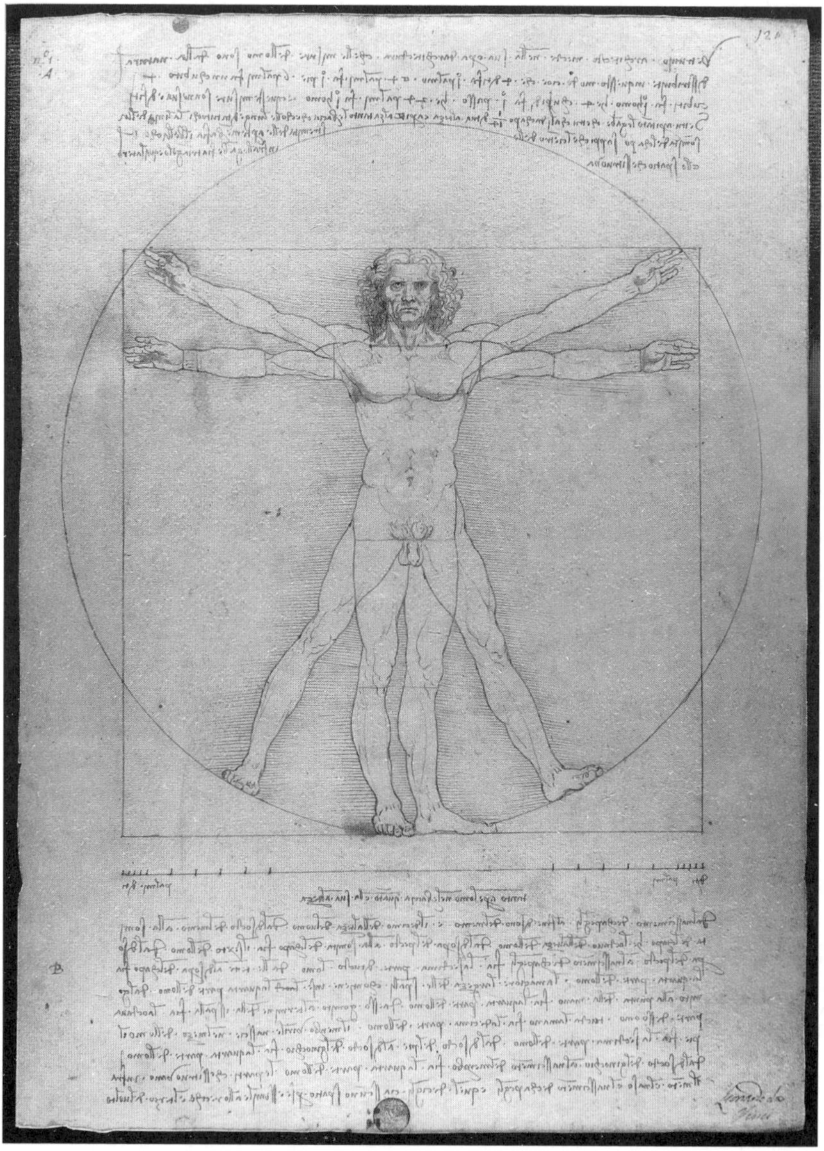

Figure 19: Leonardo da Vinci, *Vitruvian man*, drawing.

Boeoticus and *rusticus* in the case of Haller and *commun* and *servile*, in that of Falconet, where the contrast is with *élégant* and *noble*. In both writers, this attitude goes hand in hand with a rejection of the very idea of a universal canon of perfection in the human body which had been associated with the name of Polyclitus since antiquity. In Haller, this rejection is implicit, though no less definite. By denying a humoral basis for temperament, Haller disposed of the idea of temperament as mixture – the original sense of the word. He thereby removed the grounds for Galen's analogy of the balance of temperament with the *Canon* of Polyclitus – whatever the precise scope of that analogy had been. Once the temperaments were redefined in solidist terms, no balance was either possible or, given the characteristics of those possessed by Haller's muscular temperament, desirable. As has been seen, Falconet's rejection of the *Canon* was explicit. But it represents merely an extreme instance of an attitude which was increasingly prevalent. Mariette's endorsement of the non-classical and non-canonical aspects of Bouchardon's *Amour* indicates a similar position.

Winckelmann's treatment of Polyclitus and the *Canon* raises more complex issues, since the Platonic cast of his views disposed him favourably to the notion of an ideal form of beauty in the first place, unlike Falconet (see above, Chapter 2). Winckelmann's judgement of Polyclitus was, like that of Falconet, necessarily conjectural, given the lack of works by or after Polyclitus which had been securely identified at this date. Like Falconet, he was forced to rely on the authority of ancient writers. His conclusions, however, were diametrically opposed to those of the French sculptor. In the first, 1764 edition of his *History of ancient art*, the only edition published during his lifetime and under his supervision, he dealt fairly briefly with the works of Polyclitus, describing the *Diadumenos* and the *Doryphorus* as statues of 'two adolescents'. Winckelmann did not provide a source for this view, but it may well have derived from Pliny's account, where the statues are described as 'a man, yet a boy' and 'a boy, yet a man' respectively. He added that the *Doryphorus* served as a rule for all later artists, including Lysippus, quoting a passage in Cicero as his authority.[32]

In the second edition of the *History*, published posthumously in 1776, the account of Polyclitus is expanded:

> In his art he was a lofty poet, and he strove to elevate the beauty of his figures above the actual beauty of nature; hence his imagination was occupied

32. *Johann Winckelmanns Geschichte der Kunst des Alterthums* (Dresden, 1764), vol.2, p.235f. Cf. *The Elder Pliny's chapters on the history of art*, p. 43 (*N. H.*, 34:2). Winckelmann did not mention that Pliny appeared not to have identified the *Doryphorus* with the canon. For a full discussion of Winckelmann's attitude to the ideal, see Potts, *Flesh and the ideal*, *passim*.

> principally with youthful figures, so that his genius probably displayed itself in the loveliness of a Bacchus and the spiritual bloom of an Apollo more than in the strength of a Hercules or the maturity of an Aesculapius. This was the reason why those who sought to find fault with his works desired more expressiveness, that is, a more emphatic rendering of the parts of his figures.[33]

This is a free and augmented paraphrase of a text by the Roman rhetorician Quintilian:

> Polyclitus had more craftsmanship and grace than the rest; most critics award him the palm, but in order to find some fault in him, judge that he lacks 'weight', because, while he gave the human form a beauty transcending the reality, he seems not to have given adequate expression to the authority of the gods. He is said also to have avoided portraying the mature adult, never venturing beyond smooth cheeks.[34]

Ancient writers on oratory often took painting or sculpture as a point of reference when they wanted to characterise different styles of oratory. Winckelmann and others used such texts to supply the deficit of known works by the artists themselves. But the evidence to be gleaned from ancient rhetoricians on the appearance and build of Polyclitus' male figures was contradictory. As Winckelmann's Italian editor, Carlo Fea, pointed out in the edition of Winckelmann which he published in the 1783, Quintilian's testimony was contradicted by that of another, earlier authority on style, the Greek rhetorician Dionysius of Halicarnassus. Dionysius' account of Polyclitus appeared in a comparison between the styles of two famous Greek orators, Isocrates and Lysias, and it is both more extended and more detailed than that of Quintilian. Just as the literary style of Isocrates was grander and more sublime than that of Lysias, so the style of Polyclitus, according to Dionysius, was stately, sublime and dignified by comparison with that of two later sculptors, Calamis and Callimachus. In this respect Polyclitus' approach resembled that of Phidias, sculptor of the Parthenon frieze. Their style was more suited to the representation of the divine than to that of the human.[35]

33. J. J.Winckelmann, translated by G. Henry Lodge, *The History of ancient art*, 2 vols (1881), vol.2, p.199 (Winckelmann, ed. Jansen, vol.2, p.228f.). For representations of Aesculapius, the god of health, see Winckelmann, vol.1, p.385; see also Andrew Stewart, *Greek sculpture*, vol.1, p.170.
34. Quintilian, translated by Donald A. Russell, *The Orator's education* (Cambridge, MA and London, 2001), vol.5, p.285 (Quintilian 12:10).
35. Dionysius Halicarnassensis, *De Isocrate Iudicium*, 3. For Fea's comments, see Giovanni Winkelmann [*sic*], *Storia delle arti del disegno presso gli antichi, tradotta dal tedesco e in questa edizione corretta e aumentata dall'abate Carlo Fea giureconsulto* (Rome, 1783), vol.2, p.195.

Winckelmann was familiar with the minor writings of Dionysius of Halicarnassus – indeed, he had cited one of them in a different context on the previous page of his *History*.[36] Why then did he ignore his characterisation of Polyclitus? And why did he go with Quintilian's characterisation of Polyclitus rather than the testimony of Dionysius? How, too, did he cope with the *quadratus* issue, so central to Falconet's interpretation of the lost works of Polyclitus? Here, at least, we are on firmer ground, since Winckelmann devoted considerable attention to Pliny's use of that word. His interpretation of the matter became an important element of his history of style in general. He did not consider that the word *quadratus* as used by Varro and Pliny referred to the build of Polyclitus' figures at all, but to a manner of drawing which he therefore regarded as peculiar to the earlier, high style of Greek art. Such an interpretation of *quadratus* was highly improbable, as Carlo Fea pointed out. Wrong though it was, however, this interpretation of Pliny 'played a central role in Winckelmann's definition of the high style, and also in his description of the systematic changes in the style of art that came about with the advent of the beautiful phase' of Greek art.[37]

But that is not all. The type of body assigned to Polyclitus' figures by Quintilian accorded well with the type which for Winckelmann embodied the highest form of beauty. According to Winckelmann, the smoothness of the youthful body's surface endowed it with greater unity. It was as yet undisturbed by the pronounced musculature of the mature or elderly subject. He associated the beauty of youth with the aspiration of thinking beings to rise beyond the material world to the realm of ideas. The state of eternal youth was in his opinion best fitted to the representation of the immortal gods of Greek religion, not least because youthful figures of either sex were apt to ravish the senses with love and tenderness. Was it not, he added, in such rapture of the senses that human happiness was to be found – that happiness which was the true goal of all religions?[38] The possibility that the type of body preferred by

36. Winckelmann, *History of ancient art*, vol.2, p.227. In any case Winckelmann would have found Dionysius' text in the writings of Junius, whose seventeenth-century compilations of classical texts on ancient art were one of his principal sources. See Franciscus Junius, ed. and translated by Keith Aldrich, Philipp Fehl and Raina Fehl, *The Literature of classical art*, 2, *A Lexicon of artists & their works* (Berkeley, CA, 1991), p.317.

37. Potts, *Flesh and the ideal*, p.74. See also Winckelmann, vol.2, p.22f., p.27. Fea upheld Falconet's objections. He was evidently surprised that Winckelmann should have interpreted the word this way in the teeth of evidence such as that supplied by Suetonius and Celsus, not to mention Pliny's own use of the adjective to qualify the substantive *staturas* in the later passage on Lysippus (*Storia delle arti*, vol.2, p.107 note (a)).

38. Winckelmann, *History*, vol.1, p.360f., p.368f. Winckelmann was of course aware that many Greek deities, including Jupiter, ruler of the Olympian gods, were commonly represented as mature rather than youthful figures, as is clear from his expansion of the text from Quintilian (see above).

Polyclitus and taken as a canon by later generations of Greek artists was anything other than this type of youthful beauty would have introduced a note of doubt and discord at the heart of his aesthetic.

But it was not merely youth which characterised Winckelmann's ideal male body. Effortlessness of movement constituted an important aspect of the way that youthful deities were represented, whether in Homer's description of the passage of the goddess Juno from Ida to Olympus, or in the stance of the Apollo Belvedere, the soles of whose feet scarcely touch the ground.[39] Here, as in the Homeric simile which Winckelmann quoted, it was the parallel between mental and physical activity which was stressed – the physical movements of the gods had the speed and effortlessness of human thought. As the discussion unfolds, however, the emphasis shifts towards a celebration of the effortless exercise of power by gods endowed with bodies whose superhuman strength was clothed in the forms of untried adolescence. The same thought informs a later, famous description of the *Apollo*, in which Winckelmann described the statue as representing Apollo in the moment after that at which he had for the first time released an arrow from his bow in order to kill the Python. There, he stresses the lack of any discernable trace of bodily exertion in the god's limbs – only in the expression of his nostrils and eyebrows can emotional expression be discerned – that of disdain.[40] The best representations of Apollo expressed for Winckelmann the highest conception of the idea of young manhood, combining the strength of the mature god with the forms of youth in which the signs of such strength – the nerves, veins and muscles – were nonetheless suppressed. Even among representations of the mature god Hercules, Winckelmann distinguished between two statues on the basis of their physique as he interpreted it. On the one hand there was the by now familiar figure of the *Farnese Hercules* (fig.5, p.24). For Winckelmann, this was an image of the still human hero resting from his labours – hence the apples of the Hesperides – the fruit of one of those labours – which Hercules holds in the hand behind his back. This statue was distinguished by Winckelmann from the *Belvedere torso* (fig.20, p.109), which he took to be a representation of the same god in his later, divine form, resting from his labours on Olympus. In this confrontation, it was the figure of the god presumed to represent him at a later stage in his career which, paradoxically, revealed a less developed musculature than the statue of him in his earlier, human form. That was because it depicted him as a god, not as the human being who performed his labours. The distinction drawn by Winckelmann only makes sense if the marks of labour which he

39. Winckelmann, *History*, vol.1, p.370.
40. Winckelmann, *History*, vol.2, p.427-29.

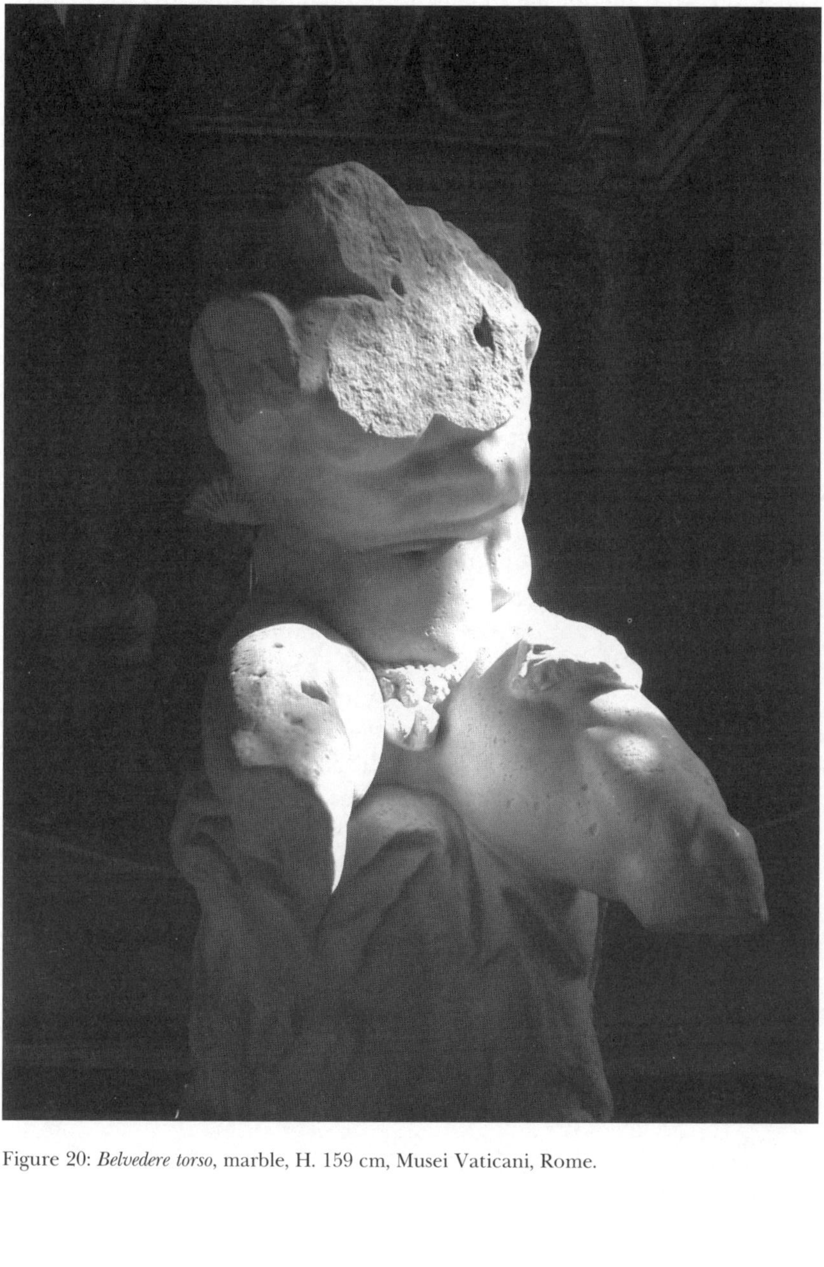

Figure 20: *Belvedere torso*, marble, H. 159 cm, Musei Vaticani, Rome.

assumes the sculptor of the *Belvedere torso* to have suppressed – the grosser parts of humanity, as he defined them in a later description of the same statue – are interpreted as deformities, insofar as they constitute a falling-off from the ideal.[41] It was not merely the youthfulness of what he regarded as the Polyclitan ideal which Winckelmann approved, but its innocence of the signs of servitude – the body untested and unmarked by experience.[42] This applied as much to the divinely rejuvenated Hercules embodied in the *Torso* as to the figures of ephebic youths which Winckelmann imagined the statues of Polyclitus to have represented. Winckelmann dealt with the question of universal canons of proportion in another chapter, in relation to Vitruvius and architecture. Unsurprisingly, given his views on the *Canon of Polyclitus*, he advised against the pursuit of a single universal canon of bodily perfection as a chimaera.[43]

The views attributed to Polyclitus by Winckelmann and his own interpretation of the difference between the two statues of Hercules recall the preference of Diderot for the body of Bouchardon's *Love* and the *Antinous* and the displeasure with which he viewed the possible effects of labour on Bouchardon's model – the transformation of its subject, in other words, into something closer to the figures of Hercules and Aesculapius, moulded and fleshed out by experience.

The question of where Polyclitus and his *Canon* should be located in the history of art – the extent to which they represented a primitive phase of Greek culture on the one hand or a lost golden age on the other – was one which had troubled eighteenth-century writers before Winckelmann and Falconet.[44] Winckelmann's view of the nature of Polyclitus' *Canon* had interesting implications for that issue, since it located the youthful ideal – that of the not as yet fully formed body – in a youthful phase of world history, the heroic and sublime golden age of ancient Greece. Bouchardon's statue inspired Diderot with fears for the brutalising effects of experience, but was it possible that something like that brutalisation had already occurred on a much grander scale in the history of the human race?

41. Winckelmann, *History*, vol.1, p.374, 382f., vol.2, p.341-43. It was Winckelmann's later comparison of the surface of the *Torso* with the unbroken surface of the sea (*History*, vol.1, p.390 – a comparison used elsewhere to describe the muscles of youth) which Diderot cited in his eulogy of Winckelmann in his *Salon of 1765* (*Diderot on art*, vol.1, p.157: see above, ch.2).
42. See also Potts, *Flesh and the ideal*, p.165.
43. Winckelmann, *History*, vol.1, p.437-42. Caylus, too, questioned the universality of the *Canon*, claiming that no statue could provide such a model except for a figure of a specific age, a position which recalls his friend Mariette's views on Bouchardon (cited by Jaucourt, *Encyclopédie*, s.v. 'Sculpture' (*sculpteurs anciens*), vol.14, p.824. For Mariette, see ch.2).
44. Potts, *Flesh and the ideal*, p.73.

A new Vitruvian man – a single figure who could embody universal canons of proportion and by implication stand as a plausible image of undifferentiated humanity – did not appear feasible for the second half of the eighteenth century. Yet a figure which laid claim to just such universality was included in one of the most significant sculptural projects undertaken in mid-eighteenth-century France. In 1755, Bouchardon's younger contemporary, Jean-Baptiste Pigalle, was commissioned to execute a monument to the reigning monarch, Louis XV, for the newly built Place Royale in Rheims. Statues of earlier French monarchs had been mounted on pedestals around which were arrayed chained slaves, symbolising defeated enemies, as in the case of Desjardin's monument to Louis XIV in the Place des Victoires (see above, Chapter 3). Such a scheme was not especially appropriate in the mid-1750s, and it rapidly became thoroughly inappropriate during the next few years, as France's largely disastrous performance in the Seven Years War led to the loss of most of France's overseas possessions. The symbolism of the earlier programmes had also been denounced by Voltaire in his *Siècle de Louis XIV*. Voltaire suggested that figures of slaves should be replaced by those of free and happy citizens. Explicitly following Voltaire's prescription, Pigalle decided to decorate the base of his statue with figures emblematic of the benefits of good government (Bouchardon had already replaced the traditional slaves with personifications of virtues on the pedestal of the equestrian statue of Louis XV for Paris, a project which was completed by Pigalle following Bouchardon's death). In a letter published in the *Correspondance littéraire* in which he asked Voltaire to compose an inscription for the statue, Pigalle explained the significance of the two human figures on the base of the statue. One, female, personified benign government. She held a rudder in one hand and with the other led an unconstrained lion by the mane (thereby indicating that 'the Frenchman, in spite of his strength, submits of his own will to benign government'). The other, male figure personified 'the happiness of peoples'. It represented the happy citizen, reposing amidst emblems of security and plenty – a cornucopia, an olive tree, bales of merchandise and an open purse. Pigalle explained that he had originally intended to depict the wolf lying down with the lamb as a symbol of the golden age, but that he had been forced to change the lamb to a child by the town government, anxious that the imagery might be interpreted by non-locals as an allusion to the proverb, 'Ninety-nine sheep and a man from Champagne make a hundred animals'. The statue as executed, however, returned to the lamb and wolf (fig.21, p.112).[45]

45. *Correspondance littéraire*, vol.3, p.465-68 (August, 1763, letter dated 23 July 1763). Pigalle tactfully omitted the word 'bêtes' (animals) from his quotation of the proverb. It is

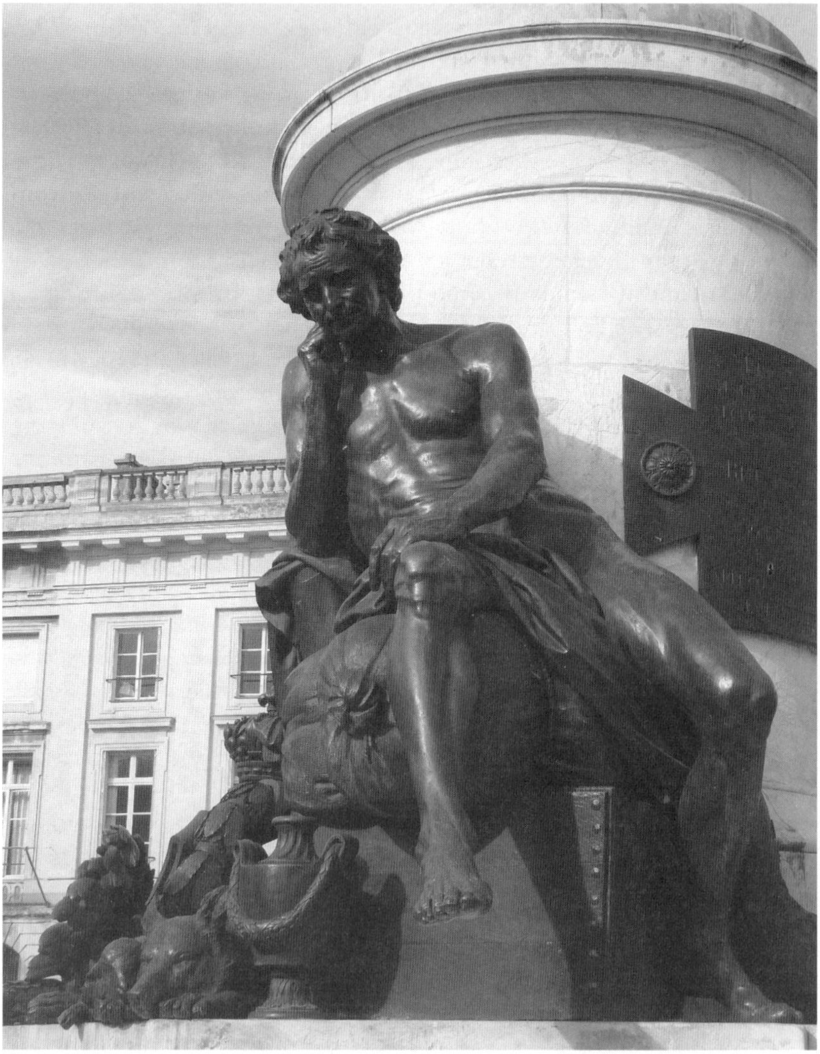

Figure 21: Jean-Baptiste Pigalle, *Monument to Louis XV*, bronze, 1765, Rheims.

According to testimony dating from the 1760s, the 'happy citizen' was a self-portrait of the sculptor himself, somewhat idealised, but recognisable. This was said to have been done at the request of the citizens of Rheims.[46]

Diderot dealt with Pigalle's statue in two extended passages, in the *Correspondance littéraire* and in his *Essais sur la peinture*, as well as in several letters. He approved of the male nude reposing on his bales of merchandise more than he did of the other components of the monument, but he failed to recognise it either as a self-portrait or as a type of the happy citizen. Instead he saw only 'a naked workman [*artisan*] seated on his merchandise, his head resting on his clenched fist and resting from his labours' (*Correspondance littéraire*) or 'a sleeping porter', 'a porter asleep on his merchandise' (*Essais sur la peinture*) which he interpreted as a personification of Commerce. He took Pigalle to task for mixing 'truth' – the exhausted workman – with allegory (the personification of good government) – ostensibly an aesthetic objection, but one with an obvious political application – in Louis XV's France, which was undergoing national humiliation in the final stages of the Seven Years War, the exhaustion was real; good government, a theoretical ideal. Diderot speculated on what might happen if the woman and the lion strayed from their side of the monument to that occupied by the dozing citizen. He offered an alternative programme with three personifications – Commerce, Agriculture and Population – the last a recurrent obsession of eighteenth-century French commentators, who believed that the population was shrinking. 'Your porter asleep on his bales – there indeed is Commerce!', exclaimed Diderot, before suggesting suitable personifications for Agriculture (a male peasant reposing on the back of a bull) and Population (a female peasant suckling a child).[47]

---

supplied by Charles Sarazin, 'La Place Royale de Reims', in *Travaux de l'Académie Nationale de Reims*, 128, année 1909-10 (Rheims, 1911), p.1-162 (61 n.3). On the commission, see, besides Sarazin, S. Rocheblave, *Jean-Baptiste Pigalle* (Paris, 1919), p.57-63, 221-39, on the political and cultural context, Crow, *Painters*, p.155-58, and on the transformation of royal monuments, Merrick, 'Politics on pedestals'. The statue of the king was removed with remarkable alacrity on 15 August 1792, a mere five days after the declaration of the Republic in Paris (Sarazin, 'La Place Royale', p.87).

46. Sarazin, 'La Place Royale', p.63, citing François-Michel Dandré-Bardon, *Le Monument de la ville de Reims* (1765). The original request no longer exists, but Tarbé, Pigalle's first biographer and his descendant, claimed to have seen it. See Paul Vitry, 'Une maquette du *Citoyen* de Pigalle', *Bulletin des Musées de France* 11 (1929), p.242-33. The architect's account of the refurbishment of the Place Royale draws on the explanation given by Pigalle, but does not identify the figure of the citizen as a self-portrait (Le Gendre, *Description de la Place de Louis XV que l'on construit a Reims; des ouvrages à continuer aux environs de cette place, et de ceux à faire dans la suite pour l'utilité et l'embellissement de cette ville* (1765), p.7).
47. *Correspondance littéraire*, vol.3, p.41-47 (July 1760); *Essais sur la peinture*, p.57-59. The emphasis on agriculture in Diderot's alternative programme points to the influence of

The tone of this passage is again ironic, but even so Diderot's scheme accords with his judgements in an earlier chapter of the *Essais*, that on expression (see Chapter 2). There, the child of the faubourg Saint-Marcel had personified the brutalising effects of the market as well as those of labour, while the savage and his wife, unspoilt by the division of labour, embodied timeless human values, like the figures of the two peasants proposed by Diderot in the present passage – the reproduction of the species by both direct and indirect means. When Grimm, the editor of the *Correspondance littéraire*, recalled Diderot's alternative programme for the monument two years later, he made explicit what had only been implied in Diderot's critique, asking ironically whether it was fitting that the security enjoyed by the citizen under Louis XV should be represented by the figure of 'a burly docker'.[48] Privately, Diderot expressed himself in similar terms to Grimm, in a letter to his friend Sophie Volland, whose brother-in-law was the architect in charge of the project. He added that Pigalle had depicted Louis XV as the protector only of the higher strata (*conditions*) of society – i.e., the wealthy merchants, rather than the low. In another letter, this time to Falconet, Diderot judged the head of the *Citizen* to be 'common' (*ignoble*).[49] Here, Diderot's preoccupation with the brutalising effects of the division of labour provided an instrument for introducing discord into the picture of an ideal French society which Pigalle's monument was designed to conjure up. But this approach was effective only because Diderot and Grimm could rely on their readers' readiness to see the figure of a mature male nude reclining against packages in a particular way; as a socially defined individual – defined, that is, in terms of his presumed habitual occupation – and not, as Pigalle intended, as an abstract personification of national identity. The praise which Pigalle's *Citizen* received as a work of art, not merely from Diderot but even from professional rivals, such as Falconet,[50] makes its general failure to convince as an image of what Crow called 'the natural everyman'[51] all the more telling. Thirty years before David and the Revolutionary committees hi-jacked the French Hercules as an image of the people, it had become difficult to find a personification of the French citizen whose identity would not be read in terms of class.

---

the contemporary Physiocrat school of political economy, who privileged agriculture rather than commerce or manufacture as the only source of true wealth. The spectre of a shrinking population haunted most eighteenth-century French political theorists.

48. Cited by Christian Michel in *Diderot & l'art de Boucher à David. Les Salons: 1759-1781* (Paris, 1984), p.526.

49. Diderot, *Correspondance*, vol.6, p.33f. and vol.6, p.304 (letters of 27 January 1766 to Sophie Volland and September 1766 to Falconet).

50. Diderot, *Salon de 1765*, p.289-91.

51. Crow, *Painters*, p.158.

What is most striking about Diderot's reaction to Pigalle's *Citizen* is his refusal even to countenance the figure's symbolic role, its universal identity. Instead, he saw it as the personification of Commerce – the porter or artisan, product of those selfish and brutalising market relations which he had stigmatised in his picture of life in the faubourg Saint-Marcel. How could he be so certain that, stripped of the social markers of dress, Pigalle's figure exemplified that role? The answer lies surely in his physique – that of the mature man, of a similar build to Leonardo's Vitruvian man (fig.19, p.104), though with somewhat elongated legs. He is the type, not quite of the *Farnese Hercules*, but certainly of an Aesculapius or a Jupiter. Yet for Diderot, this is merely the body of a porter, not a fit epitome of humanity as a whole. What classical build might have satisfied Diderot as an image of universal man? A type of universal beauty, perhaps, such as the *Apollo Belvedere* or the *Antinous*? Diderot had stigmatised the *Antinous* as a *fainéant* in comparison with the *Farnese Hercules*, which might imply possible approval for the representation of the marks of labour and experience on the mature human body. But when confronted with what he read as the body of a mature, working man in Pigalle's *Citizen*, he refused to countenance it as the embodiment of an identity which incorporated Diderot himself – that of citizen.

Diderot knew Pigalle personally, yet neither he nor Grimm acknowledged his figure of the citizen as a self-portrait.[52] If Pigalle's statue is indeed a self-portrait, it is an unusually revealing one in more than a merely literal sense. Early spectators had difficulties in interpreting the figure's distinctive pose and expression. The latter appear to be out of harmony with the emotions suggested by the role of this figure in the monument's programme. The evident lassitude of the *Citizen* was interpreted by Diderot ironically, as a sign of the docker's exhaustion. More sympathetic critics were merely puzzled. How was the spectator intended to reconcile the figure's air of dejection with the riches with which he was surrounded and on which he reposed, not to mention the protective hand which the figure of his sovereign originally extended above his head?[53] This evident discrepancy between the figure's expression and its role in the monument's programme might have arisen as a result of the sculpture's status as a self-portrait, in that a 'truthful' self-portrait as envisaged by Pigalle was somehow at variance with contentment which the figure of the *Citizen* was intended to

52. This reluctance could perhaps be explained in terms of the conventions governing the criticism of portraits of known sitters (see Halliday, *Facing the public*, p.53f.) – a reluctance presumably reinforced in the present case by the figure's nudity.

53. P. A. Dérodé-Géruzez, *Observations sur les monuments et établissements publics de la ville de Reims, sur les embellissements projétés et les améliorations dont ils sont susceptibles* (Reims, 1827), p.12, cited by Sarazin, 'La Place Royale', p.62.

embody. On the other hand, and perhaps more plausibly, it may have been these difficulties in reading the figure's expression and pose which gave rise to the tradition that this was a self-portrait in the first place. Whatever the explanation, Pigalle chose to characterise his figure in a way which went against the sense of his own programme. This becomes clear when the visual sources for the figure and its pose are taken into account. In his letter to Voltaire, Pigalle had expressed his disapproval of the use of captives on the base of royal monuments. Yet his own *Citizen* is indebted to the *Captives* on Desjardins' statue of Louis XIV in more ways than one. Most obviously, there is the pose of the lower half of the *Citizen*'s body. This is arranged after the manner of Desjardins' *Brandenburger* (fig.12, p.61) – minus the trousers, of course, and reversed. There is nothing remarkable about that. Desjardins had disposed four seated figures round the perimeter of a pedestal in a way that both holds the eye and encourages it to follow the composition round. It is unsurprising that, faced with a similar compositional problem, Pigalle should have turned to this illustrious example for his solutions. More surprising is the source for the figure's upper half, which links Pigalle's statue to Desjardins' group in a different way – as part of the tradition of personifications of the temperaments. Pigalle portrayed his *Citizen* – and perhaps himself – as the personification of melancholy – in the character of Desjardins' Holy Roman Empire, if not his pose. The upper half of the *Citizen*'s body is based on a famous and much imitated icon of temperamental character, Dürer's engraving *Melancolia I* (again reversed by Pigalle) (fig.22, p.118). This involved a radical change of pose from that of the terracotta maquette now at Orléans, for which Guilhem Scherf has suggested a date shortly after December, 1758 (fig.23, p.119).[54]

The change might therefore have been prompted by the request that Pigalle should refashion the figure as a self-portrait, if that tradition is correct. The iconography of Dürer's engraving – the sleeping dog, for example, which provided the pose of Pigalle's recumbent wolf – and more particularly the pose of Melancholia herself provided future generations with what became the definitive image of the melancholic condition, with its contorted brow, downcast eyes, head leaning on fist and clenched and hidden hands, all present in the figure of the *Citizen*.[55]

54. See *L'Esprit créateur de Pigalle à Canova. Terres cuites européennes 1740-1840*, ed. James David Draper and Guilhem Scherf (Paris, 2003), p.137 (no.52). The pose of the terracotta is adapted from that of the Barberini Faun (Vitry, 'Une maquette du *Citoyen* de Pigalle', *Bulletin des Musées de France* 11 (1929) p.242-43).

55. S. L. Gilman, 'The position of madness', in *Seeing the insane*, p.12-21. The same pose is used, for example, in an engraving by Jacob de Gheyn representing Melancholy, one of a set of four personifications of the temperaments and their related elements, illustrated in Klibansky, Panofsky and Saxl, *Saturn*, pl. 143 (fig.24), which also has a long discussion of the Dürer, p.284-373. Pigalle's use of Desjardins' figure of the *Brandenburger* as a model for

The identification of Pigalle's model inevitably prompts speculation about the reasons underlying its adoption. In his letter to Voltaire, Pigalle referred explicitly to a 'maladie considérable' from which he had suffered in the previous year and which had prevented him from working. Assuming that the figure is to be read as a self-portrait, this raises the possibility that the nature of that disease was depressive.[56] Acedia (sloth) traditionally bedevilled the melancholy condition. But melancholy was also associated with genius and creativity.[57] Thanks to the realisation that black bile was a fiction, this was by the eighteenth century the temperament furthest removed from a physical justification in humoral terms. It was thus the most amenable of the temperaments to appropriation for purely symbolic purposes – the use which Kant made of it at a similar date. Beyond the question of what immediate associations Pigalle may have intended to invoke by the adoption of this particular pose, there is that raised by his decision to cast his *Citizen*, whether a self-portrait or not, in what we can now see was a role recalling that of slaves on the bases of earlier royal statues. Is this a gesture of loyalty or rebellion, self-abasement or identification with figures set outside the social hierarchy – the sort of identification which was so attractive to eighteenth-century spectators when they encountered the figures depicted in the paintings of Pigalle's protégé, Jean-Baptiste Greuze? The nudity of the statue, a deliberate shedding of the marks of social status – all dress under the *ancien régime* was that – might support the latter view. If we accept the *Citizen* as a depiction of Pigalle himself, we are inevitably drawn into the always ambiguous realm of self-portraiture, where the spectator slithers around attempting to disentangle public from private persona, self advertisement from confessional statement. But even if this is read merely as a symbolic figure, similar problems of interpretation remain. It is ironic that we should be faced with these dilemmas in this particular case, since we know from his own words that Pigalle intended the figure of the *Citizen*, whether self-portrait or not, as a personification, an epitome in some sense of the universal human – or at least French – condition.

Diderot's and Grimm's reactions to this statue highlight one type of difficulty facing the creator of an image of universal humanity in the second half of the eighteenth century. These spectators interrogated

---

the lower half of the body appears to suggest that he identified that figure as melancholic rather than phlegmatic. See above, ch.3, n.15.

56. Rocheblave (*Jean-Baptiste Pigalle*, p.99) identifies this with the serious but unspecified sickness suffered by Pigalle in spring 1762. If so, it is likely to have been too late to have affected the composition of the *Citizen*, the plaster for which was completed in 1761.

57. See especially Wittkower, *Born under Saturn*, p.98-132, where it is noted that, according to Melanchthon, Dürer was himself melancholic (p.104).

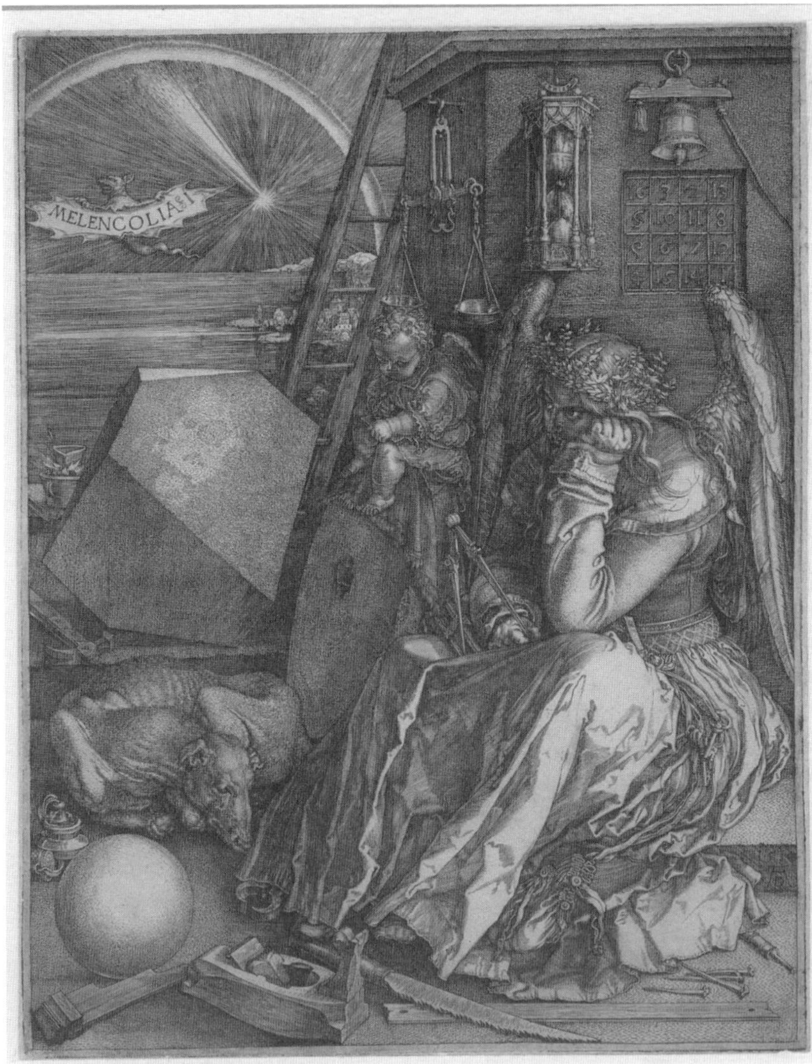

Figure 22: Albrecht Dürer, *Melancholia I*, engraving, 23.6 × 18.4 cm, British Museum, London.

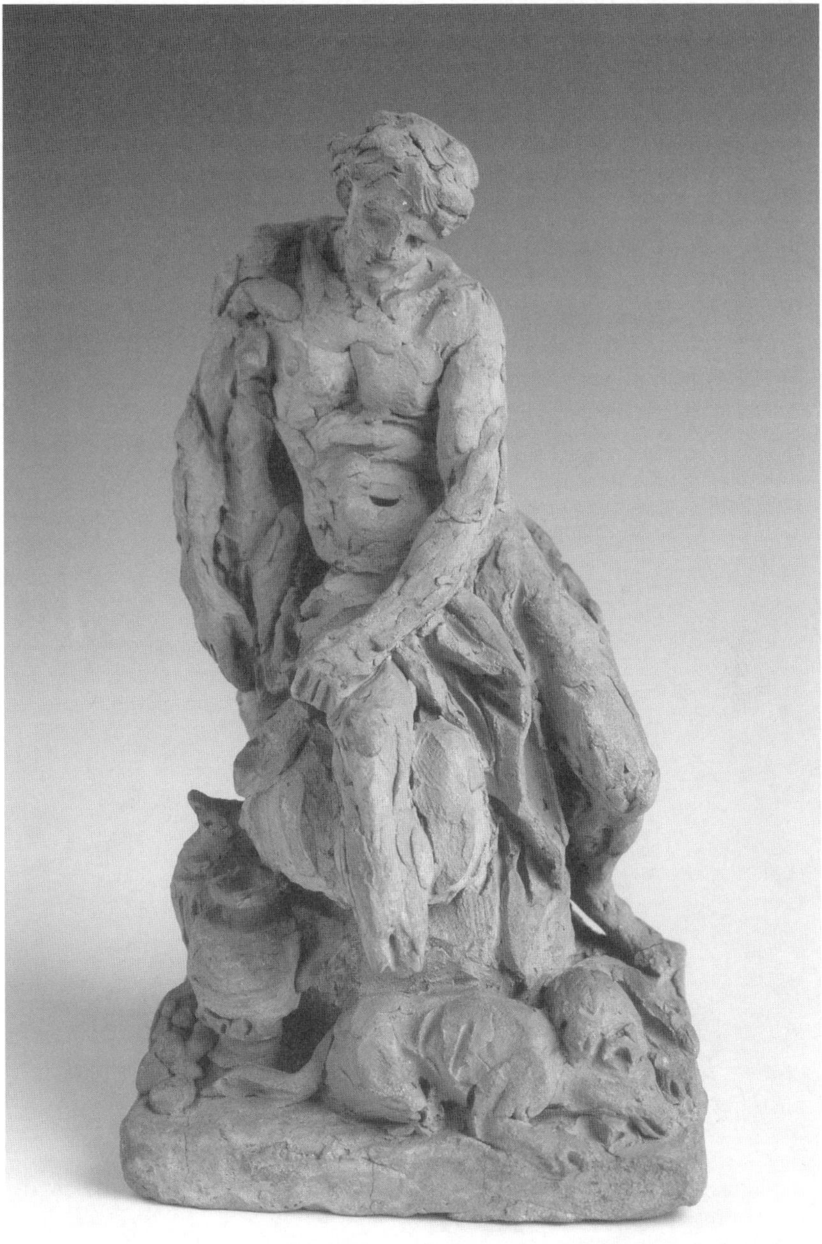

Figure 23: Jean-Baptiste Pigalle, *Le Citoyen*, terracotta, 1758, Musée des beaux-arts, Orléans.

even a deliberately 'classless' image for marks of status and social condition. Pigalle's exploitation of possibly personal reference in his portrayal of the citizen points to another area of difficulty. How could the portrayal of a specific individual represent a more general identity? This is an extension of the problem to which Mariette had already pointed in relation to Bouchardon's *Amour*. The difficulties facing the creation of a new Vitruvian man – of an icon who would embody the nation – thus seemed insuperable from two aspects. Yet that was what was going to happen in the near future, and the figure who came to embody the nation would prove to be unabashedly partisan – the French *Hercules*.

5. The citizen body: the politics of abstraction

In the 1790s, the identity and appearance of a citizen – the citizen – acquired an immediacy and relevance which would have been unthinkable to Pigalle or Diderot. The question of how the French nation should be represented came to the forefront in 1789, when the Estates-General, the traditional representatives of the kingdom, were convened by the Crown at Versailles. This was the first time that this had happened since 1614. The issues of who was entitled to participate in this newly active political sphere and how appeared relatively unproblematic at first, but they soon helped to drive French politics in radical and unforeseen directions.[1]

We are nowadays taught to think of the concepts of representative government and democracy as equivalent, or at least inextricably related. But this has not always been the case. Indeed, the relationship between the two as we now conceive them goes back no further than the French Revolution. The tensions and confusions which arose from the attempt to establish the entity we now know as representative democracy were bound up with the problems which faced successive French governments at the end of the eighteenth century. As a concept and a practice, democracy was ancient. According to European historians, it originated in the city states of ancient Greece. But the notion of representative government belonged to a more recent phase of European history. It was essentially feudal, an inheritance of the middle ages. The democracy enjoyed by Greek city states such as Athens in the fifth century BCE was direct democracy. Collective decisions were taken by assemblies of the citizenry as a whole – a body composed of adult males which excluded women, children, slaves and foreign residents. At Athens, the day-to-day administration of the state was in the hands of citizens chosen by lot or, for more important posts, such as that of general, by election at the assembly. The representative bodies of medieval Europe, on the other hand, were gatherings summoned by monarchs. They consisted originally of lords, secular or clerical, whose authority derived from those whom they represented – their vassals or subordinates. In France, this body was known as the Estates-General and its membership was divided

1. The literature on the events of 1789 is vast. Readable introductions in English with suggestions for further reading can be found in Georges Lefebvre, translated by Elizabeth Moss Evanson, *The French Revolution from its origins to 1793* (London, 1962; 2001), p.93-139; William Doyle, *The Oxford history of the French Revolution* (Oxford, 1989) (and later), p.86-135; Colin Jones, *The Great nation: France from Louis XV to Napoleon* (London, 2002), p.378-448.

into three orders – the clergy, the nobility and the so-called Third Estate or *Tiers*, which represented commoners – that is, those who were excluded from the other two orders. Representation – and this was where it differed most obviously from democracies past and future – operated by mandate. In other words, those elected to the Estates were expected to act according to the interests and the expressed will of those who chose them. They had no authority except as representatives of others. Even when assembled together, they did not represent the nation as a whole, except as the agglomeration of its component parts and in relation to its sovereign, the king.

Mandated representatives had little or no power to negotiate. The restrictions which this placed on the actions of the Estates proved unsatisfactory to the Crown in particular, since they precluded modification by negotiation or bullying. It was partly for this reason that the Estates-General had not been convoked by the king for so long. During the seventeenth and eighteenth centuries the absolute powers of the Crown had been gradually consolidated. When the Estates assembled once more in 1789, they were summoned by the king, Louis XVI, in an attempt to solve a longstanding crisis of the state's finances. The representatives were chosen in the traditional fashion, according to order, although the mode of election had to be refashioned to take account of the numbers of voters, especially in the case of the Third Estate. There, a two-tier system prevailed with eligible voters (male taxpayers over twenty-five) meeting to elect two representatives per hundred households who then met in electoral assemblies to choose their deputies.

The twelve hundred deputies – half of them from the Third Estate – assembled at Versailles on 5 May, at the start of what would prove to be a summer of widespread social unrest, especially in the countryside. Germaine de Staël, the daughter of Necker, Louis XVI's principal minister, later recalled this occasion as both imposing and mysterious. The deputies appeared to represent a 'new kind of authority in the state, of which neither the nature nor the strength was as yet known'. Their appearance was still distinguished by costumes appropriate to their orders – priests and bishops in clerical vestments according to their rank in the church, the nobility with feathers in their hats and swords (the wearing of swords in public was a right restricted to nobles) and the Third Estate in modest black. As Lynn Hunt has pointed out, this arrangement appeared to revive and reinforce more ancient sumptuary legislation, which had purported to govern individual dress according to rank.[2] But such distinctions did not convince. However splendid their

2. Lynn Hunt, 'Freedom of dress in revolutionary France', in *From the royal to the republican body: incorporating the political in seventeenth- and eighteenth-century France*, ed. Sara E. Melzer and Kathryn Norberg (Los Angeles, CA, 1998), p.224-49 (228).

show, the first two orders no longer commanded the respect which had once been their due, as Staël explained:

> The higher clergy had lost a portion of its influence with the public, because a number of prelates had been irregular in their moral conduct, and a still greater number employed themselves only in political affairs. The people are strict in regard to the clergy, as in regard to women; they require from both a close observance of their duties. Military fame, which is the foundation of reputation to the *noblesse*, as piety is to the clergy, could now only appear in the past. A long peace had deprived those noblemen who would have most desired it of the opportunity of rivalling their ancestors, and the great lords of France were now illustrious obscures [*d'illustres obscurs*].
>
> The nobility having fallen from its splendour by its courtier habits, by its intermixture with those of recent creation, and by a long peace; the clergy possessing no longer that superiority of information which had marked it in days of barbarism, the importance of the deputies of the *Tiers Etat* had augmented from all these considerations. Their imposing numbers, their confident looks, their black cloaks and dresses, fixed the attention of the spectators. Literary men, merchants, and a great number of lawyers, formed the chief part of this order.[3]

The three Orders did not retain their separate identities for long. The deputies of the Third Estate constituted only half of the representative body, but they represented the overwhelming majority of the population numerically. From the start, they were critical of the terms under which the Estates-General were expected to deliberate and vote – terms which accorded disproportionate power to the other two orders. On 17 June 1789, following an unsuccessful appeal to the representatives of the other orders to join them, the deputies of the *Tiers* declared themselves to be a National Assembly – the representatives, not of the Third Estate merely, but of the nation as a whole. There were rumours that Louis XVI was about to dissolve the Estates. The rumours were unfounded but plausible, since the will of the king was known to be dominated by those of his queen, Marie-Antoinette, and his younger brothers, who were all more or less openly hostile to these developments. When the members of the newly self-proclaimed National Assembly found themselves excluded from their meeting hall on 20 June, they therefore considered themselves the victims of a royal lock-out and convened in a disused tennis court

3. The Baroness de Staël, *Considerations on the principal events of the French Revolution* [...] *translated from the original manuscript* (1818), p.185-87. All italics are the translator's, including '*d'illustres obscurs*' in parenthesis. (The translator evidently preferred the sonority of Staël's original phrase to its sense ('obscurely illustrious'), as did Shelley, when he purloined the phrase for his preface to *Adonaïs*). For criticism of the distinctions of dress made by representatives of the *Tiers* at the time and their subsequent suppression, see Richard Wrigley, *The Politics of appearances: representations of dress in revolutionary France* (Oxford, 2002), p.62.

nearby. There they took a famous oath, refusing to disband on orders from the king, or until they had agreed a new constitution. The oath was renewed in defiance of the royal will at a session of the Estates presided over by the king three days later. On 27 June, the king capitulated, commanding the deputies of the clergy and the nobility to join the newly constituted National Assembly. At the same time he released all the deputies from the mandates imposed on them by the terms of their election to the Estates-General.

The representation to which the National Assembly now laid claim was clearly on a very different basis to that traditionally accorded to the Estates-General. The very constitution of such an Assembly was beyond anything envisaged by those who had elected the Estates-General only a few months earlier. The deputies had been mandated to propose, at best to legislate – not to govern (though day-to-day government would remain in the hands of the king and his ministers for another three years). How in any case could a National Assembly established by the Third Estate represent the nation as a whole, including the other two orders, not to mention the nation's head, the king?

The idea of political representation which underlay the formation of the National Assembly owed much to the earlier writings of one of its number, the abbé Sieyès. Though a priest, Sieyès had been elected as a deputy for the Third Estate. He was already famous for two pamphlets, his *Essay on Privileges* and, especially, *What is the Third Estate?* (*Que'est-ce que le Tiers Etat?*). Sieyès' answer to his own question in the latter case had been that, though the Third Estate was everything to the nation economically, it was, politically, nothing. He had set forth a new definition of the nation, based on the 'utility' of its citizens, not on the hierarchy of the three orders, which had been grounded in distinctions of privilege. The principle of sovereignty could reside only in the nation as a whole – no individual or body of individuals could exercise authority which did not derive from it. (This view would soon find expression as Article Three of *The Declaration of the Rights of Man and the Citizen* which the Assembly formulated in August 1789.) Only the will of the nation as a whole – the 'general will' – could constrain the actions of a free citizen. At this date, no-one – least of all Sieyès – envisaged France without its king. Sieyès' system was thus designed to supply two forms of political representation at the same time – elected representatives and the sovereign as representative of the nation as a whole. Three years later, when France became a republic following the suspension of royal power on 10 August 1792, sovereign power was held solely by the nation.[4]

4. Michel Pertué, 'La Représentation des citoyens dans les institutions révolutionnaires', in *La Révolution française et le processus de socialisation de l'homme moderne (Colloque international de*

The representative system thus conceived meant that power resided exclusively in the citizens' representatives, not in the citizens themselves, individually or collectively. The latter exercised their power only by 'delegation'. But what the voters delegated was no longer their mandate – it was merely an expression of confidence in the representatives for whom they voted. Thus the deputies became not so much representatives of the national will as its creators. But even they could only exercise this role collectively, not individually. Sovereign power was held 'indivisibly' by the whole nation – the 'Republic One and Indivisible', as it would become following the abolition of the monarchy. Sieyès endowed the Assembly of the representatives with a quasi-organic identity. He stipulated that its membership should be renewed or 'regenerated' by one third only at a time rather than by general elections, thereby bolstering the fiction of its existence as an unfragmentable entity.[5] This new model of representation had one drawback which became increasingly clear. It left no room for opposition. The general will was assumed to be by its very nature indivisible. This led to fatal results as irreconcilable conflicts of interest emerged in the coming years among citizens and their representatives alike – conflicts which the unitary concept of the general will prevented from being articulated or resolved acceptably. Nonetheless, this provided the basis for the representative democracy which prevails in Western societies today. It has been adapted to deal with the advent of party politics. It has even accommodated universal adult suffrage, even if 'the increasing role of the people in decision-making has not been proportionate to the role they have played in official discourse'.[6]

Such a view of representation presupposed an abstract and therefore somewhat generalised model of the individual citizen. The emphasis was on sameness and equality between citizens, not individuality and distinction. Indeed, the rhetorical 'other' against whom the citizen was defined in Sieyès' pamphlets was the man (or woman) of privilege – the *privilégié* – enjoying particular and exclusive rights under the feudal structures of the *ancien régime* and typically (though not necessarily) belonging to the two higher orders. Those rights were themselves abolished during a momentous sitting of the National Assembly on the night

Rouen 13, 14 et 15 Octobre 1988), ed. Claude Mazauric (Paris, 1989), p.85-93. For a discussion of Sieyès' often complex theories in English, see Michael Sonenscher's introduction to his edition of Emmanuel Joseph Sieyès, *Political writings including the debate between Sieyès and Tom Paine in 1791* (Indianapolis, IN, Cambridge, 2003).

5. Antoine de Baecque, translated by Charlotte Mandell, *The Body politic. Corporeal metaphor in revolutionary France, 1770-1800* (Stanford, CA, 1997), p.98-100 (originally published in French in 1993 as *Le Corps de l'histoire* (Paris, 1993).

6. Michel Pertué, 'Représentation', p.91.

of 4 August 1789. Henceforth, it would only be the citizen's universal qualities, those which he [*sic*] shared with others, which counted, at least in the public sphere. His other qualities, those whereby he differed from others, belonged only to private life. As Sieyès had already explained:

> The right to be *represented* belongs to citizens only in respect to what they have in common and not to what serves to differentiate them. Those assets and advantages that serve to differentiate citizens among themselves fall *beyond* the quality and character of citizenship. Inequalities of property and industry are like inequalities of age, sex, height, colour, etc. These do not infringe upon civic *equality*, because rights of citizenship cannot be attached to such differences. [...] Those interests by which citizens resemble one another are therefore the only ones that they can treat in common, the only ones by which and in whose name they can demand political rights or an active part in the formation of the social law. They are therefore the only ones that make a citizen someone who can be *represented*.[7]

This did not mean that *all* citizens were entitled to political rights. The most notorious aspect of Sieyès' views found expression in the Constitution which was eventually agreed in 1791 and according to which the first elections to the National Assembly were held in the same year. This was the restriction of those eligible to vote to 'active' citizens – that is, adult males who were property holders. (Only relatively wealthy men – those who paid the equivalent of a *marc d'argent* in taxes – were allowed to become deputies.) Women, children, servants, soldiers and the propertyless were denied the vote. They were known as 'passive' citizens. They enjoyed the civil rights of citizens without being allowed to exercise political rights – that is, they were entitled to equal treatment before the law and to the protection of their 'natural' rights of life, liberty and property, but they were excluded from voting or holding office. To that extent, the 'inequalities' of age and sex singled out by Sieyès *did* dictate exclusion from active citizenship, but not from citizenship in general. There was nothing exceptional about this distinction in terms of eighteenth-century political thought, nor about the limitation of political rights to property holders, since they were presumed to have a stake in the commonwealth to which the propertyless could lay no claim. Given Sieyès' abstract view of the content of representation – 'the right to be represented belongs to citizens only by virtue of the qualities which they have in common, and not those which differentiate them' – an 'active' citizen was already a 'representative' in that he represented what was 'common to him and his fellow citizens'.[8] Moreover, with the abolition of mandated power, the question of who was eligible to vote had become

7. 'What is the Third Estate?' in Sieyès, translated by Sonenscher, *Political writings*, p.155f.
8. Brian C. J. Singer, *Society, theory and the French Revolution* (London, 1986), p.153.

irrelevant, at least from Sieyès' point of view, insofar as individual citizens could be represented only indirectly, as components of a nation whose collective will could be pronounced only by its elected representatives. It was thus only as a member of the nation and by the nation's permission that the citizen exercised the function of elector. This was expressed very clearly by Barnave, a dominant figure during the first two years of the Assembly's existence: 'The quality of elector is merely a public function, to which no-one has a right, but which society allots according to its interest.'[9]

Sieyès contrasted this representative system favourably with the democracies of antiquity. Like Hume, he considered that the institution of slavery disqualified ancient democracy of a truly popular character. By virtue of slavery, the free citizens of ancient cities had themselves constituted a privileged élite. Their participation in government could thus be interpreted as a sort of social division of labour – the sort of development which Sieyès himself was increasingly to favour in relation to the political arrangements of French society. He regarded the distinction between active and passive citizens – between those who enjoyed full political rights and those entitled merely to civil rights of citizenship – as the more humane contemporary substitute for the ancient institution of slavery.[10]

Although the question of universal suffrage was not seriously considered at any stage of the Revolution, these principles, endorsed by the National Assembly, resulted in a franchise whose extent was unparalleled in modern times. The proportion of adult males eligible to vote under the Constitution of 1791 has been estimated at an unprecedented 60 per cent.[11]

The emphasis on equality among citizens instead of hierarchies of difference transformed the way in which the individual citizen could be conceptualised and represented. The idea of the citizen presented by Sieyès may appear excessively abstract when judged by everyday perceptions of society. But in some respects it was the very abstractness of the qualities attributed to him which helped to make the citizen a concrete and plausible figure in the eyes of Sieyès' contemporaries.

9. *Arch. Parl.*, 1ère série, 29:356, cited by Pertué, 'Représentation', p.90.

10. Pierre Rosanvallon, *Le Sacre du citoyen. Histoire du suffrage universel en France* (Paris, 1992), p.78-88. See also Sonenscher, *Political writings*, p.xxix; Sieyès, 'Notes et fragments inédits', in Emmanuel-Joseph Sieyès, *Ecrits politiques*, ed. Roberto Zapperi (Brussels, 1994; 1985), p.63, and 'Observations sur le rapport du Comité de constitution sur la nouvelle organisation de la France', p.262. Theremin, who was Sieyès' mouthpiece in the Councils of the Directoire, would use a similar argument ten years later when he argued that ancient democracy was incompatible with modern capitalism. See below, ch.7.

11. Colin Jones, *Great nation*, p.428. For figures for those eligible for the franchise under the later Constitutions, see below.

The social role allotted to the private citizen in *What is the Third Estate?* was that of consumer and producer in an exchange economy – someone who, as both buyer and seller, was constrained to emphasise the qualities which he had in common with others in the market and to minimise those which divided him from them. It was precisely in the context of the market that the notion of equality of status had been formulated and set at a premium.[12] Just as in the processes of production and exchange which created the nation's wealth, so in the nation's political constitution, it was what individuals had in common which qualified them as citizens, not what differentiated them.

The figure of the citizen on Pigalle's monument to Louis XV at Rheims (fig.21, p.112) turns out to have been a plausible avatar of the citizens of 1789 when viewed in these terms – the embodiment of undifferentiated mercantile activity. This had served to identify Pigalle's citizen with the private activities of the civil sphere rather than with the political. The latter were symbolised by the protective figure of the king which stood above him. In 1765, it had been taken for granted that the former could only flourish under the benevolent tutelage of the latter. Sieyès' account of society largely reversed those roles. For Sieyès, the citizen's private activities – his *travaux particuliers* – formed the base of society, of which the *fonctions publiques* embodied in the king were merely a consequence.[13]

At first, the traditional model of a people united under its monarch continued to prevail in public consciousness. Symbolic representations of the new nation accorded pre-eminence to the person of the king, much as Pigalle's monument had done. Thus, for example, prints celebrating the union of the representatives of the three orders in June 1789 still credited the king, together with Necker, as the architect of the *rapprochement*.[14] Such a version of events accorded ill with the actual historical record, but it was ideologically appropriate, if not inevitable. How else could that power in the nation which represented its united interest have been exercised, and how could it have been depicted if not with reference to its monarch? But this tradition was already beginning to fade. In prints where the nation itself was personified as being composed of representatives of the three orders, the person of the king was significantly absent, as observed by Colin Jones.[15] France was still a monarchy, and would remain so until the storming of the Tuileries Palace on 10 August 1792 led to the suspension of the king's powers and the establishment of the first French republic. But the notion of the monarch as part of the national representation – a

12. Pertué, 'Représentation', p.87.
13. Singer, *Society, theory*, p.93.
14. *L'Image de la Révolution française*, ed. Claudette Hould (Quebec, 1989), p.189.
15. Jones, *Great nation*, p.401f.

notion to which Sieyès himself continued to adhere – was already becoming redundant in popular imagery.

This transformation implied a fundamental shift in perceptions of how the nation was constituted. It would have momentous consequences. As Brian Singer has explained, the eclipse and abolition of the monarchy entailed the invention of society as an independent concept. No longer was 'society [...] made present to itself through the representation of a supra-social principle', the existence of a Christian God and his representative on earth, the king. To some extent, this was merely a further stage in a process which had been taking place for over a century. The rivalries among the nobility of the *ancien régime* and between the Crown and the nobility had exposed the fictitious nature of power as a quality which flowed down from heaven above in a preordained, symbolic manner. Sieyès had already acknowledged that real power rested on the power to govern, not on distinctions: 'it supposes a superiority of functions, not of persons'.[16]

But where did that leave the representation of the national identity? Surely nowhere but in the persons of its citizens – the representatives, at first, of the three Estates, but from June onwards of the third of those Estates as the embodiment of the nation. The representative of the Third Estate rapidly became the abstract 'new man' of contemporary rhetoric, destined for freedom and regeneration as a result of the Revolution[17]. But how exactly was he to be represented? The figure of the citizen executed by Pigalle in the 1760s had exhibited some of the qualities which would be attributed to the citizen of 1789. As has been seen, the supposedly universal character of the citizen – symbolised by his nudity and lack of distinguishing marks of status – was equated by Pigalle with a specific form of social activity – commerce. But precisely what commercial function was this particular personification of the citizen meant to be performing? What was the Citizen's relationship to the bales of merchandise on which he sprawled? What was the precise significance of the citizen's pose and appearance? To what extent did this personification of commercial activity represent the merchant class, and to what extent those who laboured for that class, the true producers of the nation's wealth by another, more stringent measure than that which Diderot or for that matter Sieyès chose to apply? This was unclear, and the ambiguity was seized on at the time, notably by Diderot and

16. In his *Essai sur les privilèges* (in Sieyès, *Ecrits politiques*, *ed. cit.*, p. 103), cited by Singer, *Society, theory*, p.59; see also p.55.

17. On the 'new man' of 1789, see Antoine de Baecque, 'L'homme nouveau est arrivé. La 'régénération du Français', *Dix-huitième Siècle* 20 (1988), p.193-208, and *The Body politic*, p.131-56.

Grimm.[18] The uncertainty was only compounded by the figure's nudity and the lack of marks of external distinction.

The reactions of Diderot and Grimm to Pigalle's statue already pointed to the increasing difficulty of seeing any individual citizen as an embodiment of the nation as a whole – that is, of the people – in the second half of the eighteenth century. This issue is explicitly addressed in Jaucourt's entry on *peuple* (people) for the *Encyclopédie*. Besides commenting on Diderot's use of the word,[19] Jaucourt observed a more general change in the meaning given to *peuple*. It had formerly been used to designate the nation as a whole, but was now increasingly applied to a restricted class (*classe*) within that nation, comprising manual workers and peasant farmers ('les ouvriers et les laboureurs') – that is, implicitly excluding the bourgeoisie and the first two orders on the one hand, and the unrespectable poor – the *populace* or *bas peuple* – on the other.[20] At the same time, Diderot's more restricted and unequivocally pejorative usage was also clearly gaining ground. These trends are borne out by the ways in which the term *peuple* was used in political and historical discourse. It was used positively in descriptions of the democracies of antiquity – that is, when applied to those free citizens who for Sieyès had constituted a privileged élite in the ancient city state – but less so in relation to the urban poor – the *populace* – of ancient Rome; the so-called *turba forensis*, who, hanging around the public places, had constituted a potential threat to the peace and property of the better off.[21]

This was not an isolated development. As we saw in Chapter 3, it is clear from the terms in which Haller, Kant and Lavater reformulated temperament theory that there was an increasing preoccupation among the propertied classes with social differentiation in general and with the

18. See ch.4, n.46.
19. See above, ch.2.
20. *Encyclopédie*, s.v. 'peuple'. See above, ch.2, n.42. See also Jean Fabre, 'L'article "Peuple" de l'"Encyclopédie" et le couple Coyer-Jaucourt', in Centre Aixois d'Études et de recherches sur le dix-huitième siècle, *Images du peuple au dix-huitième siècle (Colloque d'Aix-en-Provence 25 et 26 octobre 1969)* (1973), p.11-24. The practice of other eighteenth-century writers, such as Rousseau and Condorcet, was similar (Isabelle Vissière, 'L'émancipation du peuple selon Condorcet' in *Images du peuple*, p.205). See Gérard Fritz, *L'Idée de peuple en France du XVIIe au XIXe siècles* (Strasbourg, 1988), for the question as a whole. It was during these years that the term 'classe', associated with the vocabulary of natural history, came to be used to describe abstractly defined groups differentiated in terms of wealth or relationship to production. See Marie-France Piguet, *Classe, histoire du mot et genèse du concept des physiocrates aux historiens de la Restauration* (Lyons, 1996). Piguet cites the example of Necker, who, writing on the market in grain in 1775, divided society into three classes – the proprietors, the merchants and 'the people' (p.68).
21. Jean Fabre, 'L'article "Peuple" de l'"Encyclopédie" et le couple Coyer-Jaucourt', in *Images du peuple au dix-huitième siècle*, p.16. Diderot's disquiet at the implications of Bouchardon's *Amour* had been couched specifically in terms of the urban poor – the inhabitants of the faubourg Saint-Marceau.

distancing of the labouring classes in particular. These developments are in line with evidence about contemporary social patterns. In Paris, in particular, the habits and lifestyles of rich and poor, even within the same neighbourhood, were increasingly distanced socially, radically affecting traditional models of community life.[22] The ambiguity of the word *peuple* – between the old meaning (a synonym of *nation*) and its increasingly prevalent use to designate a specific and at times even a despised class of men – emerged in the debates of 1789. It became an issue at the meetings of what was to become the National Assembly in June, when the deputies of the old Third Estate set about defining their new relationship to those who had elected them. Mirabeau, the outstanding orator of the new body, proposed that they should call themselves the 'assembly of representatives of the people'. This suggestion prompted a debate during which Mirabeau's choice of words was questioned by another deputy, Thouret, who based his criticism on the ambivalence of the word *peuple* in current usage.[23] In the event, the word was discretely dropped, and Sieyès' preferred term, 'national assembly', was adopted.

At first there appears to have been a tendency to ignore the more pejorative meanings of the word *peuple* in political debate, or at least to subsume them under the more general and old-fashioned use of the term as a synonym for *nation*. It was as yet only disaffected figures on the right of politics, such as the journalist and poet André Chénier, who challenged this consensus. Chénier protested at the extent to which even the nation's legislators so ignored their language as to extend the holy name of 'people' to a horde of lazy troublemakers – a view on which he was challenged by his brother, the more populist M. J. Chénier, who explicitly refused to exclude the poor and the propertyless from consideration as citizens, since they constituted the vast majority in the nation.[24] Such singling out of the *bas peuple*, whether in positive or

22. David Garrioch, *Neighbourhood and community in Paris, 1740-1790* (Cambridge, 1986), p.205-56.
23. See Edna Hindie LeMay, '"Peuple" dans le discours des Constituants 1789/91', in *Peuple, plèbe, populace. Idées, représentations, quotidien de l'ancien régime au temps des Girondins. Actes du colloque de Bordeaux, Revue française d'histoire du livre* 66-67 (1990), p.203-12.
24. Cited respectively in Michèle Sicault and Marc Bouloiseau, 'La notion de "peuple" dans la correspondance de Blin de Sainmore avec la grande-duchesse Marie-Feodorovna 1787-1791', in *Images du peuple au dix-huitième siècle*, p.47, and in Jean Fabre, *André Chénier. L'homme et l'œuvre* (Paris, 1955), p.81. See also Jacques Guilhaumou, 'Le peuple est-il divisible en classes? A propos du débat sur "la division des intérêts de classe" (1789-1793)', in *Peuple, plèbe, populace*, p.161-71. For the not always unsympathetic but increasingly distant attitude of the propertied to the poor and propertyless of Paris in the eighteenth century, see Daniel Roche, *The People of Paris. An essay in popular culture in the 18th century*, translated by Marie Evans in association with Gwynne Lewis (Leamington Spa, 1987), p.36-63.

negative terms, was however as yet rare. Sieyès' identification of the civic body as property-owning, adult and male was tacitly accepted by his colleagues in the Assembly and by the press. But how plausibly could such a view be equated with that of a nation encompassing an undifferentiated 'people'? How long, for that matter, would the enthusiasm of the new democrats for an inclusive notion of national identity survive the social realities of late eighteenth-century France? A hint of future disagreements came on 27 April 1791 in a debate on eligibility for membership of the National Guard. Only active citizens were eligible for the Guard, a bourgeois militia established in 1789. The left-wing deputy Robespierre proposed the abolition of any property qualification, claiming that membership should be available to all, even the 'people'. He chided his fellow-deputies for daring to blaspheme against 'the people, your sovereign' by insisting on a property qualification at all. Another deputy picked him up on this usage – surely the term *peuple* embraced the totality of citizens? Robespierre agreed, excusing his earlier expressions on the grounds that he was at a loss for any other term to denote collectively those presently excluded from the National Guard.[25]

Perhaps predictably, it was images of the new citizen in the mould defined by Sieyès who were used to personify the Third Estate in the caricatures which were published to celebrate the reconciliation of the three orders in the aftermath of the events of 20 June 1789. Whether they celebrated the fusion of the three orders or the ascendancy of the *Tiers* over the two privileged Estates, these images usually presented the personification of the Third Estate in something like the form of dress assigned to the representatives of the *Tiers* at the opening session of the Estates-General at Versailles in May 1789 – coat, waistcoat, breeches (*culottes*) and stockings – the form, though not the colour. Black was traditionally identified with the clergy of the First Estate. In some images the dress is hard to distinguish from the uniform of the National Guard, whose uniform was standardised in the following year, a circumstance which reinforced the social distinction implied in the form of the dress itself.[26] This respectable, middle-class representative of the Third Estate appeared not merely in the many optimistic images published in the early months of the Revolution which show the three orders united in friendship, but also in what has come to be perhaps the best known caricature on this subject, *The Awakening of the Third Estate* (fig.24, p.133). This shows representatives of the two privileged orders, a noble army

25. *Œuvres complètes de Maximilien Robespierre*, 7 vols (Paris, 1910-1967), vol.7, p.265. See also the discussions in Fritz, *L'idée de peuple*, p.5, and Annie Geffroy, 'Le peuple selon Robespierre', in *Peuple, plèbe, populace*, p.213-16.
26. On the uniform of the National Guard, see Wrigley, *Politics*, p.64-68.

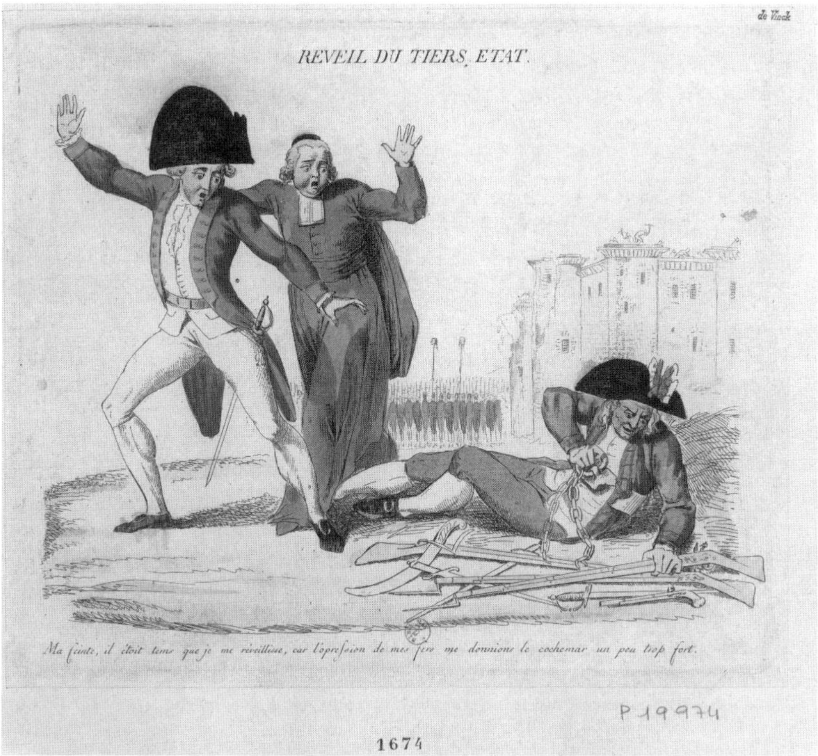
de Vinck
REVEIL DU TIERS ETAT.
Ma ſainte, il étoit tems que je me réveillise, car l'opreſsion de mes fers me donnions le cochemar un peu trop fort.
P 19974
1674

Figure 24: Anonymous, *Le Réveil du Tiers État* ('Awakening of the Third Estate'), coloured etching, 1674, 20.1 × 24.5 cm, De Vinck Collection, Bibliothèque nationale de France, Paris, Qb 14 juillet 1789, M 98807.

officer (all commissioned officers were required to be of noble birth under the *ancien régime*) and a priest, who flee in horror as the embodiment of the *Tiers* wakes from his slumber to break the chains of servitude and reach for a gun. A hint of his capacity for effective action is given by the scene in the background, which shows the demolition of the Bastille, the royal prison and fortress which was successfully stormed by a Parisian crowd on 14 July 1789. This print has become a favourite with historians, doubtless because its more threatening elements – the fear of the priest and the nobleman and the menacing pose of the commoner – appear to presage the revolutionary violence to come.[27] Unlike Pigalle's *Citizen*, this anonymous artist's personification of the *Tiers* is clothed, but it derives from a painted nude whose aggressive pose, like that of Pigalle's figure, originally indicated a state of melancholy – the figure of the mad Rakewell in the final scene of Hogarth's *Rake's progress*, set in Bedlam (1733-1734, London, Sir John Soane's Museum) (fig.25, p.135). The pose and the nudity of Hogarth's figure in turn derive from the statue of *Melancholy Madness*, one of the two representations of naked madmen by Caius Gabriel Cibber which once decorated the portals of the Old Bethlehem (Bedlam) Hospital in London.[28]

There are cases in which the personification of the Third Estate was not a bourgeois, as when the symbolism of chain-breaking demanded that the representative of the *Tiers* be cast as a blacksmith (fig.26, p.136).[29] There is also a group of widely diffused images in which the *Tiers* was personified by a very different figure – that of the honest peasant, here represented with features intended to recall those of Henry IV, first French king of the Bourbon dynasty and the only king to attain the status of a popular figure under the *ancien régime*.[30] But these images, were

27. *De Vinck*, 1674. The characterisation of the representative of the *Tiers* in this caricature has been related to a specific passage in Sieyès' *What is the Third Estate?* in which the Third Estate is likened to 'a strong, vigorous man whose arm is still in chains' (*French caricature and the French Revolution, 1789-1799*, ed. James Cuno (Chicago, IL, 1988), p.156 no. 27). The same imagery appears in other contemporary pamphlets. See de Baecque, *Body politic*, p.145.
28. Now in Bethlem Royal Hospital, Beckenham, Kent. Cf. Gilman, *Seeing the insane*, p.54. The figure in the caricature derives from Hogarth's painting (or a pirated engraving of it, since the figure in the caricature is in the same sense as that in the painting) and not from Hogarth's own engraving, in which the gesture of the Rake's arm was altered, yielding a pose which corresponds rather with Cibber's other Bedlam figure, that of Raving Madness, as observed by David Kunzle ('Plagiaries-by-Memory of the *Rake's progress* and the genesis of Hogarth's second picture story' in *The Journal of the Warburg and Courtauld Institutes* 29 (1966), p.311-48 (341). Cf. Ronald Paulson, *Hogarth's graphic works* (1989), no.139 (p.98).
29. De Vinck 2072, ill. James Cuno, *French caricatures and the French Revolution*, p.160 no.34.
30. See François Pupil, *Le Style troubadour ou la nostalgie du bon vieux temps* (Nancy, 1985), p.470-81. In this instance, the choice of a peasant to personify the Third Estate is consistent with Jaucourt's identification of the *peuple* with the figure of the *laboureur* (see above, n.19).

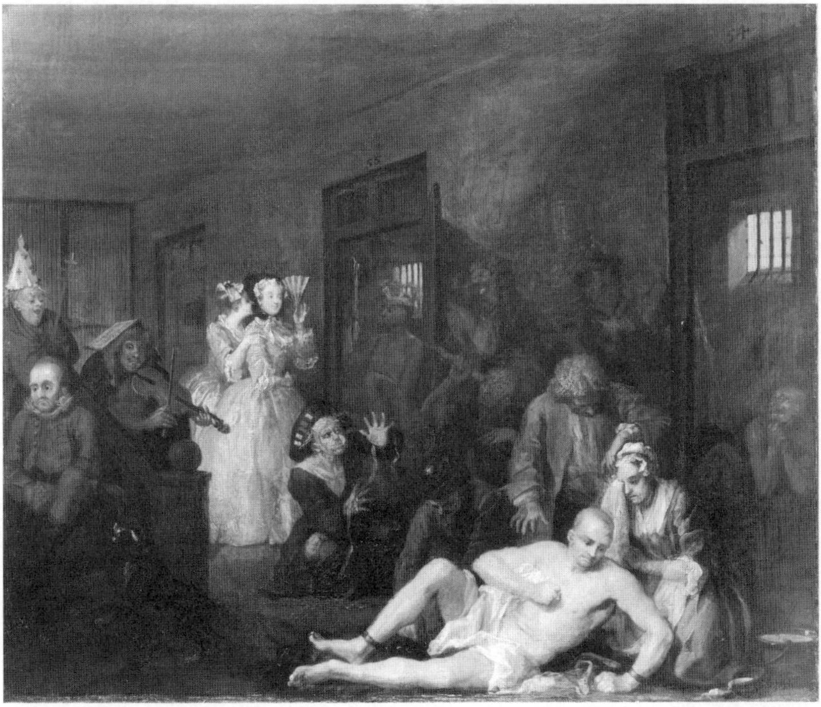

Figure 25: William Hogarth, *Rake's progress: Bedlam*, oil on canvas, 1733-34, 62.5 × 75.2 cm, Sir John Soane's Museum, London.

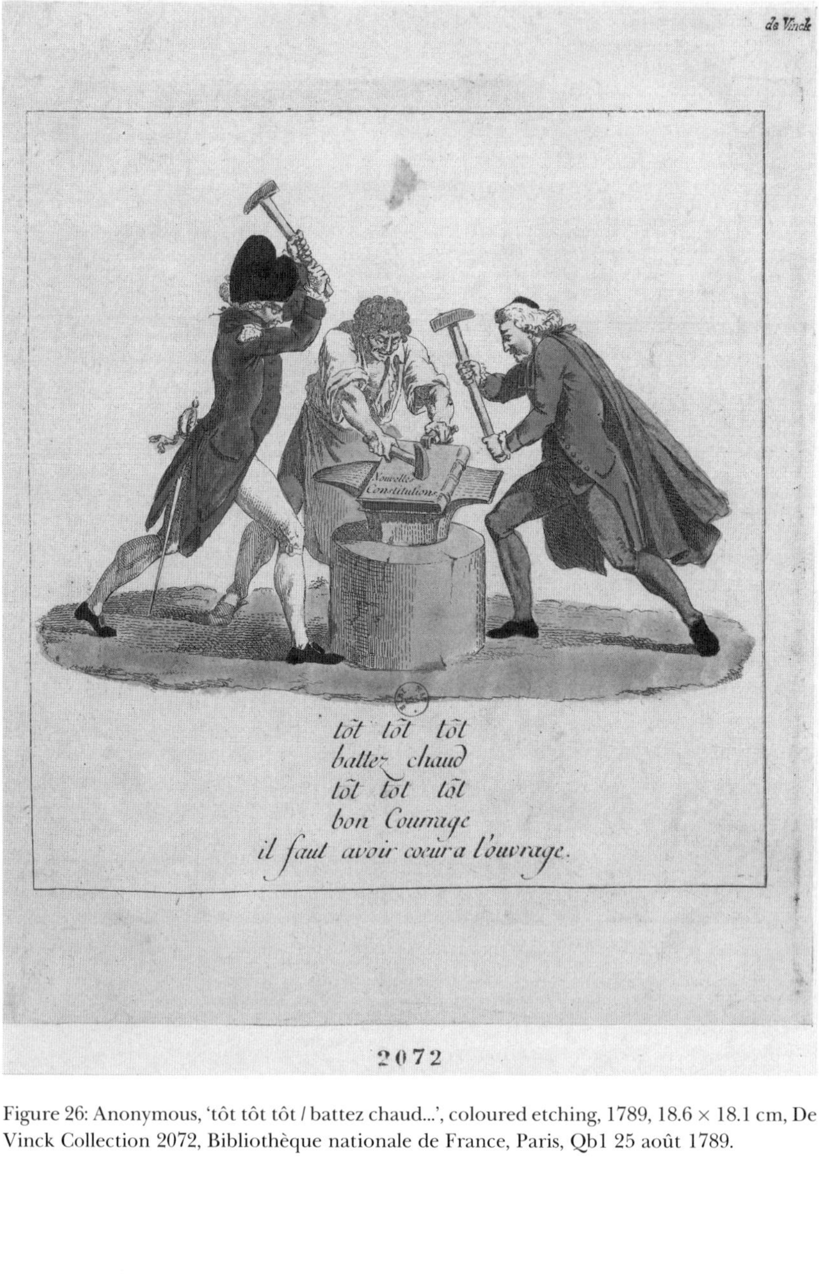
de Vinck
Nouvelles Constitutions
tôt tôt tôt
battez chaud
tôt tôt tôt
bon Courage
il faut avoir coeur a l'ouvrage.
2072

Figure 26: Anonymous, 'tôt tôt tôt / battez chaud...', coloured etching, 1789, 18.6 × 18.1 cm, De Vinck Collection 2072, Bibliothèque nationale de France, Paris, Qb1 25 août 1789.

designed to make a specific political point. In each, personifications of the two privileged orders ride on the back of a personification of the *Tiers*, while pendants show a happy peasant riding on the backs of the representatives of the clergy and the nobility. In one such pair of images, the representatives of the three orders are women. These caricatures all allude to the feudal dues, taxes and game laws which fell especially on the rural poor and some of which were abolished by the Assembly on the night of 4 August 1789.[31] Where representation was at issue, the *Tiers* was represented by a bourgeois; where it was a question of taxes, by a peasant. This is clear from a sheet of caricatures in which the twinned 'peasant' images form a triptych with a central caricature in which the three orders embrace each other in celebration of their new-found unity. In the latter, the representative of the Third Estate is no longer the peasant, but a respectably accoutred bourgeois (even though his short jacket, in contrast with the nobleman's tailcoat, resembles the popular *carmagnole* of a few years later).[32] This example appears to indicate that in cases where political representation was at issue, the Third Estate was personified as a respectable bourgeois, even when, as in this case, an alternative characterisation appeared on the same sheet.

The personification of the Third Estate as a bourgeois becomes comprehensible if the social background of those who constituted the market for caricatures at this date is taken into consideration. These were chiefly the more affluent commoners – citizens who may thus have found in such caricatures a mirror of their own new identity as elements in an unprecedented social, cultural and political entity – the Third Estate as Nation which Sieyès had proclaimed.[33]

By far the most ambitious attempt to represent the nation in the persons of its representatives was David's painting of the oath sworn in the Versailles tennis court on 20 June 1789, which Antoine de Baecque has described as 'an incarnation of the body politic of the new National Assembly' (fig.27, p.138).[34] David's project was officially undertaken at

31. *De Vinck*, 2795, 2796. See Claudette Hould, *op. cit.*, p.192f.

32. *L'Image de la Révolution française*, ed. Claudette Hould (Quebec, 1989), p.94 (no. 25). The popularity of the *carmagnole* appears to date from 1792. See Aileen Ribeiro, *Fashion in the French Revolution* (London, 1988), p.86. On *sans-culottes* and the fashion for *sans-culotte* dress in general, see Wrigley, *Politics*, p.187-227.

33. Michel Melot, 'Caricature and the Revolution', in *French caricature and the French Revolution*, ed. Cuno p.25-32.

34. *Body politic*, p.192. Philippe Bordes, *Le Serment du jeu de paume de Jacques-Louis David* (Paris, 1983), is the definitive work on David's enterprise. See also the entries in Antoine Schnapper and Arlette Sérullaz, *Jacques-Louis David 1748-1825* (Paris, 1989), p.242-75. David, like the caricaturists, suppressed any reference to the monarchy, although, as de Baeque points out in his imaginative and insightful account of the *Oath of the tennis court*, the oath itself had explicitly referred to the duty of the deputies to 'maintain the true

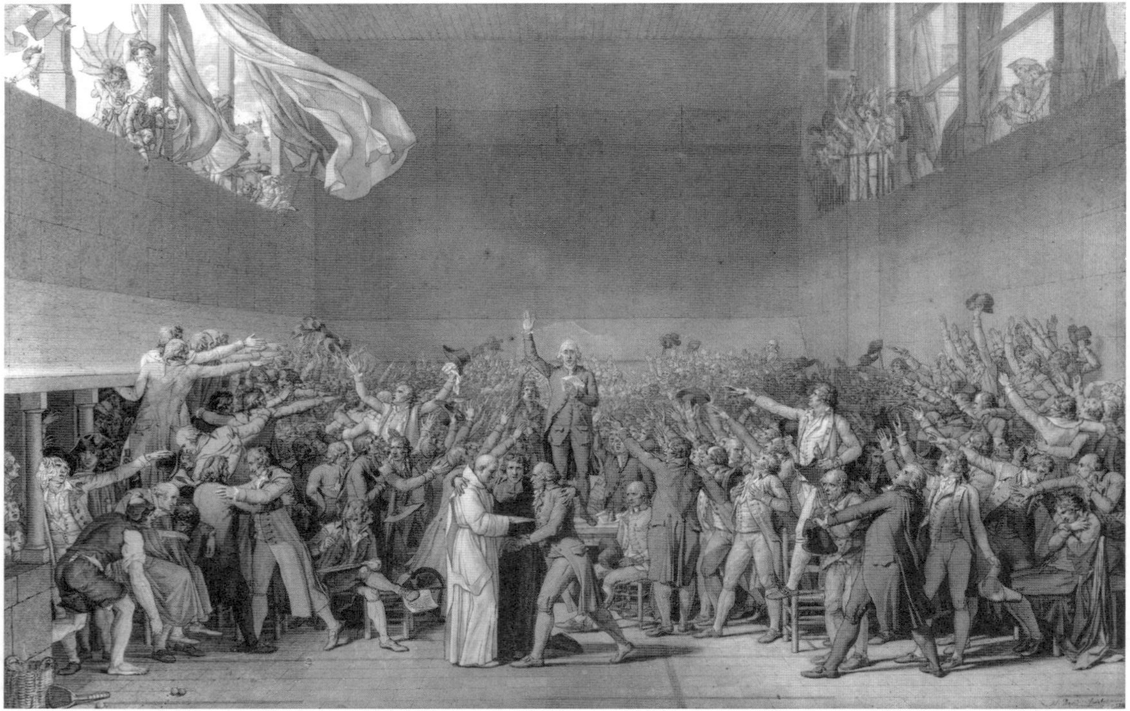

Figure 27: Jacques-Louis David, *Oath of the tennis court*, pen and brown ink, with black ink, heightening and pencil, 66 × 101.2 cm, Versailles, Musée nationale du château: on deposit from Cabinet des Dessins du Louvre, RF 1914, MV 8409.

the instigation of the deputy Dubois-Crancé on 28 October 1790. Dubois-Crancé made his proposal, not in the National Assembly, but in the so-called *Société des Jacobins*, or Jacobins' club, one of several influential political clubs formed during the early years of the Revolution. Dubois-Crancé, who was evidently speaking at the prompting of the artist, proposed that David be called upon to immortalise the oath, as the founding moment of the Revolution. The idea of a history painting which commemorated an event in contemporary French politics was novel. Since the mid-eighteenth century, history paintings had regularly been exhibited in public at the Salon. They had almost invariably been commissioned (and eventually paid for) by the Crown and were geared to the enlightenment and edification of the public in ways consonant with royal policy. They took their subjects for the most part from classical antiquity – a 'modern' history painting was regarded as one which illustrated a post-classical (usually medieval) subject. But it was not merely the contemporary subject matter of David's projected painting which was unusual. Even more so was the means proposed for financing it – a subscription for an engraving of the painting to which it was hoped that three thousand citizens would contribute. It was thus an enterprise which embodied the values of the new order not merely in its subject but in the way in which it was to be realised – as an expression of the collective will, if not of the nation as a whole, then at least of a significant body of its supporters. It was at the same time an expression of faith in their commitment to the encouragement of high art.[35] In the event, the subscription numbers were disappointing. In September, a finished drawing for the composition appeared at the Salon. On 28 September, only two days before the dissolution of the first Constituent Assembly following the elections of that year, the influential deputy Barère successfully proposed that the project be taken over by the National Assembly itself, and that the finished painting should hang in its meeting place, a perpetual reminder of the glorious circumstances of its birth, 'the first monument to the Revolution'.[36]

The painting was not completed. The surviving portion of the canvas contains the centre and right-hand side of the composition (fig.28, p.140). The figures of the deputies are all nude. This is not particularly remarkable in an unfinished work. Given the emphasis on drawing from

principles of the monarchy' (p. 192). Other, more traditional allegorical or quasi-allegorical commemorations of the Revolution by history painters did accord a place to the king, or at least to his effigy, and David himself accepted a commission for a painting of the king indicating to the dauphin his acceptance of the new constitution (see Bordes, *Serment*, p.56f, p.77-80).

35. For precedents, see Bordes, *Serment*, p.33-38.

36. Bordes, *Serment*, p.53f.

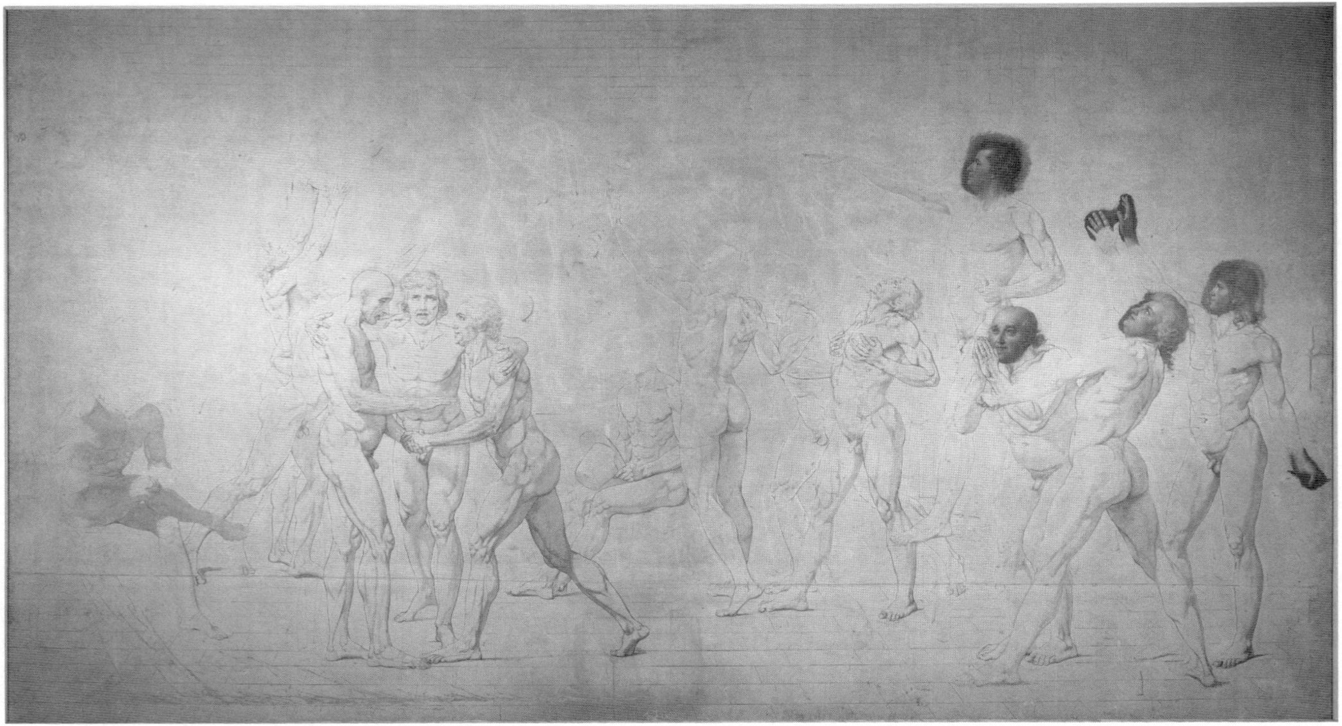

Figure 28: Jacques-Louis David, *Oath of the tennis court*, oil on canvas (unfinished), 358 × 648 cm, Versailles, Musée nationale du château: dépôt Cabinet des Dessins du Louvre, MV 5841.

life in academic training, it was recommended that an academically trained artist should sketch out a history painting with unclothed figures, if only to insure anatomical verisimilitude in the final painting, and it was not unusual for them to do so.[37] The drawing exhibited at the Salon of 1791 also contains instances of nude underdrawing which remain visible, notably in the toes of figures in the right foreground. In the painting, the chalk outlines of the original nude figures are still clearly visible, as are suggestions of clothing lightly brushed in with grey paint. What is unusual and puzzling is that David, having already sketched in their clothing, recreated some of the nudes in grey paint lightly shaded with bistre over the first versions of the same figures.[38]

It has been suggested that the reworking of the nudes points to an attempt by David to salvage the *Oath of the tennis court* as an exemplary history painting shorn of its subject, a decision which would have indicated that he had abandoned the hope of completing the work in its intended form.[39] Philippe Bordes has provided convincing arguments for rejecting this view. But as Bordes has also recognised, David's procedure seems to indicate a reluctance to engage with the clothed figure as readily and fully as with the nude, as witness the absence in this case of any drapery studies such as those which he had produced for earlier history paintings (the execution of the drapery itself was usually consigned to assistants).[40] The use of modern dress in high art (as against the lower genres such as portraiture or scenes of everyday life) was a debateable issue in the eighteenth century. There was a well-established view that modern dress was aesthetically inferior to that of antiquity, especially when used in works of art. The clothing of different parts of the body in separate garments was held to be less true to the forms of nature and less grateful to the eye than the harmonious folds of classical drapery.[41] During the 1780s, David had become the most successful and admired history painter in France as a result of a series of works exhibited at the Salon, all of which had represented classical subjects and therefore classical dress. But during the same period there were calls by critics for more patriotic and upbeat modern dress subjects, which Régis Michel has interpreted as in part symptoms of a 'resistance' to

37. See Martial Guédron, *De Chair et de marbre: imiter et exprimer le nu en France, 1745-1815* (Paris, 2003), p.58, f.140.
38. On the question on nudity and completion, see Mathias Bleyl's review of Philippe Bordes, *Le Serment du jeu de paume* (1983), *Kunstchronik* 38 (1985), p.384-88.
39. Horst W. Janson, 'Observations on nudity in neoclassical art', in *Stil und Überlieferung in der Kunst des Abendlandes. Akten des 21 Internationalen Kongresses für Kunstgeschichte in Bonn 1964* (Berlin, 1967), vol.1, p.198-207 (206).
40. Janson, 'Observations', p.183 f.
41. Quatremère de Quincy, *Considérations sur les arts du dessin en France* (Paris, 1791), p.41. For a succinct and comprehensive overview of the issue, see Bordes, *Serment*, p.101 (n.99).

David and his success.[42] David's identification with the classical rather than the contemporary pole in this discourse may have made him reluctant to embark on the detailed design of modern drapery in the the *Oath of the tennis court.*

Reluctance to engage with modern dress in a full-scale history painting may have been born out of more than academic precept and studio practice. In identifying modern as against classical subject matter with patriotic sentiments, the critics discussed by Michel were implicitly endorsing one aspect of the policies pursued by the comte d'Angiviller, the *Directeur des Bâtiments*, Louis XVI's official in charge of the arts. D'Angiviller had commissioned an impressive quantity of history paintings and sculptures from academicians on behalf of the Crown. Some of the paintings, among them works by David, had been of classical subjects, but others had represented 'modern' (that is, post-classical) subjects which specifically related to the achievements of the French Crown and nobility.[43] The sculptures were modern in the same sense. They were free-standing figures of great men of the nation (*Grands Hommes*), many of whom had exhibited loyalty to the Crown under adverse conditions, and all of whom were considered to have acted disinterestedly in the service of the nation. They were intended to decorate a gallery in the Louvre which was never realised. Ostensibly, therefore, the sculpture project looked back to the practice of the ancients, who had set up statues of great men in public places both to honour them and to encourage others to match their example. The question of the clothing to be adopted in these statues led to differences between d'Angiviller and the sculptors. Privately commissioned statues of contemporary great men had adopted classical nudity or drapery in evident homage to classical tradition. These included a statue of Buffon by Pajou which had been commissioned by d'Angiviller himself prior to his appointment as *Directeur des Bâtiments*.[44] From the start, however, the overtly national and propagandistic pur-

42. In R. Michel, *David e Roma* (Rome, 1981), p.138.

43. See Jean Locquin, *La Peinture d'histoire en France de 1747 à 1785* (Paris,1912; 1978), p.282-86; Crow, *Painters*, p.186-209; see also Régis Michel, 'Diderot and Modernity', *Oxford art journal* 7 (1985), p.36-51; Berthélemy Jobert, 'The "Travaux d'encouragement": an aspect of official arts policy in France under Louis XVI', *Oxford art journal* 10 (1987), p.3-14.

44. Completed 1776, Paris, Muséum National d'Histoire Naturelle. See James David Draper and Guilhem Scherf, *Augustin Pajou royal sculptor 1730-1809* (New York, 1998), p.280-89, no. 112. Two other statues were of Voltaire, one, nude, by Pigalle (Paris, Louvre) (the immediate precedent for Pajou's *Buffon* (p.286) as well as for the pose of Clodion's first statue of Montesquieu) and the other, in quasi-classical drapery and classical diadem, by Houdon, 1781 (Paris, Comédie-Française) (see Anne L. Poulet and Guilhem Scherf, *Houdon Sculpteur des Lumières 1741-1828* (2003), p.167-72, no.26). On Lecomte's statue of d'Alembert (Louvre), see Guilhem Scherf, 'La Galerie des "Grands Hommes" au cœur des salles consacrées à la sculpture française du XVIIIe siècle', in *Revue du Louvre* (1993), p.58-67.

pose of the *Grands Hommes* project precluded such treatment.[45] Instead, these heroes of specifically French history were portrayed in dress appropriate to the era in which they had lived, thereby emphasising their relationship to the nation and the Crown they had served. Several had flourished in the age of Louis XIV, the so-called *grand siècle* of French history. The sculptors followed d'Angiviller's wishes, even though this resulted in unfavourable critical responses to the finished statues. Critics belittled the civilian figures in particular as representations of mere courtiers (which of course they had been) rather than great men. Partly for that reason, perhaps, d'Angiviller's dress code was flouted by one sculptor, Clodion, who had been awarded the commission for a statue of the political theorist Montesquieu. As President of the law court (*Parlement*) of Guyenne, Montesquieu had held high magisterial office under the Crown, but his posthumous fame was as a writer, not as a lawyer. It was therefore as a writer that Clodion chose to portray him, partially nude and in quasi-classical drapery, thereby recalling ancient practice. He submitted a plaster to the Salon of 1779 which portrayed Montesquieu gesturing dramatically to an open folio which presumably contained his great work, *L'Esprit des lois* – a hero for the human race, not merely the Crown of France. Reactions to the pose and dress of the figure were divided, but it was evidently the use of modern dress which chiefly roused d'Angiviller's disapproval. The marble for the final statue was withheld, apparently until the costume had been changed to that of a magistrate.[46] The original plaster disappeared, presumably destroyed, and the final, marble version, exhibited four years later, presented the writer swathed in the swirling robes of his *parlementaire* office (fig.29, p.144). It was observed by one critic that pose and costume now suggested the magistrate composing a judgement rather than the philosopher.[47]

45. See Locquin, *Peinture d'histoire*, p.48-53; *Correspondance de M. d'Angiviller avec Pierre*, ed. Marc Furcy-Raynaud, NAAF, 3e série, 21 (1905) and 22 (1906); Furcy-Raynaud, 'Inventaire des sculptures exécutées au XVIIIe siècle pour la direction des Bâtiments du Roi', *AAF*, nouvelle série, 14 (1927); Francis H. Dowley, 'D'Angiviller's *Grands Hommes* and the significant moment', *Art bulletin* 39 (1957), p.259-77; Andrew McClellan, 'D'Angiviller's great men and the politics of the Parlement', *Art history* 13 (1990), p.175-92.
46. See the documents from Furcy-Raynaud (1906), cited in Anne L. Poulet and Guilhem Scherf, *Clodion 1738-1814* (Paris, 1992), p.278-86.
47. Cited by Gisela Gramaccini, 'L'image de l'homme nouveau [.] exemples de la sculpture publique à la fin de l'Ancien Régime et à l'époque révolutionnaire', in *La Révolution française et les processus de socialisation de l'homme moderne* (Rouen and Paris, 1989), p.675-89 (678), an article to which this account is substantially indebted. The little drawing by Gabriel de Saint-Aubin (Stockholm, Bibliothèque Royale) is the only known record of the appearance of the destroyed first version of Clodion's statue. Although the plaster came in for criticism, much of this was evidently ideologically fuelled (as was that of the final marble). It may therefore be somewhat incautious to conclude, as Scherf does ('La galerie des "Grands Hommes"', p.58-67), that the plaster was inferior aesthetically to the marble which replaced it, or to the works by Moitte and Julien discussed below.

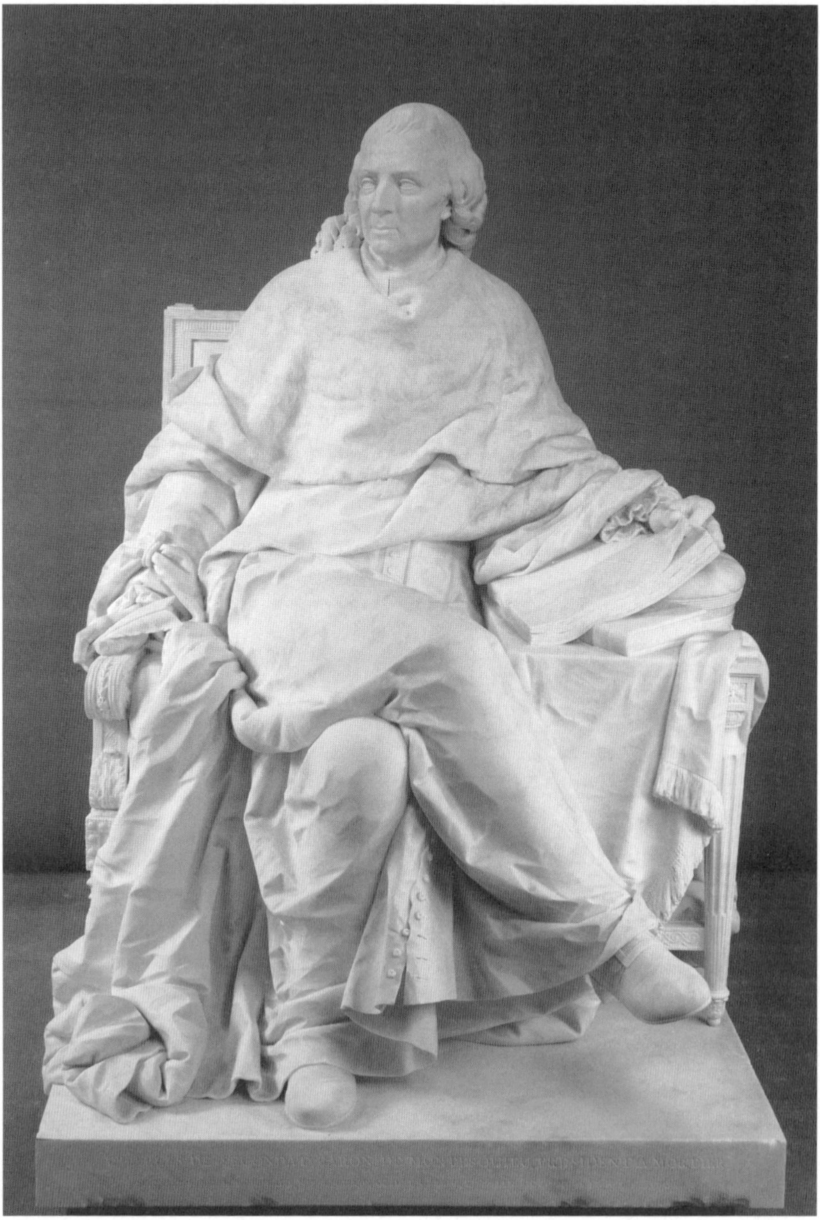

Figure 29: Clodion, *Montesquieu*, marble, 164 × 122 cm, Salon de 1783, Musée du Louvre, Paris.

It was not until 1789 that two other sculptors dared to use classical dress for figures in the same series. Once again, the statues – that by Moitte, Pigalle's pupil, of the seventeenth-century astronomer and mathematician Cassini (fig.30, p.146) and Julien's of the painter Poussin (fig.31, p.147) – represent civilian, not military figures.

Cassini and Poussin had enjoyed the patronage of the French Crown – hence their inclusion in the *Grands Hommes* series. In viewing Julien's *Poussin* the spectator was asked to imagine that the painter had risen from his bed in the middle of the night, inspired with the idea for his *Testament of Eudamidas*, the work for which he was then most famous (fig.32, p.148), the outline of which he has traced on the tablet he is holding. This anecdote was used to excuse the use of quasi-classical drapery – in the heat of creation, the painter was presumed to have paused only to throw a cloak about his person as he left his bed.[48] The drapery of Moitte's *Cassini* makes more concessions to seventeenth-century dress, notably in the form of his shirt collar, but the cloak which envelopes him is given a thoroughly classical hang, while his tight doublet barely disguises the torso beneath, as witness the visible outline of Cassini's nipple (through what must be assumed to be two layers of clothing) – a device which recalls the classical convention of so-called 'wet drapery', but which is patently contrived in this context. The two sculptors' attempts to palliate the use of classical conventions by such subterfuges failed to satisfy d'Angiviller. Documents published by Gisela Gramaccini demonstrate that the *Directeur des Bâtiments* punished the sculptors and obstructed the completion of their statues as he had in the case of Clodion's *Montesquieu*, this time by allocating unworkable blocks of marble to them. It was only with the Revolution and the fall of d'Angiviller that the two men were eventually able to demand and obtain the means to bring their statues to completion.[49]

The appropriateness of classical drapery to the representation of Poussin and Cassini is obvious. Both had been patronised by the French Crown in the seventeenth century, but by 1789 their achievements had acquired a fame which transcended national boundaries and those of time. The expansion of print media – books and engravings – had furnished them with a public which extended far beyond the confines of any available court audience, just as it had in the case of Montesquieu

48. *Explication des ouvrages de peinture, sculpture, architecture et gravure, des Artistes vivans, exposés au Musée Napoléon, le 1er jour Complémentaire, An XII de la République française* (An XII/1804), p.97, no.642.

49. Gramaccini, 'L'image de l'homme nouveau', p.678. The 1789 plaster version of Moitte's *Cassini* is preserved in the former *hôtel de ville* at Clermont (Oise); the marble, completed 1810, is in the Paris Observatoire. The marble of Julien's *Poussin* dates from 1804 (Paris, Louvre). See Guilhem Scherf, in *Pierre Julien 1731-1804*, ed. Gilles Grandjean and Guilhem Scherf (Le Puy-en-Velay, 2004), p.63-65.

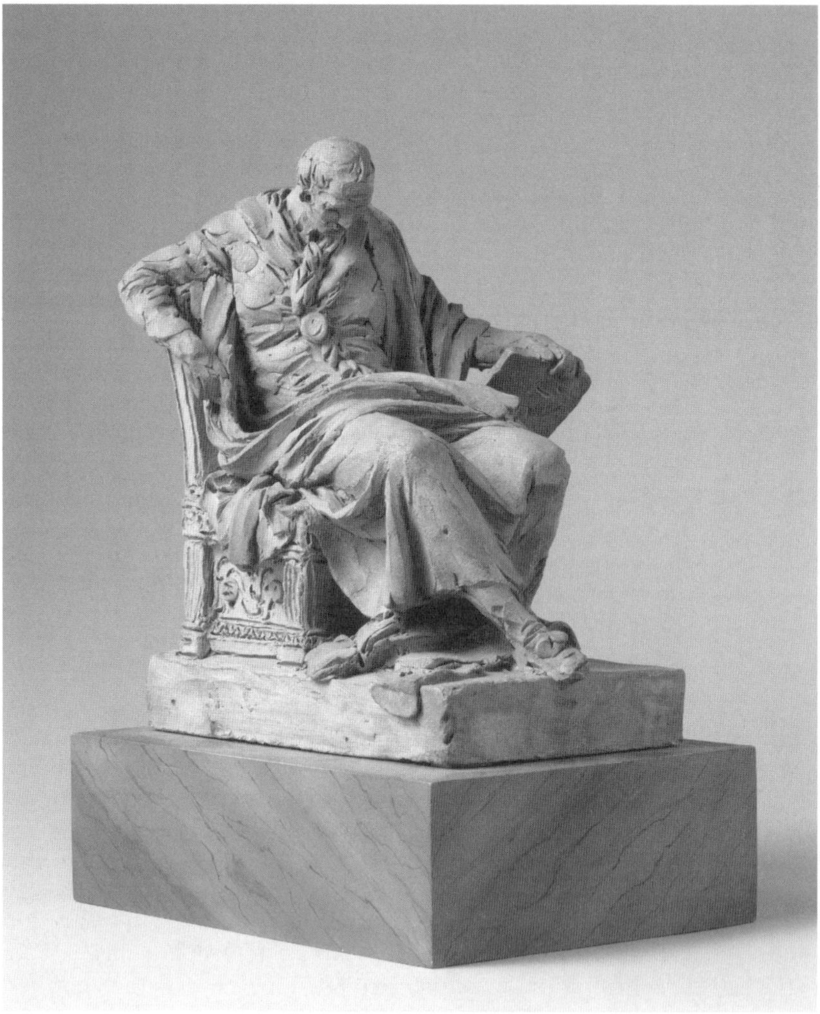

Figure 30: Jean-Guillaume Moitte, *Cassini*, marble, 1810, Observatoire, Paris (Plaster at 1789 Salon).

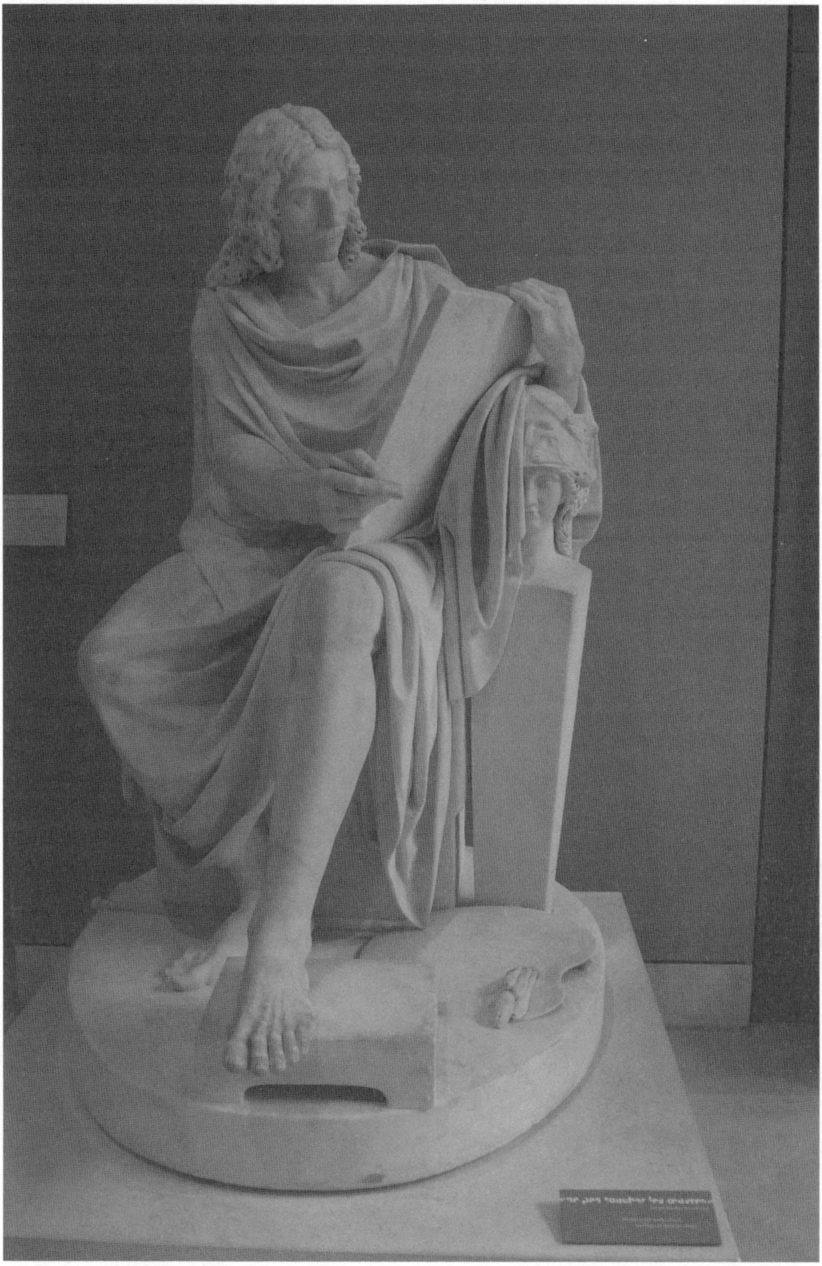

Figure 31: Pierre Julien, *Poussin*, marble, 164 × 101 cm, Musée du Louvre, Paris, RF 2984.

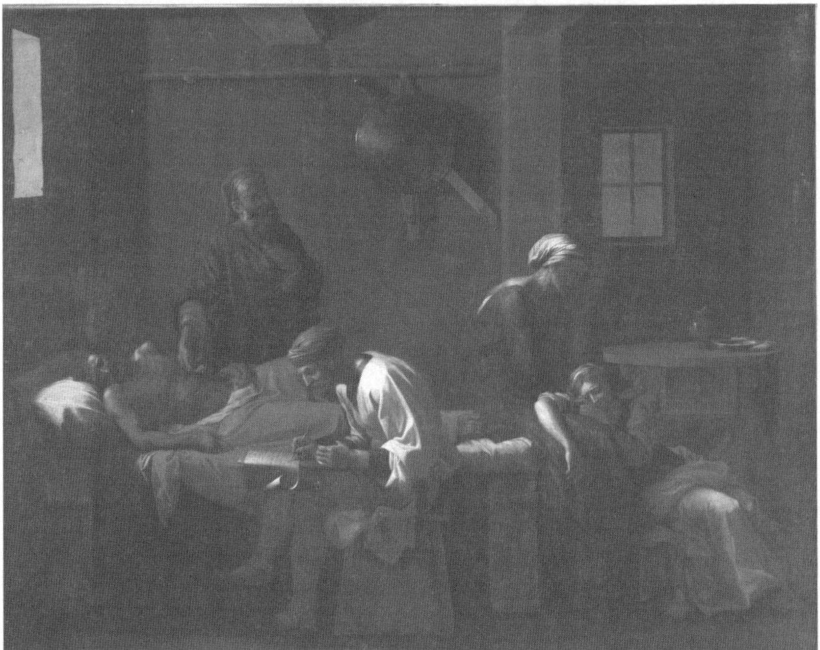

Figure 32: Nicolas Poussin, *Testament of Eudamidas*, oil on canvas, 110.5 × 138.5 cm, *c.* 1643-1644, Statens Museum for Kunst, Copenhagen.

or, for that matter, the English novelists read and admired by Kant.[50] It was fitting, then, that both Poussin and Cassini were represented absorbed in inner activity and lost to their immediate world. Moitte and Julien endowed these two *grands hommes* with the *personae* of creators, not courtiers. By the 1780s, the model of the artist as a producer who worked for the market and the greater public was gaining ground over that of the artist-courtier, pursuing advancement through the honours system attached to the hierarchy of the Royal Academy of Painting and Sculpture. It matched a new model of professionalism at variance with that offered by the academies of the *ancien régime*, one which Colin Jones has described as 'transcorporative, egalitarian, "horizontal" where its predecessor had been "vertical", internalist and hierarchical'.[51] Such was the path which painters and even some sculptors such as Clodion[52] were starting to follow in the pre-revolutionary decades, to the active displeasure of d'Angiviller. It was also that which David had himself followed in the 1780s. Although the most successful history painter of the decade, he had refused to seek promotion within the Academy's ranks above the most junior level – the minimum qualification which enabled an artist to exhibit at the Salon. During the early years of the Revolution he became a leading figure in the campaigns first to reform and then to abolish the Academy.[53] The treatment which Clodion, Julien and Moitte received at the hands of d'Angiviller was symptomatic of an attempt to reimpose court values on an art world increasingly directed at a broader public of consumers – the public, in fact, which David hoped would finance his *Oath of the tennis court*. The treatment of the sculptors had a particular irony in the case of Julien's *Poussin*, since Julien accepted the by then prevalent view that Poussin had been driven to seek refuge from French indifference in Rome, where he had produced his best work, not for a court which despised and neglected him, but for a select public of enlightened art lovers.[54] Now Poussin's sculptor appeared also to have fallen victim to the hostility of a French court.

50. See ch.3, n.79.

51. Colin Jones, 'Bourgeois revolution revivified: 1789 and social change', in *Rewriting the French Revolution*, ed. Colin Lucas (Oxford, 1991), p.69-118 (96). See also Halliday, *Facing the public*, p.141.

52. See Poulet and Scherf, *Clodion*, p.278.

53. See Jean-Pierre Mouilleseaux, 'David: a classical painter against the Academy and a teacher of the French school', in *The French Academy: classicism and its antagonists*, ed. June Hargrove (Newark and London, 1990), p.131-39.

54. *Explication des ouvrages*, p.97. See also Taillasson, *Observations sur quelques grands peintres, dans lesquelles on cherche à fixer les caractères distinctifs de leur talent, avec un précis de leur vie* (Paris, 1807), p.95. On the evolution of Poussin's reputation, see Nathalie Heinich, *Du peintre à l'artiste. Artisans et académiciens à l'âge classique* (Paris, 1993), p.122-29; for interest in Poussin's career in the 1780s, see Crow, *Painters*, p.211, and *Commemorating Poussin: reception and intrepretation of the artist*, ed. Katie Scott and Genevieve Warwick (Cambridge, 1999).

Thus a tradition was already establishing itself within which modern dress in sculpture was linked with the representation of the servant of the Crown and the use of the nude or classical drapery with that of another type of cultural producer, one who served the public sphere through the medium of the newly emerging market. There had also been a recent incident in which two of David's colleagues in the Royal Academy of Painting and Sculpture had apparently been victimised by the Crown for adopting classical rather than modern dress. But a new, revolutionary discourse on dress and the body was also evolving in the years during which David was at work on the *Oath of the tennis court*. The distinctions of dress which Germaine de Staël had described on the occasion of the opening of the Estates-General had already become redundant in the days leading up to the Tennis court oath, when the representatives of the *Tiers* had reconstituted themselves as the National Assembly. They were soon abolished altogether, and in 1790 all decorations based on distinctions of birth were also prohibited. Dress remained the primary index of social distinction all the same. In 1794, the pro-revolutionary Société populaire et républicaine des arts mounted a campaign for reforms which would have imposed uniform dress on all citizens in the name of equality. For them, all forms of dress were a regrettable if necessary interference with the integrity of the naked body:

> Nature, who destined man [*sic*] for activity and work, built him with those splendid proportions which constitute at once his strength and his beauty. Clothes, which he is constrained to use in order to protect himself from the effects of weather, must fulfill that task without going against nature, without impairing the development of his limbs, without hampering their movements, without spoiling their beautiful forms.[55]

In terms which recall the eighteenth-century philosopher Rousseau, the report went on to blame distinctions of dress and superfluous decorations on a corrupt and ageing civilisation. Preoccupied with securing equality among citizens in appearance at least, the Committee of Public Safety of the Jacobin government took up the Society's proposals and David himself was called upon to provide designs for the new, revolutionary costumes, uniform for all citizens, which he did.[56]

55. 'Considérations sur les avantages de changer le costume français, par la Société Populaire et Républicaine des Arts', in *Aux armes et aux arts! Peinture, sculpture, architecture, gravure. Journal de la Société républicaine des arts, séante au Louvre, Salle du Laocoön, Rédigé par Détournelle, Architecte. Première partie* (An II/1794), p.315 f. (session of 26 germinal). On the *Société populaire et républicaine des arts*, see Jules Renouvier, *Histoire de l'art pendant la Révolution, considéré principalement dans les estampes* (Paris, 1863), p.15f.

56. See Antoine Schnapper and Arlette Sérullaz, *Jacques-Louis David*, p.296-302 (with references). As Madeleine Delpierre has pointed out ('A propos d'un manteau de représentant du peuple de 1798 récemment offert au Musée du Costume' in *Bulletin du Musée Carnavalet*,

The implications of such developments for readings of the *Oath of the tennis court* can be seen most clearly in relation to the group of three men embracing in what was originally the painting's central foreground. These are three clerics – a monk, a Catholic priest and a protestant minister. The composition of the group clearly derives from well-known revolutionary caricatures celebrating the union of the three Estates.[57] The dress which would have distinguished the three men according to vocation and denomination now hovers spectrally beneath the re-inscribed lines of their naked bodies. Of course, such distinctions of dress continued to prevail among ministers of the Christian churches, as they still do. But by 1794 the nudity of the three clerics could have been read as attesting to the men's common humanity in civil society at least, triumphing over the divisions of religion which their clothing had denoted. Had the painting been completed, dress would inevitably have re-imposed that difference, as may be seen in the drawing of 1791. If David was reluctant to embark on adding contemporary clothing to the deputies in his painting, it may have been because this necessary step could only have reminded spectators of distinctions of dress, both past and, as in this case, present, and would thereby have drawn attention to increasingly anachronistic features of the act whose timeless significance the painting was intended to celebrate. There is a sense in which the nudity of David's figures was becoming that of the new man, the public man of a new age.

The marks of distinction conferred by clothing may have disappeared from David's painting, but there remains a marked variety of bodily types among David's figures, each visibly shaped by individual habits of life. They range from the ascetic and spindly monk, Dom Gerle, on the left of the central trio, to the well-fleshed figure of Mirabeau or the Apollonian Barnave above him on the right. David's concept of the citizen body deliberately encompasses a wide range of age, physical health – note, in the drawing (fig.33, p.152), the figure of the infirm Maupetit de la Mayenne being carried in from the left (the corresponding portion of the canvas is missing) – and even political allegiance, in the dissenting figure of the deputy Martin Dauch, slumped with his arms folded across his chest who occupies a similar position at the opposite edge of the composition. (Antoine De Baecque has likened David's procedure in

1972, p.13-23), David's designs are highly eclectic and not particularly classical in inspiration. Nor, as Lynn Hunt observed, do they resemble the dress of the *sans-culottes* ('Freedom of dress in revolutionary France'), *From the royal to the republican body: incorporating the political in seventeenth- and eighteenth-century France*, ed. Sara E. Melzer and Kathryn Norberg (Los Angeles, CA, 1998), p.224-49.

57. See *French caricature and the French Revolution, 1789-1799*, ed. James Cuno (Chicago, IL, 1988), p.157-67.

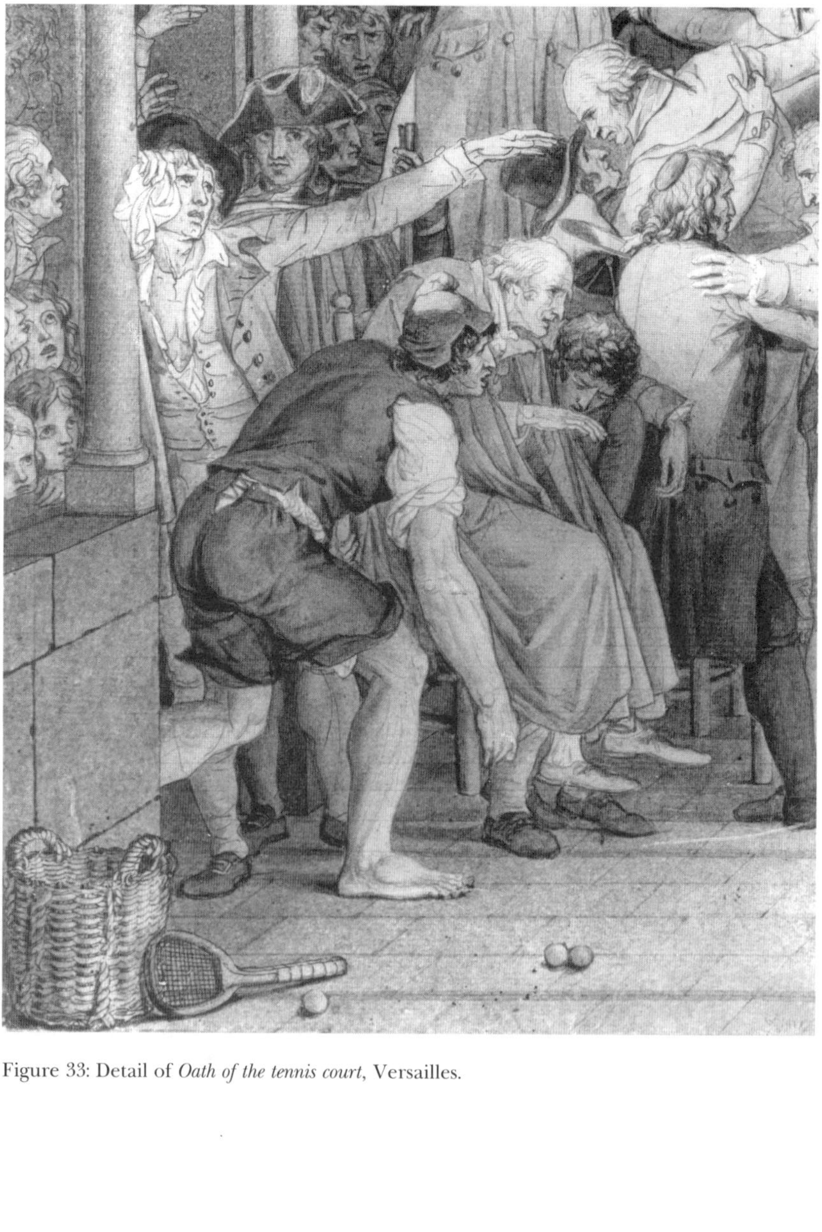

Figure 33: Detail of *Oath of the tennis court*, Versailles.

putting together his image of the body politic to that of the Greek painter Zeuxis in the construction of the selective *beau idéal*)[58]. Yet however varied according to age, condition and commitment to the cause, this group of men is animated by a single movement, identified by de Baecque as the 'Idea of the oath', expressed quintessentially in the gesture of Barnave, but echoed across the canvas 'according to a directing principle, elevation'.[59] These bodies perform a series of variations on the pose of the *Apollo Belvedere*, a source which their present state of nudity only reinforces. Expression and willed effort are concentrated in the face – in this case, according to de Baecque, the mouth – as they were in Winckelmann's description of the *Apollo*.[60] Nudity also makes visible that effortlessness of body which was the salient characteristic of the *Apollo*'s pose for Winckelmann. Like Winckelmann's god, these men appear to be about to rise from the ground. Even the bulky Mirabeau, with his feet so firmly and widely placed, looks ready to take off. In this respect, David's vision of the new body politic gives concrete expression to Sieyès' imaginings. It may indeed have a head (Bailly, who is shown administering the oath from atop the central trestle) and a heart (the three clerics immediately beneath him),[61] but it lacks working limbs. Even with no clothes to distinguish it, this is visibly a bourgeois body. Only two figures in the entire composition are engaged in purposeful strenuous physical activity. They are also the only two who are precluded from the collective activity of the Assembly. Their gestures do not partake of the general elevation. Instead, their task draws them down to earth. They glance upwards at the activities of their social superiors, who are also their representatives. They do not belong in this body. They are the porters carrying Maupetit in from the left.

As Philippe Bordes has demonstrated, David's own political position, at least at the outset of this project, was relatively moderate, like that of the Jacobin club itself. This is borne out by the prominence which was still accorded to such figures as Mirabeau, Barnave and above all Sieyès (seated with a hat on his lap to the right of the central table, his gaze fixed on the central trio of his fellow clerics). But David's position was soon to change. In 1792 he was himself elected to the Assembly, henceforth generally known as the Convention. There, he was increasingly identified with the powerful faction of Jacobins known as the Mountain (because its members occupied the higher ranks of seats in the hall where the Convention met) and with its leader, Robespierre. In mid-1793, the Jacobins gained undisputed ascendancy in a Convention torn with

58. De Baecque, *Body politic*, p.197.

59. De Baecque, *Body politic*, p.188. See ch.2.

60. See ch.4.

61. De Baecque, *Body politic*, p.193.

factional fighting. David now served on one of the powerful revolutionary committees which monopolised government, the Committee of General Security. He was already a member of the Committee of Public Instruction. By this stage, many of the men who figure most prominently in the *Oath tennis court* were dead, discredited or, in several cases, both. Many died on the scaffold in the Reign of Terror orchestrated by the government. David himself was twice imprisoned following the fall of Robespierre in the coup d'état of 9 Thermidor in the second year of the newly instituted republican calendar (27 July 1794). He was lucky to have escaped with his life. All these circumstances conspired against David's attempt to complete the *Oath of the tennis court* project later in the decade, although the decisive factor is likely to have been the runaway inflation of the Republic's paper currency, which rendered the original subscriptions virtually worthless. But the picture it presented of the citizen body had lost credibility long before that.

6. A body one and indivisible: Jacobin representations of the people

David's *Tennis court oath* was a casualty of the fact that the Revolution did not turn out in the way that the painting appeared to predict. The Assembly pitifully failed to achieve that organic unity and oneness of purpose with which Sieyès had striven to endow it. More importantly, its claim to represent the people was repeatedly challenged by events from 1792 onwards. This was a circumstance for which it was ill-prepared, as Germaine de Staël observed:

> The Constituent Assembly always thought, but very erroneously, that its decrees possessed something of magic power, and that the people would stop in everything exactly at the line which it had traced. Its authority in this respect may be compared to that of the ribband suspended in the garden of the Tuileries to prevent the people from approaching the palace: so long as public opinion was in favour of those who had caused this ribband to be strung, it was respected by every one; but, as soon as the people would no longer have a barrier, it was not of the slightest use.[1]

The Assembly's internal feuds were increasingly conditioned and their outcome decided by the actions of others outside it who considered that they too had a claim to represent the people. These included political clubs, such as the Jacobins, whose memberships were largely drawn from the same social élite as the deputies themselves, but also, decisively, a broader and more numerous division of the population of Paris. The squabble over representation in the National Assembly between the privileged orders and the Third Estate largely ignored what Colin Lucas has called 'the primary articulation in Ancien Régime society', the distinction 'between those for whom manual labour provided their livelihood and those for whom it did not'.[2] This was a division which the fusion of the representatives of the three Estates into a single Assembly in June 1789 only served to clarify, as did the franchise set under the Constitution of 1791. Power was no longer parcelled out among a host of privileged bodies and individuals under the nominal authority of the Crown. Instead it was placed in the hands of the

1. Baroness de Staël, *Considerations on the principal events of the French Revolution* [...] *translated from the original manuscript*, 3 vols (1818), vol.1, p.414f.
2. Colin Lucas, 'Nobles, bourgeois and the origins of the French Revolution', *Past and present* 60 (1973), p.84-126 (87f.).

property owners of France as a group.[3] But by the same events a collective identity became potentially available to the non-franchised and the propertyless, the so-called passive citizenry. A social institution capable of articulating or at least laying claim to that identity already existed. This was the 'purposive crowd' of the *ancien régime*.[4]

In practice, the crowd already identified the people as *nation* with the people as the *bas peuple*. The activity of urban crowds – riots and demonstrations intended to manifest grievances and secure redress – had been a regular feature of life in France before 1789, just as it was throughout Europe under the *ancien régime*. From the outset of the Revolution, the authorities set out to control and circumscribe the activities of the urban crowd. It was to this purpose that the National Guard and new forms of municipal government were set up following the disturbances of mid-1789 in Paris and elsewhere. The Revolutionary fêtes which replaced the religious festivals of the *ancien régime* can themselves be interpreted as a strategy for control of the crowd.[5] What distinguished the revolutionary crowd from its predecessors under the *ancien régime* were its organisation and leadership, which alike emanated from the assemblies of the newly created Parisian *sections* or districts. The location of the popular movement in these assemblies gave it a powerful tinge of direct democracy. The first 'really organised *journée*' on which the crowd manifested its power was 10 August 1792, when the Tuileries Palace was stormed and the royal family were forced to take refuge in the National Assembly.[6] This led directly to the abolition of the monarchy and the proclamation of the Republic on 21 September. But it also paved the way for the first phase of the Terror with the 'September massacres', when crowds invaded the prisons of Paris to mete out popular justice and death to many of the inmates. By this stage the future of the Republic was doubtful. The government was under attack from royalists within (especially in the West) but also from a coalition of foreign powers intent on restoring the monarchy. It willingly allied itself with the popular movement in the Parisian sections. From the winter of 1793-1794, it was obvious that political power inside the Assembly was held by whoever could best harness the power of the crowd outside it. This meant those who could most plausibly present themselves as speaking and acting in the interests of the 'people' as embodied in the militants of the clubs and

3. Lucas, 'Nobles', p.123-26.
4. Colin Lucas, 'The crowd and politics between *ancien régime* and Revolution in France', in *The Rise and fall of the French Revolution*, ed. T. C. W. Blanning (Chicago, IL, and London, 1996), p.199-235 (originally published in *The Political culture of the French Revolution* (Oxford, 1988), p.259-85.
5. Lucas, 'Crowd', p.224f., 229, 232.
6. Lucas, 'Crowd', p.227.

the sections.[7] This was the period of the ascendancy of the Jacobins under Robespierre and the Reign of Terror.

Who made up this urban crowd? Its individual embodiment was soon known, notoriously, as the *sans-culotte*, from a distinctive if negative feature of male dress – men who did not wear the knee-breeches and tight stockings of the better-off. But as Aileen Ribeiro has observed, 'it is easier to define what the *sans-culottes* wore, than what they were' in the still pre-industrial society of eighteenth-century Paris.[8] Defining the *sans-culottes* in terms of social profile and political interest or ideology constituted a major element in twentieth-century histories of the Revolution. It remains an area of disagreement. On the face of it, the label might appear to have distinguished those who belonged to the *peuple* in either of the more restricted social senses given to the term by Jaucourt in the *Encyclopédie* – *les ouvriers et les laboureurs* or *le bas peuple* – from those above them in the social hierarchy. The *sans-culottes* combined participation in trade with the practice of manual crafts. Whatever their precise social station as individuals, they collectively occupied the fundamental frontier of French society – that between those who supported themselves by means of manual work and those who did not.[9]

The iconography of the *sans-culotte* is relatively unequivocal, whether it is provided by caricatures or by what purport to be more documentary records of political events (as Richard Wrigley has observed, even celebratory representations of *sans-culottes* possess a caricatural character[10]). *Sans-culotte* men were represented in a dress which closely resembles that of the two men carrying in the ailing deputy Maupetit in the drawing of David's *Oath of the tennis court* (fig.33, p.152). The similarity extends beyond dress to the type of activity in which they are engaged – strenuous labour – and the physical quality – robustness – most appro-

7. See François Furet, *Interpreting the French Revolution* (Cambridge, 1981) (original French edition, *Penser la Révolution française* (Paris, 1977)), p.50-56. 'The 'people' was not a datum or a concept that reflected existing society. Rather, it was the Revolution's claim to legitimacy, its very definition as it were; for henceforth all power, all political endeavour revolved around that founding principle, which it was nonetheless impossible to embody' (Furet, p.51).
8. Ribeiro, *Fashion in the French Revolution* (London, 1988), p.85.
9. Lucas, 'Nobles', p.88. For a summary of views, see Patrice Higonnet, 'Sans-culottes', in *Dictionnaire critique de la Révolution française*, ed. François Furet and Mona Ozouf (Paris, 1988), p.418-24. For a characterisation of the essentially Parisian culture of the *sans-culottes* (and for the origin of the term), see Michael Sonenscher, *Work and wages: natural law, politics and the eighteenth-century French trades* (Cambridge, 1989), p.328-62. On the representation of the *sans-culottes*, see Richard Wrigley, *Politics of appearances*, p.187-227. For a recent social history of the *sans-culottes*, see David Andress, *The French Revolution and the people* (London, 2004).
10. Wrigley, *Politics*, p.210. And now Michael Sonenscher, *Sans-culottes: an eighteenth-century emblem in the French Revolution* (Oxford, 2009).

priate to it. This is especially evident in caricatures where the *sans-culotte* was elevated to the status of a national stereotype to be played off against the nation's enemies. These enemies were, by 1793, principally the English, personified by the spindly Pitt and his obese master George III, as in *Le Charlatan politique*, an officially sponsored caricature by the sculptor Antoine-Denis Chaudet, a pupil of David (fig.34, p.159).[11] The period of the crowd's ascendancy was brief. It saw the introduction of a new constitution based on universal adult male suffrage – a constitution which was endorsed by a national referendum and then put on hold. But as external threats to the future of the Republic receded, Robespierre and the Jacobin government moved to consolidate the power of central government. By the end of 1793, they had intervened successfully against the leaders of the popular movement both in the Assembly and outside it and had brought a halt to dechristianisation, generally regarded as the popular movement's most obvious cultural manifestation. Thereafter, until the fall of Robespierre himself in the following summer, the crowd was reduced to a relatively passive role. Jacobin ideology was sharply reoriented away from the endorsement of popular involvement and towards an ideal of centralised government.[12] The final attempts at popular interventions in the Revolution were in the months of germinal and prairial of the year IV (April and May 1795), following the fall of the Jacobins in thermidor of the previous year. They were violently suppressed by the government. But the period of the crowd's ascendancy helped to change the attitudes of the élites not merely to the behaviour of the crowds, but to the character of those who composed them.

The contradictions in the Jacobin position following the distancing of central government from the sections – the fragmentation of the unity imposed on the multiple senses of the word 'people' – are evident in the next great enterprise in which David conjured up an image of the new nation. This was a work very different in almost every respect from the *Oath of the tennis court*, except that it, too, was not brought to completion. The *Triumph of the French people* survives as a drawing (fig.35, p.160). It is

11. De Vinck, 4388. See the discussion of the *sans-culotte* in caricature in Wrigley, *Politics*, p.209-14.
12. The shift can be documented from Robespierre's own speeches. On 16 June 1793, he endorsed the principle of direct democracy to the extent of repudiating the use of 'representative' in favour of 'mandatory' to describe the powers of deputies, but by 5 February 1794 was propounding a scheme of government under which 'the citizen would submit to the magistrate, the magistrate to the people, and the people to justice' – where the 'justice' which constitutes the supreme authority is evidently that of the government itself. See Annie Geffroy, 'Le peuple selon Robespierre', in *Peuple, plèbe, populace. Idées, représentations, quotidien de l'ancien régime au temps des Girondins*, Actes du colloque de Bordeaux, *Revue française d'histoire du livre* 66-67 (1990), p.213-26.

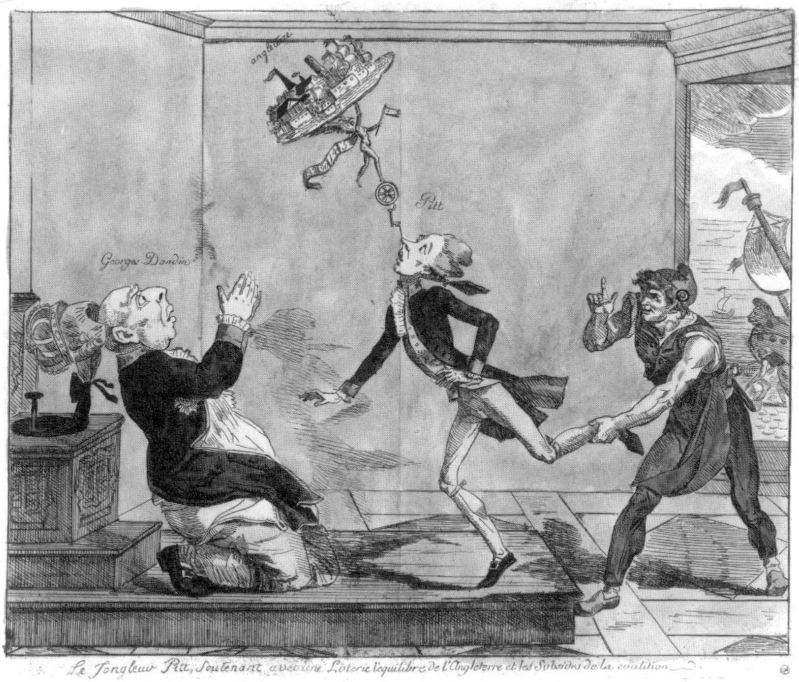
Georges Dandin
Pitt
Le Jongleur Pitt, Soutenant avec une Loterie l'equilibre de l'Angleterre et les Subsides de la coalition

Figure 34: Antoine Denis Chaudet, *Le Charlatan politique, ou le léopard apprivoisé* ('The Political charlatan or the leopard tamed'), etching, first half of 1794, 46.1 × 60.3 cm, De Vinck Collection, vol.26, no. 4388, Département des arts graphiques, Bibliothèque nationale de France, Paris.

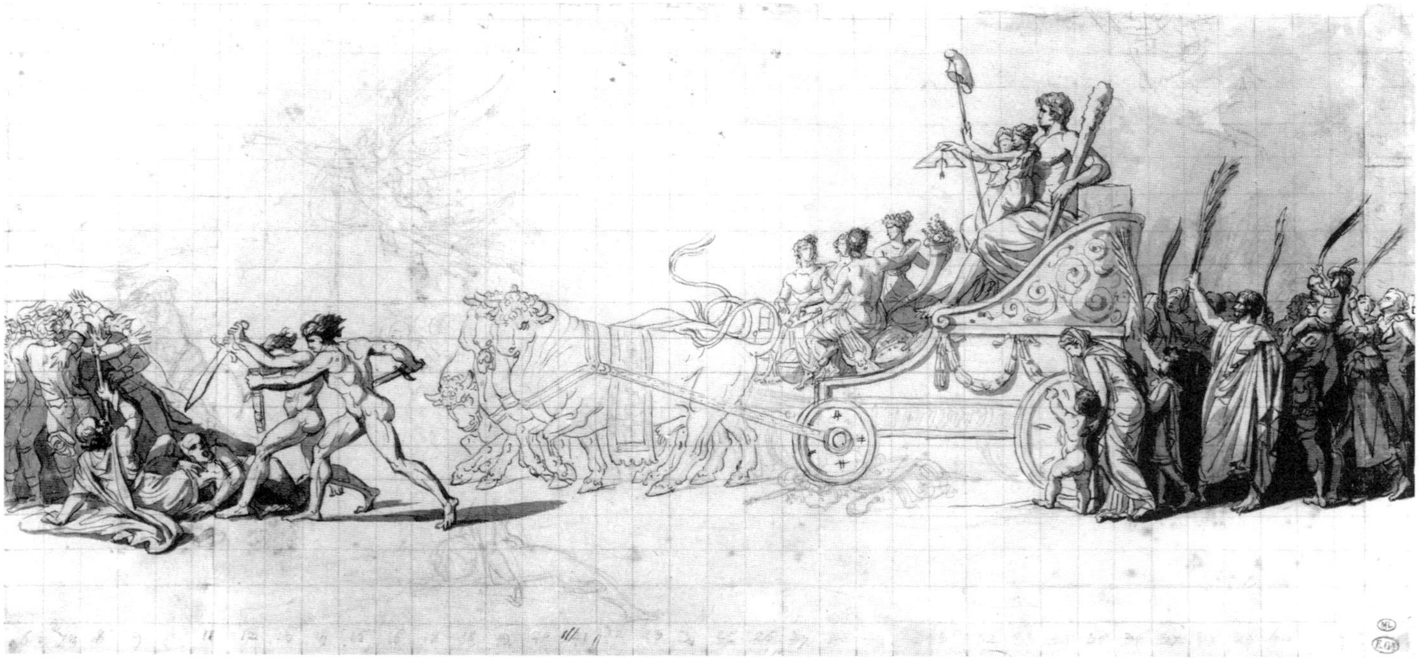

Figure 35: Jacques-Louis David, *Triumph of the French people*, pencil, pen and ink, grey wash, 21.1 × 44 cm, Département des arts graphiques, Musée du Louvre, Paris, Inv. RF 71.

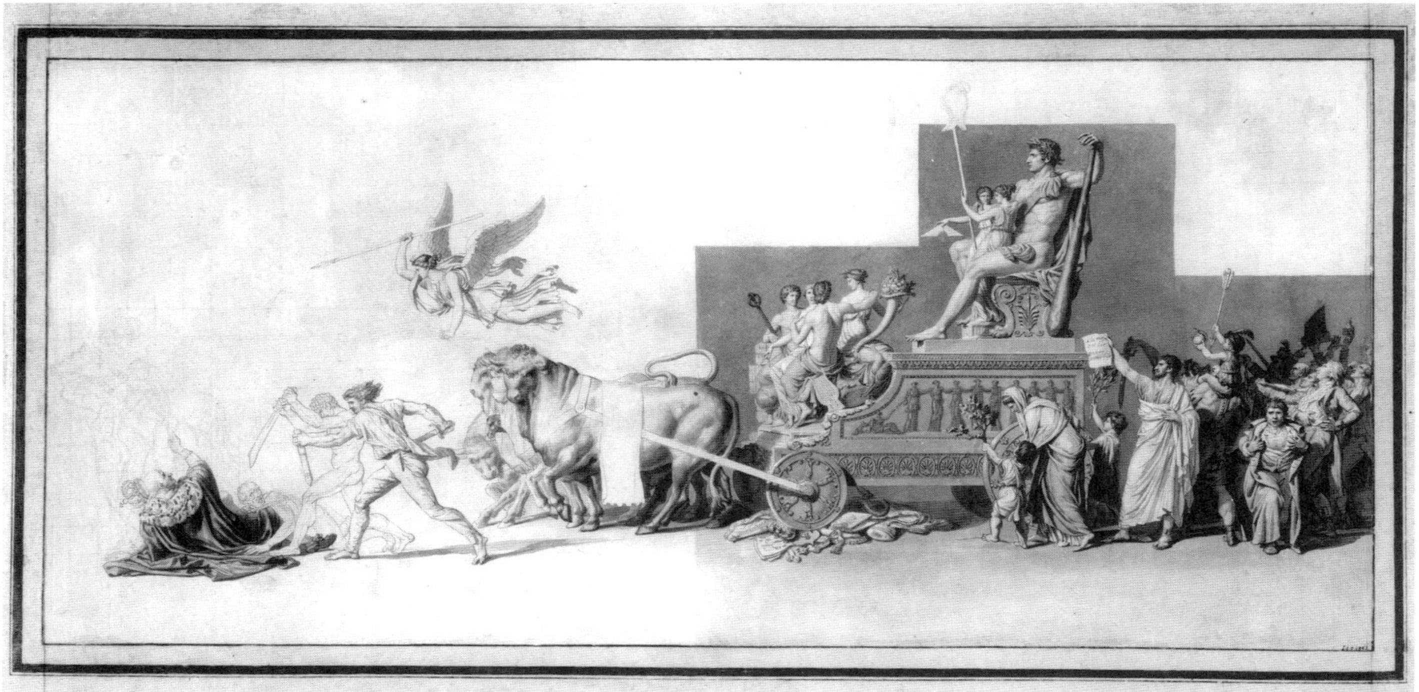

Figure 36: Jacques-Louis David, *Triumph of the French people*, pencil and grey wash, 1794, 38.6 × 71 cm, Musée Carnavalet, Paris, Inv. I.E.D 4856.

said to have been a project for a curtain at the Opéra, and has been convincingly dated to the spring of 1794. The French people are personified by the colossal figure of Hercules riding a chariot which is meant to resemble that used by the victorious general in a Roman triumph. Between his legs stand smaller, female personifications of Liberty and Equality. Other female figures personifying Science, Art, Commerce and Plenty ride in front of the main group. The chariot crushes symbols of tyranny as it advances. From the right, a procession of martyrs of Liberty and the Revolution follows, the latter displaying their wounds or the instruments of their deaths. Among them are the figures of Lepelletier de Saint-Fargeau and Marat, two deputies who had been assassinated in the previous year and whom David had already commemorated in two posthumous portraits which now hung in the Convention. Alone among the martyrs, Marat turns his gaze, not to the People personified on the chariot to his left, but to us, the people as spectators. He breaks rank to bare his chest in a gesture of arresting theatricality which Philippe Bordes has interpreted as a call for vengeance. On the other side of the triumphal car, in the left foreground, two well-built males, one naked and the other clothed, bear down with swords on a personification of monarchy and another figure (perhaps intended to personify religion before the government put an end to the dechristianisation movement in the previous autumn). Above them, a winged Victory brandishing a spear swoops down on a group of lightly sketched naked figures fleeing to the left. Victory replaces a less aggressive personification of Fame who appeared in an earlier version of the composition, now in the Louvre. Who would these fleeing figures have represented in the finished project? Bordes has suggested that their identity may be explained by an entry in the register of the Cabinet des Estampes of the Bibliothèque nationale for 5 April 1794, which records that David had borrowed a selection of portrait engravings. The portraits included those of some of the figures who appear among the martyrs on the right of the *Triumph of the French people*, but also those of some, such as Mirabeau, who had been posthumously identified as counter-revolutionaries by the Jacobins, and others of deputies more recently identified as 'enemies of the Republic' and executed accordingly under the ongoing Reign of Terror – men such as the Girondin deputies and Danton. The naked figures on the left of the composition (in the earlier drawing they were clothed) could thus have been intended to represent those who had conspired against the Republic fleeing in terror at the advance of the French people, a counterpoise to the martyrs of Liberty on the other side of the composition. The earlier, Louvre drawing had been a relatively straightforward allegory of the overthrow of the monarchy by popular action on 10 August 1792. But in the later project this was evidently being transformed into an allegory of the Reign of Terror in its final and most sanguinary phase.[13]

The French People is personified as the colossal Hercules riding in triumph, but the two figures who fall so ferociously on the personification of tyranny in the left foreground also embody the people since they represent the *sans-culottes* – the heroes of the 10 August 1792. In the earlier Louvre drawing both these figures were nude, but in the Carnavalet version David added unmistakeably *sans-culotte* clothes to the man who is closer to the spectator (fig.36, p.161).

His clothing has been classicised in keeping with the elevated character of allegory, the shirt and pantaloons being given the appearance of classical 'wet drapery', as in Moitte's statue of Cassini (fig.30, p.146). But neither the classicising treatment of the drapery nor the classical source for these two figures (an ancient relief of two men attacking a lion in the circus) mitigate the energy with which their actions are portrayed. As Bordes has pointed out, the notion of the 'People' has been given two contradictory personifications – one idealised, the other bestialised – in the same composition.[14] There is thus a sharp contrast with the martyrs of the Revolution who follow the chariot which the two *sans-culottes* precede – not merely in terms of dress and the social affiliations which that implies, but even more in comportment, which in the latter group recalls the refined and effortless exaltation of the deputies in the *Tennis court oath.* The People, whose unity had so recently been celebrated in the speeches of Robespierre, were once again split into two, mutually contradictory entities – the people as Nation and the people as class. This was, as it turned out, the final phase of the Jacobin dictatorship, the period in which Robespierre's colleague Saint-Just famously observed that the Revolution had been 'put on ice'. What is most striking in the personification of the people as *sans-culottes* is the single-minded ferocity with which they are portrayed, a chilling contrast with the strength and rude heartiness of the *sans-culottes* in Chaudet's caricature.

But what of the other, dominant personification – the people as Hercules? This identification derived from a very different and more venerable tradition. The second-century Greek prose writer Lucian wrote a short treatise on a god of the Gauls called Ogmius, whom he

13. Philippe Bordes, '"Brissotin enragé, ennemi de Robespierre": David, conventionnel et terroriste', in *David contre David [.] Actes du colloque organisé par le service culturel au musée du Louvre du 6 au 10 décembre 1989*, ed. Régis Michel (Paris, 1993), p.321-47. See also the entries on the two drawings by Arlette Sérullaz, in Antoine Schnapper and Arlette Sérullaz, *Jacques-Louis David*, nos. 123 and 124, p.292-95. The composition of David's drawings has evident affinities with that of the *morceau de réception* of a younger artist, Carle Vernet, *Le Triomphe de Paule Emile*, exhibited at the Salon of 1791 (no.217) (Metropolitan Museum of Art, New York), which itself draws on (presumably engravings after) Mantegna's *Triumphs of Caesar*.

14. Bordes, '"Brissotin enragé"', p.339f. See also Wrigley, *Politics*, p.209.

described as the 'Gallic Hercules', since he fulfilled a similar role among the Gauls to that played by Hercules in the Greek and Roman pantheon. He was also, like the Roman Mercury, the god of eloquence and persuasion – an intellectual Hercules.[15] This tradition was exploited in sixteenth-century France, when the Gallic Hercules appeared on medals and other propaganda. It was a cult associated with the person of the king, and in particular with Henry IV, the founder of the Bourbon dynasty.[16] It was even claimed that Henry was an actual descendant of the (Greek and Roman) Hercules.[17] This connection was maintained in the iconography of Henry's successors. Thus, for example, the statue of Louis XIV in the Place des Victoires whose base was surrounded by Desjardins' four captives (see above, Chapter 3) depicted the king with the club of Hercules at his feet. Bouchardon's *Love making himself a bow from the club of Hercules*, commissioned by Louis XV, had for a time graced the Salon of Hercules at Versailles.[18] Hercules had also been pressed into the service of Louis XVI, predictably enough.[19]

Following the overthrow of the monarchy in August 1792, the Assembly at first opted for female personifications of the new Republic (as Pigalle had done for the figure who personifies benign government on his monument in Rheims). But a festival on 10 August 1793 organised by David to celebrate the first anniversary of the fall of the monarchy featured a colossal statue of the People armed with the attributes of Hercules. In this case, the symbolism carried a specific political charge. The colossus was represented in the act of smiting the personification of the counter-revolution – a reference to the civil war which had broken out in western France against the royalists and elsewhere against the federalists. The iconography exploited representations of the mythical Hercules' defeat of the many-headed monster, the Hydra.[20] The figure of

15. Lucian, *Hercules gallicus*.

16. See Corrado Vivanti, 'Henry IV, the Gallic Hercules', *Journal of the Warburg and Courtauld Institutes* 30 (1967), p.176-97; Marie Veillon, 'L'iconographie métallique d'Hercule dans la France du seizième siècle', *The Medal* 46 (2005), p.31-40.

17. Jean Seznec, *La Survivance des dieux antiques. Essai sur le rôle de la tradition mythologique dans l'humanisme et dans l'art de la Renaissance*, Studies of the Warburg Institute, XI (London, 1940), p.29.

18. On Hercules and the French and Spanish monarchies, see Gérard Sabatier, *Versailles ou la figure du roi* (Paris, 1999), p.215-38. For Louis XV and the cult of Hercules, see Katie Scott, 'Under the sign of Venus: the making and meaning of Bouchardon's *L'Amour* in the age of the French Rococo', in *Manifestations of Venus: art and sexuality*, ed. Caroline Arscott and Katie Scott (Manchester, 2000), p.83.

19. See J. A. Leith, 'Allégorie et symbole dans la Révolution française', in Hould, *L'Image de la Révolution française*, p.95-113.

20. See the account in Lynn Hunt, *Politics, culture, & class in the French Revolution* (Berkeley, CA and London, 1984), p.87-119. The club of Hercules had already been used on medals struck to celebrate the storming of the Bastille on 14 July 1789 (Jean-Charles Benzaken,

Hercules was adopted as the official personification of the French people in November, following David's proposal for the erection of another, more permanent colossus on the site of the by then destroyed equestrian statue of Henry IV on the Pont Neuf. It was to stand on a pile of statues of former sovereigns – the statues of kings and prophets which had decorated the façade of the cathedral of Notre-Dame. The decision to adopt the figure of Hercules on the official seal of the Republic came at the height of the crisis over dechristianisation – the last phase of the ascendancy of popular militancy in Paris. It has been interpreted by Lynn Hunt as a ploy 'to represent radical aspirations, while at the same time curbing them'. How this could work is immediately apparent from the figure's gender, which implicitly excludes the women whose role in the urban crowd was so prominent and, from the Jacobins' point of view, unwelcome. Hunt has also pointed to the essential ambiguity of the figure of Hercules as symbol of the people – on the one hand, an emblem of the people's power, but on the other, an image of the people as perceived and defined by the people's representatives rather than the people themselves. The symbolism of the statue proposed by David for erection on the Pont Neuf as an 'emblem of the people' is particularly revealing of the role which the Jacobins envisaged for the people. Its parts were inscribed with words denotive of the people's function as at once the nation's moral police and labour force, but not, by implication, its government – 'light' (*lumière*) on the forehead, 'nature' and 'truth' on the chest, 'force' on the arms and 'work' (*travail*) on the hands.[21]

In the *Triumph of the French people* the Jacobins' syncretic model of the people and their strength was resolved into its component terms – the backward-looking symbol of the sovereign Nation personified as the French Hercules on the chariot against the newer, social characterisation of the people as dynamic but dangerous *sans-culottes* – feared, but also necessary, since they alone are capable of clearing the path of the Revolution of its enemies.[22] For the scenographers of the Revolution –

'Hercule dans la révolution française (1789-1799) ou les "nouveaux travaux d'Hercule"', in *Les Images de la Révolution française. Actes du colloque 25-27 octobre 1985*, ed. Michel Vovelle (Paris, 1988), p.203-14. Hercules himself appeared on the certificates issued to the 'Conquerors of the Bastille' and on the certificates and some banners of the National Guard (Leith, 'Allégorie', p.103). The female personification of Liberty was not eclipsed during this period. Leith has argued that she continued to symbolise the goal of the Revolution while the personification of the people as Hercules represented the means whereby that goal was to be realised (p.105).

21. Hunt, *Politics*, p.99f., 106. Cf. D. and G. Wildenstein, *Documents complémentaires au catalogue de l'œuvre de Louis David* (Paris, 1973), no.666, p. 70.
22. On the use of allegory in the *Triumph of the French people*, see Philippe Bordes, 'Le recours à l'allégorie dans l'art de la Révolution française', in *Les Images de la Révolution française*, ed. Michel Vovelle (Paris, 1988), p.243-49 (247f.).

'these seekers after pure presence', as Mona Ozouf described them – the symbolic was always suspect, possibly implying the intention to deceive, to be reduced as far as possible to abstract allegory.[23] It was the second of these two fantastic visions, that of the people as bloodthirsty *sans-culottes*, which was the more avowedly lifelike. It was certainly closer to the image of the people which would prevail in the consciousness of government and the governing class after the fall of the Jacobins, as will be seen in the next chapter.

The festival of 10 August 1793 had been the first of three designed by David, of which only two, that of 10 August and the Festival of the Supreme Being held on 20 prairial of year II/8 June 1794, took place. The third of these festivals would have occurred on 10 thermidor/28 July of the same year, but was overtaken by events. In a coup d'état on the previous day Robespierre and his closest associates were arrested. They were guillotined on the tenth. Had it gone ahead, the festival would have presented the nation with yet another ideal embodiment of its virtues, one very different from those provided by the French Hercules and Herculean *sans-culottes* of the *Triumph of the French people*. The festival had been planned to celebrate two more martyrs of the Revolution, the boy heroes Bara and Viala, who had been killed, aged fourteen and thirteen respectively, in the previous year. Bara, sole support of his mother and younger siblings, had died at the hands of royalists in the civil war being waged in the Vendée in western France. This was reputedly because he insisted on shouting 'Vive la République' when ordered to say 'Vive le Roi'. Viala had been killed by federalist insurgents near Avignon when he attempted to sabotage their advance by cutting the rope of a river ferry. The cult of Bara was instituted by Robespierre in a speech to the Convention on 8 nivôse of the year II/28 December 1793 in which he called for the honours of burial in the Pantheon for the boy's remains. At the same time, he called on David to organise the fête to accompany this event. David, who was present, accepted enthusiastically. On 18 floréal/7 May 1794 Robespierre again extolled Bara and also Viala in a speech in which he inaugurated a religious revival to centre on the cult of the Supreme Being, celebrated in the fête which David organised on 20 prairial. The fête celebrating the Pantheonisation of Bara and Viala should have occurred ten days later, but was postponed for some unknown reason until 10 thermidor.

The cult planned for the two boys was to have been a very different affair from those of Lepelletier, Marat and the other revolutionary

23. Mona Ozouf, translated by Alan Sheridan, *Festivals and the French Revolution* (Cambridge, MA, and London, 1988) (French edition, 1976), p.205-12 (207); Lynn Hunt, *Politics*, p.117, and, on the revolutionaries and the use of symbols, Brian C. J. Singer, *Society, theory and the French Revolution* (London, 1986), p.136f.

martyrs who appeared in the *Triumph of the French people*. Robespierre's speech on 18 floréal was designed to redirect the ideology of the Revolution along new, more religious and more authoritarian lines. Much of the speech was taken up with his justification of the actions taken against erstwhile rivals in the Convention both to the right and to the left of the Jacobins – those 'enemies of the people' who, following Bordes' hypothesis, were intended to figure in the group on the left side of the *Triumph of the French people*. According to Robespierre, irreligion had characterised all these opponents, whether it was the secularism preached by the followers of Enlightenment philosophy or the iconoclasm practised by the dechristianising leaders of the popular party, the *Enragés*. Henceforth, the Republic would devote itself to the cultivation of virtue and justice. Nature encouraged these sentiments in humanity, but Nature alone was not strong enough to ensure that men would live just and virtuous lives, as witness the course of history. It would take the fear inspired by faith in the Supreme Being and the immortality of the soul to achieve that. (Robespierre did not explain why such faith had hitherto failed to achieve this goal.) As part of a programme for moral regeneration, he set forth a plan for future national festivals. These fêtes would celebrate the virtues conducive to private and public moral wellbeing, but also the lives of those whose achievements were fit to inspire the emulation of future generations – heroes such as Bara and Viala.

Bara and Viala were carefully chosen embodiments of national unity. As victims of the two most formidable manifestations of internal opposition to the Jacobin government, the Vendéen royalists and the federalists, they testified to the republic one and indivisible at a time of what was effectively civil war. At the same time, clad as they were in the innocence of childhood, they could offend no-one.[24] They provided the nation with a new type of hero. Robespierre's invocation of the 'gloire' proper to Republicans implied a contrast with the type of military hero celebrated under the *ancien régime*. In David's speech of 23 messidor, this contrast became explicit. The artist scoffed at the courtiers and effeminate sybarites who had formally been honoured for their valour – perhaps an allusion to the statues of military leaders such as Tourville and Turenne which had been commissioned by d'Angiviller for his series of *Great men*.[25] Of course, Bara and Viala had not been courtiers, unlike these heroes of the *grand siècle*. But they had not been leaders either – merely two children who had come to sticky and premature ends in the

24. M. Vovelle, 'Child heroes of the Revolution', *FMR* 39 (1989), p.51-64 (64).

25. Both Robespierre's and David's speeches are reprinted in M.-P. Foissy-Aufrère, J. Cl. Martin, R. Michel, E. Pommier and M. Vovelle, *La Mort de Bara* (Avignon, 1989), p.143-54 and 158-61 respectively.

chaotic conditions of post-revolutionary France. According to David, they had died like flowers of the field cut down by the blade of the plough. If they provided role models, it could only be for boys as young and powerless as themselves – the cannon fodder of the wars which France was now fighting against a coalition of massed European powers. But the speeches of Robespierre and David suggest that they were intended to be much more than that – figures who would help forge the already fractured unity of the regenerated republic of virtue which France was supposedly striving to become: 'In according honours to the young Bara, you accord them to all the virtues, to heroism, to courage, to the love of children for their parents, to the love of the Fatherland.'[26] In David's painting of the dying Bara (fig.37, p.169), the young hero is depicted much as David himself described him in his speech to the Convention of 23 messidor: 'He falls, pressing to his heart the tricolour cockade; he dies to live again forever in the calendar of history.'[27] The cockade, symbol of the republic, indicates the values for which Bara had sacrificed his life. He also clutches a letter. The writing is no longer legible, but it may have contained the orders which he was obeying or a testimony to his devotion to his mother.[28] He is naked. The significance accorded to his nudity depends to some extent on whether or not the painting is regarded as finished. If it is unfinished, there is the possibility that clothes would have been added to the figure at a later stage, as in the case of the *Tennis court oath.* But other explanations have also been offered. According to one view, Bara's nakedness indicates that his clothes have been stolen by his killers, whose shadowy forms can be glimpsed disappearing into the distance in the rear left of the painting. Alternatively, nudity might have been adopted to avoid the embarrassment which attached to the depiction of uniform in the context of a civil war, where both sides wore what purported to be 'national' French uniforms, whether royalist or republican.[29] But such anecdotal explanations are improbable given the exalted tone of the speeches by Robespierre and David. It is more likely that the nudity is symbolic, transforming Bara's death into what Richard Wrigley has described as an apotheosis. That David viewed his task in this light is suggested by his evocation of Bara's place in 'the calendar of history'. The nudity would then be emblematic of that virtue which Robespierre and David had so

26. Robespierre in his speech of 8 nivôse An II (28 December 1793), reprinted *Mort de Bara,* p.142.
27. Foissy-Aufrère et al., *Mort de Bara,* p.159.
28. Foissy-Aufrère et al., *Mort de Bara,* p.68.
29. See the discussion, Foissy-Aufrère et al., *Mort de Bara,* p.67f. See also Philippe Bordes, *David* (Paris, 1988), p.69.

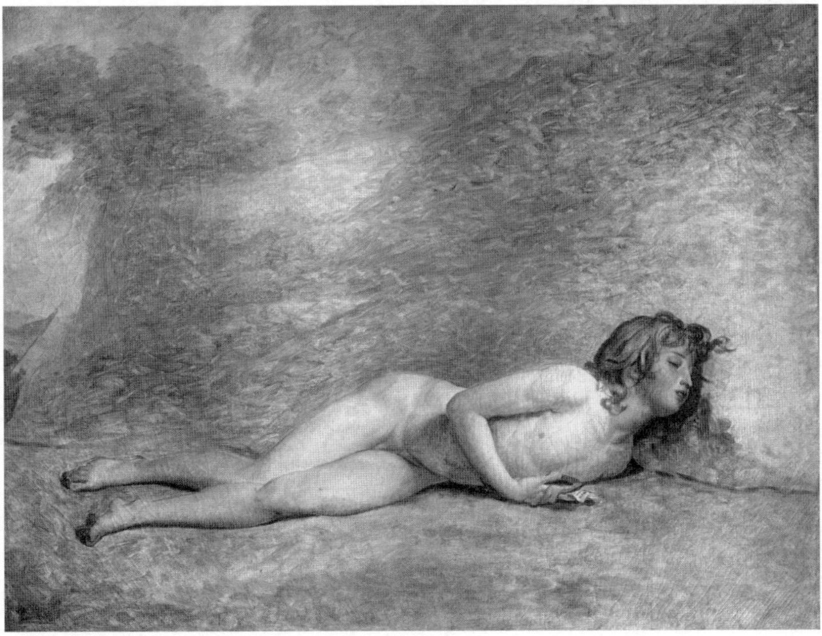

Figure 37: Jacques-Louis David, *The Death of Bara*, oil on canvas, 119 × 156 cm, 1794, Musée Calvet, Avignon.

insistently associated with the young hero in their speeches to the Convention. It is the nudity of the ideal.[30]

Uncertainty over the function of Bara's nudity – anecdotal or emblematic – is compounded by the absence of evidence about the intended function of the painting itself. Such a lack is surprising, given the abundance of information which survives about the Bara cult and about the attitude and intentions of its prime movers, Robespierre and David. Various hypotheses have been put forward to account for the painting's existence. It has been suggested that it was designed to serve as the basis for an engraving. Such an engraving was certainly envisaged. When Robespierre first demanded Bara's Pantheonisation on 8 nivôse, another Jacobin deputy, Barère, had called on David to provide an image, engravings of which should be hung in every primary school of the Republic. But the very scale of David's painting – it is almost two metres across and may originally have been even larger[31] – is enough to indicate that this cannot have been its only or even its primary purpose. Images of earlier martyrs of the Revolution had already been given important positions in public spaces. David's own paintings of Lepelletier and Marat hung in the Convention itself. But Lepelletier and Marat had themselves been members of the Convention over whose meeting place their images now presided. Bara had no such claim. Yet the painting is on a similar scale to the *Lepelletier* and the *Marat* and must therefore have been intended for some sort of public display. It is difficult to imagine an appropriate permanent public setting for this painting of a naked dying boy.

Régis Michel has provided the most convincing hypothesis. He has drawn attention to documents relating to two banners in distemper painted for the fête of the Pantheonisation of Bara and Viala by two of David's favourite pupils, Gérard and Serangeli. The banners remained unused in David's studio in the nave of the former Feuillants church after the cancellation of the festival. The two artists petitioned, initially for remuneration, but then for restitution of their canvases and the red serge which presumably framed them. Might not David's *Bara* have been intended to serve a similar purpose?[32] As has been seen, the artist was already at work on one piece of ephemeral display art – *The Triumph of the French people*, designed as a curtain for the Opéra. Such a purpose would explain the unusual facture of the painting. It has generally been assumed, even by David's pupils, that the painting was unfinished – an

30. See Wrigley, *Politics*, p.116, Foissy-Aufrère et al., *Mort de Bara*, p.68.

31. A second version (Lille), evidently a copy, shows a more extended scene to the left. See Foissy-Aufrère et al., *Mort de Bara*, p.66.

32. Foissy-Aufrère et al., *Mort de Bara*, p.61-66.

underpainting or *ébauche*. But if so, it displays a remarkable consistency of overall finish. The effect of the background is close to that of the lightly scumbled backgrounds of portraits which David produced at about this time, of which the best known is that of *Madame Trudaine* (*Madame Chalgrin*) (Louvre).[33] Although it is clear from *The Triumph of the French people* that David at least planned other paintings of an ephemeral nature, no such completed work by him survives, which means that it is not possible to say how his attitude to the finish required in such work resembled or differed from that which he adopted in other, more conventional genres. If the painting were designed for display in public and in the open air, to be viewed from a variety of oblique angles and under variable light conditions, the lightly scumbled background and the lack of recession would have made good sense and the loose overall handling would have added vibrancy to the surface even at a distance. These qualities would thus have functioned as strengths, not peculiarities which require explaining away on the assumption that the painting is unfinished. Régis Michel's hypothesis has not found general acceptance, but it has the not inconsiderable merit of making sense of the appearance of the painting as it stands. It also provides the only fully plausible explanation of why it should exist at all.[34]

Like the *Triumph of the French people*, the *Bara* appears to have been intended for a mass audience, but the manner in which it seeks to impress that audience recalls the practices of high art, and in particular a

33. Some of these have also been considered unfinished, but similar background treatment appears in other portraits known to have been regarded as finished (because delivered to the patron who commissioned them and therefore presumably paid for), such as the *Catherine-Maire-Jeanne Tallard* (also Louvre) or, for that matter, the upper right hand area of the *Marat* (Brussels, Musées Royaux des Beaux-Arts; see also Détournelle's strictures on the backgrounds in David's *Lepelletier* and *Marat* (*Aux armes et aux arts*!, p.110)). I have suggested elsewhere (*Facing the public*, p.37) that the use of such scumbled backgrounds in portraits should be related to exhibition conditions.

34. But see Udolpho van de Sandt, 'The death of Bara', *FMR* 39 (1989), p.51-57, where it is suggested that David's painting was intended as 'a votive icon' on an outdoor altar set up in front of the Pantheon; a spiritual counterpart to the presumably more anecdotal banners provided by Gérard and Serangeli for the procession itself. The painting's horizontal format, which differs from that of surviving portable banners and makes it less likely to have functioned as such (verbal information from Stephanie Brown), would also favour this suggestion, although there is no evidence that such an image was called for, as Antoine Schnapper has emphasised (Schnapper and Sérullaz, *Jacques-Louis David*, p.290, where further interpretations are mentioned). The public destination of the work would also explain why the genitals are hidden. At a time when the nudity of the statues in the gardens of the Tuileries Palace, now open for the first time to the public, was already giving offence, the public exhibition of a painting without such modification would have been unthinkable. David would himself be forced to paint over the visible male genitals in his own *Intervention of the Sabine women* a few years later, even though that work was visible only as part of a paying exhibition under conditions which were thus, strictly speaking, private. See below, ch.8.

number of highly emotive male nudes of dead or dying classical or biblical figures, both in marble and oils, which had been exhibited in recent years. These were not commissioned works, but prize pieces, produced to fulfill academic requirements. In the case of the sculptures, these were chiefly *morceaux de réception* – the works which young artists had to submit in order to gain admission to the Academy, but also in most instances their first opportunity to launch a career with a work of art displayed to the public. At the Salon of 1779, where the ill-fated plaster version of Clodion's *Montesquieu* was shown among the life-size statues, two smaller figures of this type were displayed upstairs in the Salon itself, among the paintings, where they attracted particular comment. Like David's *Bara*, they both depicted mortally wounded figures expiring. One, by the Swedish sculptor, Sergel, was awarded a gold medal. It represented Othryades, a Spartan warrior who, wounded at the battle of Thyreia, returned, carrying trophies of the defeated enemy, to die at Sparta (fig.38, p.173). The other was Julien's *morceau de réception*, a *Dying gladiator* (fig.39, p.174). Both sculptors had lived and worked in Rome, and these two small works recall the famous, life-size classical statue of a dying Gaul, then known as the *Dying gladiator*, in the Capitoline Museum (fig.40, p.175), of which Julien had made a marble copy, now in the Louvre.[35] Julien's own *Dying gladiator* differs from its ancient prototype, not merely in its compactness, but also in the introversion of its subject. The spectator is mutely invited to reconstruct the dying man's inner thoughts as, steadying himself against final collapse, he looks down at the laurel crown which has cost him his life. In spite of the struggle against physical dissolution which informs the composition, Julien's *Gladiator* is a study in psychological interiority. Echoing the wording of Winckelmann's account of the *Apollo Belvedere*, one contemporary critic described it as 'all soul'.[36] This was the sort of response that such sculptures were calculated to provoke. Such *morceaux de réception* enjoyed a fate similar to that of the rediscovered masterpieces of ancient sculpture, in that their only destination was exhibition in public or private collections. Their purpose was to function as museum pieces – to secure and hold the interest of spectators when placed in competition with other perhaps not dissimilar works. It was predictable that they should invite and receive the sort of response from contemporaries which the surviving masterpieces of ancient art had elicited from Winckelmann. Some of Winckelmann's most famous descriptions had been of sculp-

35. Guilhem Scherf and Gilles Grandjean ed., *Pierre Julien 1731-1804* (Le Puy-en-Velay, 2004), no.1, for the sculptures at the Salon of 1779, p.32-37.

36. Cited Scherf and Grandjean, *Pierre Julien*, p.34. Compare Winckelmann's description of the Apollo, *Histoire de l'art chez les anciens*, 2 vols (Paris: H. J. Jansen, An II/1794-An XI/1803), vol.2, p.427.

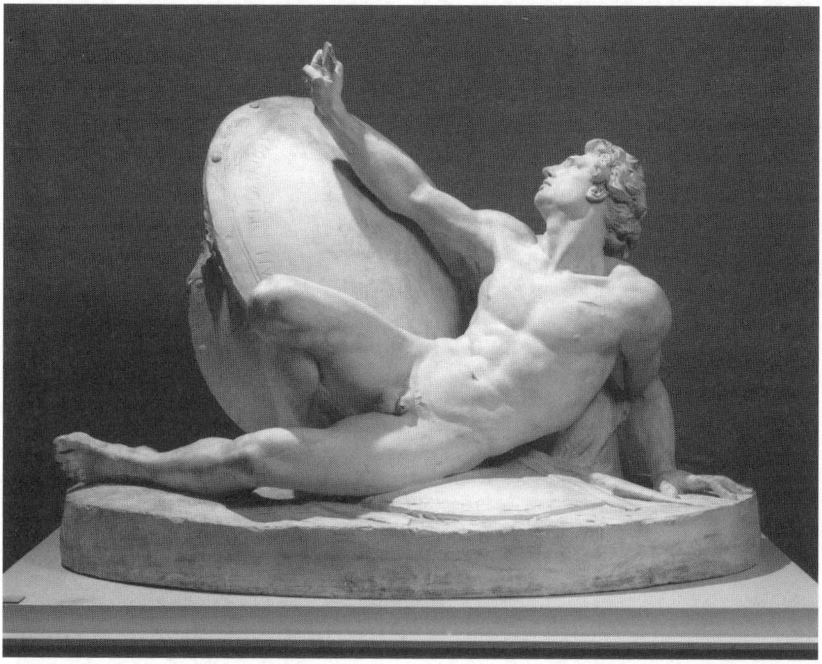

Figure 38: Johan Tobias Sergel, *Othryades the Spartan dying*, terracotta, 1779, 92 cm, NM Sk 454.

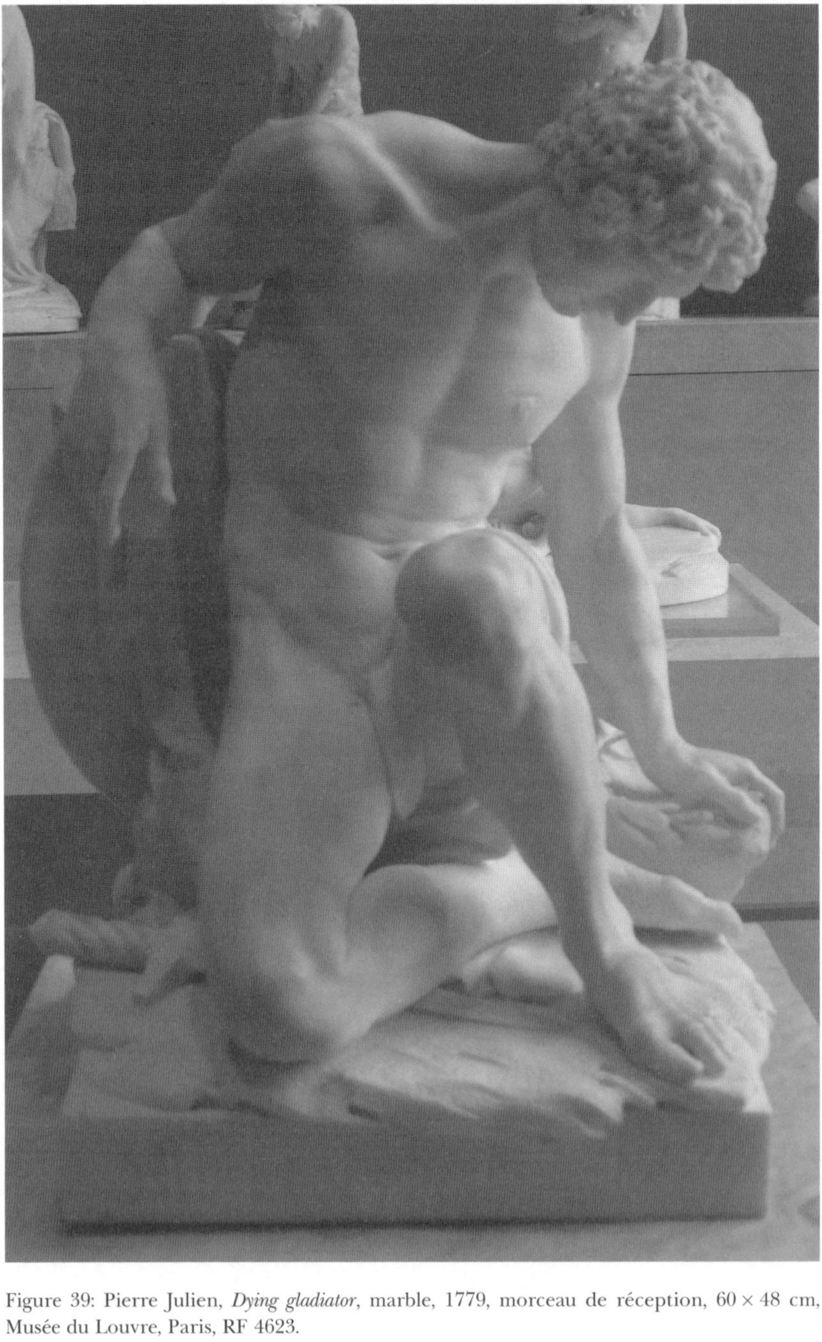

Figure 39: Pierre Julien, *Dying gladiator*, marble, 1779, morceau de réception, 60 × 48 cm, Musée du Louvre, Paris, RF 4623.

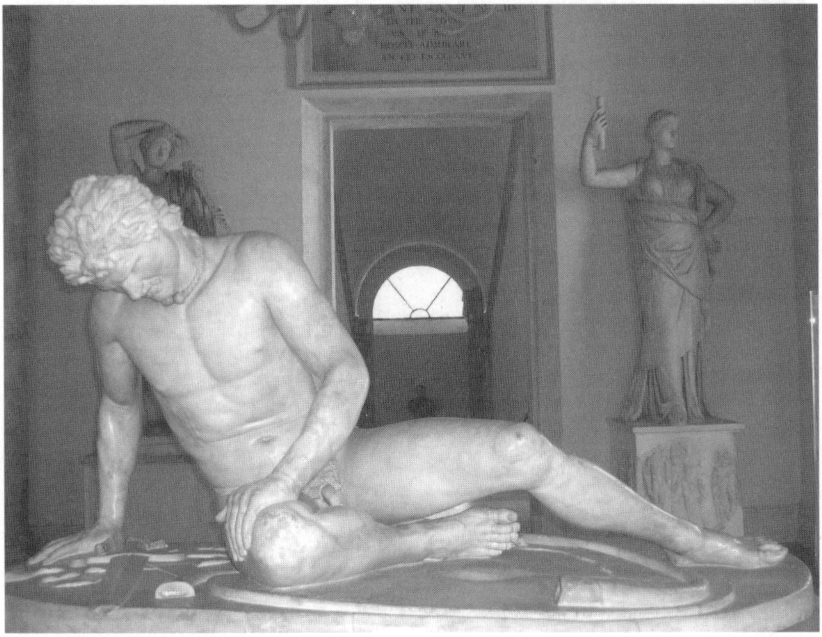

Figure 40: *Dying Gaul*, marble, 93 × 186.5 cm, Musei Capitolini, Rome.

tures which represented subjects in similar states of pain, such as the Laocoön or Niobid groups.[37] In this respect they resembled much of the art produced by foreign artists resident in Rome during the 1770s, where they were often responding to the opportunities presented by the first international art scene of modern times.[38]

As was recognised by Alvar Gonzalez-Palacios, an even closer precedent for the *Bara* is provided by another *morceau de réception*, J.-B. Stouf's *Dying Abel* (*Abel expirant*) (fig.41, p.177) shown at the Salon of 1785.[39] This, too, depicts a dying adolescent. It evokes a similar pathos to David's painting by similar means. Abel's youthful vulnerability, like that of Bara, is underlined by the abject position of his body. In each case, a dying breath parting the lips and a final grasp of the hand are employed to indicate a not yet completely departed consciousness, just as they were in David's *Marat*. But there is one respect in which Stouf's image of a dying adolescent differs markedly from David's. Although Abel and Bara appear to be of a similar age, their youth is characterised physically in very different ways. Whereas Bara's body is harmoniously proportioned and gracefully disposed, Stouf's *Abel* appears to be deliberately angular and awkward, exhibiting such marks of the adolescent transition to adulthood as the disproportionately large hands and feet which Cochin had identified in Bouchardon's *Love making himself a bow from the club of Hercules*. The pose of the dying youth and the treatment of the hips and torso in particular emphasise vulnerable immaturity. His right elbow and hand are twisted over so that the arm lies clear of the body, exposing the skinniness of the chest with its clearly visible ribcage. Together with the arrangement of the legs, this pose helps thrust upwards the jutting profile of the pelvis which shows clearly through the right hip, the

37. Winckelmann, *Histoire*, vol.1, p.424-26. Winckelmann's descriptions of such statues as the *Apollo*, the *Torso* and the *Laocoon* were already widely circulated and admired. See Édouard Pommier, 'Winckelmann et la vision de l'antiquité classique dans la France des Lumières et de la Révolution', *Revue de l'art* 83 (1989), p.9-20. The statues described by Winckelmann had originally been executed with a view to a variety of different purposes and settings.

38. On the artistic milieu in Rome, see Nancy L. Pressly, *The Fuseli circle in Rome* (London, 1979), and Alison West, *From Pigalle to Préault: neoclassicism and the sublime in French sculpture, 1760-1840* (Cambridge, 1998), p.62-74. David also painted a male *académie* based on a rear view of the *Dying gladiator* while he was in Rome in the 1770s, the so-called *Patrocle* (Cherbourg, Musée Thomas Henry, see Schnapper and Sérullaz, *David*, no.37, p.102f.). On David's painted *académies*, see Antoine Schnapper, 'Les académies peintes et le "Christ en croix" de David', *Revue du Louvre* 6 (1974), p.381-92, and on the growth of a market for drawn and painted *académies*, see Guédron, *De Chair et de marbre*, p.136f., 162 (n.5). Among painted *académies* which have been linked to the *Bara* are two important works produced by pupils of David, Fabre's *Death of Abel*, 1791 (Montpellier, Musée Fabre) and Girodet's *Endymion*, 1793 (Louvre). See Foissy-Aufrère et al., *Mort de Bara*, p.69-74.

39. 'La grammatica neoclassica', *Antichità viva* 4 (1973), p.29-55 (36). Stouf, too, had been in Rome, where he had been an associate of Sergel. See Pressly, *Fuseli circle*, p.26.

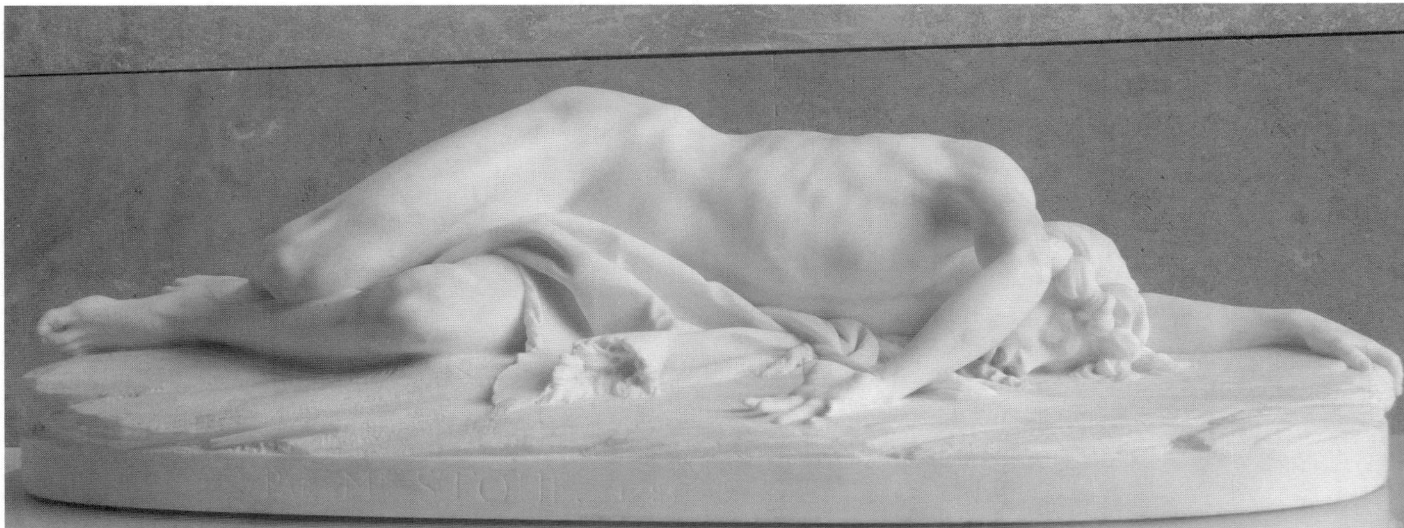

Figure 41: Jean-Baptiste Stouf, *Dying Abel*, marble, 1785 morceau de réception, 30 × 102 cm, Musée du Louvre, Paris, MN 80.

most elevated point in the sculpture. This arrangement emphasises the awkwardness of the early adolescent body – its provisional and unfinished character – to great pathetic effect, but it was a resource that David was to avoid in his *Bara.*

The emphasis on the particularity of adolescent physique in Stouf's figure is obviously intended to infuse in the spectator an added sense of loss – a recognition that this is not merely a life cut short, but one whose full development had yet to be realised. The incomplete state of bodily development in Bouchardon's *Love* had made Diderot apprehensive about how the subject might turn out, but Stouf's *Abel,* lacking any indication of future labours such as those which were present in the earlier statue, only fills the spectator with regret for a future which will never be realised. In fact, the question of the physical and mental effects of labour on the body and that of the division of labour are central issues in the narrative which Stouf's *Abel* was designed to illustrate and this appears to have determined his decision to interpret Abel's adolescent build in the way that he did. Stouf's literary source was not the biblical narrative (Genesis 4), but a poem which the Swiss poet Salomon Gessner based on it. Though now largely forgotten, Gessner's poem enjoyed as great a popularity during the second half of the eighteenth century as any other work of contemporary literature, inspiring numerous works of art in various media.[40]

Gessner's *Death of Abel* was faithful enough to the relatively brief account in the book of Genesis to be acceptable to protestants and Catholics alike, but it added significant layers of emphasis and interpretation of its own. It is reasonable to assume that its immense popularity owed something to the success with which these, the novel aspects of Gessner's work, answered the preoccupations of his Europe-wide readership. The characters and relationship of Cain and Abel were fleshed out in ways which a twentieth-century readership might not expect. As in the book of Genesis, Cain, Adam and Eve's first-born, murdered Abel, his younger brother. But Gessner presented the first murder as a more or less direct consequence of the first division of labour, set up between the brothers themselves on the basis of their different ages. Cain, the older and therefore the stronger of the two, was bred to till the fields. Abel, out of consideration for his youth, was given the less arduous task of minding (and, when necessary, slaughtering) sheep. This division of responsibilities gave Abel the leisure to cultivate

40. On Gessner, see John Hibberd, *Salomon Gessner. His creative achievement and influence* (Cambridge, 1976), esp. p.127 ff.; Fernand Baldensperger, 'Gessner en France' in *Revue d'histoire littéraire de la France* 10 (1903), p.437-56. For works inspired by Gessner's poem which were exhibited at the Salon, see Sylvain Laveissière, *Prud'hon. La justice et la vengeance divine poursuivant le crime* (Paris, 1986), p.65.

social accomplishments, chiefly the composition of hymns to the Deity, for which his older brother had neither the time nor, perhaps, the inclination. Cain repeatedly scorned Abel's effeminacy (a term which as yet had no specific connotations of sexual orientation) and rejected occupations which were not to his own rough tastes: 'Can the towering eagle adopt the flight, or the cooing [,] of the fearful dove?'[41]

When Adam fell sick, it was Abel, with time on his hands as usual, who prayed to God. He was rewarded with a visit from an angel who indicated the 'restorative herbs' which would cure his father's ailment. On Adam's recovery, Abel basked in the gratitude of heaven and earth. Cain, meanwhile, complained bitterly that the angels had ignored him, sweating away in his fields:

> The bright messengers of heaven did not appear to me: they pass me by with contempt: they shew no regard to my supplications. While I exhaust my strength in the tillage of the field: while I earn my bread by the sweat of my brow, under the scorching sun, the angels hold fellowship with him, whose delicate hands are not bedaubed by labour; who lies idle tending his flocks, or, with female softness, is shedding tears because the shining dew glitters on the grass and herbage, or the setting sun tinges the clouds with purple. Happy favourite! all nature smiles on thee, I only feel the care: I only am obliged to spend my strength in the labours of the field. The whole weight of the Divine curse falls on my miserable head. I am in everything wretched.[42]

When the brothers were commanded to offer sacrifices of their produce to the Deity, Abel responded by slaughtering the youngest and tenderest of his lambs, but Cain had only fruit and vegetables to offer. Accepting the lamb with pleasure, God scorned Cain's vegetarian option. Cain's resentment at this slight was exploited by an evil demon, Anamalech, who sent him a dream in which Cain foresaw the future of the human race – a future in which his descendants would be attacked and enslaved by those of Abel. The latter would continue to live in ease and plenty, exploiting the forced labour of the sons of Cain. It was on awakening from this dream that Cain, greeted by his brother, clubbed him to death.

Gessner was a devout Christian, and there is no suggestion in his poem that God was being unfair to Cain in all this. There is an attempt, however, to introduce some degree of psychological verisimilitude into the brothers' behaviour. This is largely achieved by recourse to temperament. Cain is repeatedly described, by himself and others, as melancholy. The question of how much Cain's attitude was determined by the nature

41. *The Death of Abel. In five books from the German of Mr. Gessner of Zurich, in Switzerland. A new translation* (1764), p.15.
42. *Death of Abel*, p.95.

of his occupations and how much by temperament is a recurring preoccupation of the characters in the poem. Conversely, Abel's youth is made to account for his innocence and trust of others, including Cain. Gessner does not indicate whether an Abel grown to maturity might have fulfilled Cain's nightmare, but the role assigned to conditioning in the debates over Cain's personality makes this a pertinent question for a reader to ask in relation to Abel as well. How far should innocence of the deforming effects of labour and moral innocence be equated? The two brothers are the first inhabitants to be born into a postlapsarian world in which neither happiness nor goodness can be taken for granted. The emphasis on youthfulness in Stouf's figure thus picks up on fundamental issues in Gessner's poem. It relates to differences between the two brothers, whether of occupation or of consciousness – differences which would be perpetuated among the progeny of the seed of Adam – the human race. The potential sensitivity of an eighteenth-century spectator to suggestions of such future development is attested by Diderot's response to Bouchardon's *Love*, which represents a boy of similar age and physical development to the youth portrayed by Stouf, but one apparently fated by the nature of his labours to follow a career more akin to that of Cain.

David's *Bara* may be indebted to Stouf's *Abel*, but the physique of the boy portrayed in the painting is very different. In its timeless perfection *Bara*'s body is not merely innocent of labour, like Abel's, but foreign – immune in death – to any hint of its deforming and brutalising effects. As several commentators have observed, David's idealising treatment of Bara's body suggests parallels with Winckelmann. In particular, the rounded contours of his limbs might have been designed to recall Winckelmann's claim that the ideal beauty of form given to their gods by the ancients was that of youth, unmarred by the pronounced musculature of maturity.[43] As has been seen, Winckelmann's construction of that ideal was itself informed by considerations beyond the merely

43. It thus corresponded with the canon of Polyclitus as interpreted by Winckelmann. The *Bara* has been linked to other passages in Winckelmann as well, including his description of the third or 'comic' grace in art, associated with the representation of a child. See above, ch.2, n.9. On the *Bara* and Winckelmann, see Foissy-Aufrère et al., *Mort de Bara*, p.68; Edouard Pommier, 'Rêver devant l'antique un Winckelmann à la main', in Foissy-Aufrère et al., *Mort de Bara*, p.78-81; Alex Potts, 'De Winckelmann à David: l'incarnation des idéaux politiques', in *David contre David*, ed. R. Michel, p.647-69; *Flesh and the ideal*, p.230-36. Potts' closely argued discussion of the painting in relation to questions of gender and desire and in particular his argument that 'David's Bara might be seen as straddling the differently gendered roles of female symbolic ideal and male public hero' (p.236) are not issues with which I would wish to disagree. If I have not taken them up here, that is a consequence of constraints of space and because, like Gessner in his treatment of the myth of Cain and Abel, I have different priorities.

historical or aesthetic (see above, Chapter 4). The function of the ideal in David's *Bara* is similarly related to more than merely aesthetic considerations. The Bara of Jacobin myth symbolised the unity of a nation involved in something very like civil war. But in his nakedness David's *Bara* symbolised something more – a unity which glossed over the division at the heart of the French society, that between the propertied and those who lived by the fruits of their labour.

Jacobin ideology depended on the myth of the erasure of social distinction from civil society as from the political sphere. Whereas Sieyès and his followers had postulated a general will which existed only at the level of national representation, in a National Assembly, the Jacobin amalgam of direct democracy with representative government presupposed that the general will possessed unity prior to its representation, in civil society itself, and that the task of representation was 'not to produce a unified political will above society, but simply to mirror the larger unity of purpose present within a politicised social totality'.[44] Germaine de Staël pinpointed the consequences of such policies for the world of representation: 'Something abstract was wanted in authority, that everybody might be thought to have a share in it.'[45]

The representation of work and workers in Jacobin ideology was ambiguous, and increasingly so following the Jacobins' curbing of popular activity in December 1793. In the previous July, Robespierre had frankly admitted the limited benefits which had accrued from the Revolution to the labouring poor during a speech in which he presented to the Convention the educational reforms drawn up by the now martyred Lepelletier: 'The revolutions of the past three years have done everything for the other classes of citizens, but almost nothing yet for what is perhaps the most necessary class, the proletarian citizens, whose only property is in their work.'[46] In his speech of 18 floréal, however, he used what he characterised as the happy state of the labouring classes to differentiate republican France from the rest of Europe: 'In Europe, a farmer, an artisan is an animal trained to serve the pleasures of a noble; in France, the nobles seek to transform themselves into farmers and artisans and fail to attain even that honour.'[47]

The evocation of labour in the festivals was pervasive but abstract. As has been seen, the statue of the people as Hercules which David proposed for the Pont Neuf had the word *travail* (work) inscribed on

44. Singer, *Society, theory*, p.158.
45. Baroness de Staël, *Considerations on the principal events of the French Revolution* [...] *translated from the original manuscript*, 3 vols (London, 1818), vol.2, p.142.
46. *Projet de decret sur l'éducation publique*, in *Robespierre. Ecrits*, ed. Claude Mazauric (Paris, 1989), p.265.
47. Cited in Foissy-Aufrère et al., *Mort de Bara*, p.144.

its hands. Work was also exalted (and *otium* stigmatised) in the Festival of 10 August 1793, but by similarly abstract means. Representatives of different trades marching under a banner which read 'Behold the service which an untiring people renders to humanity' were followed by tumbrils containing the attributes of monarchy and aristocracy under another banner inscribed 'People, behold what has always made the unhappiness of human society'.[48] In that respect it serves the incorporation of the child martyr into the Jacobin pantheon in a way which accords with the Jacobin appropriation of popular power.

Acceptable approaches to the portrayal of the bodies of the poor and labouring classes played a prominent role in the deliberations of those whose job it was to represent democratic bodies – the artists themselves. They figured as a topic of debate at meetings of the Société populaire et républicaine des arts during the spring and early summer of 1794, the months in which Robespierre, David and Barère delivered their speeches about the Bara cult in the Convention. The issue was raised as a consequence of a protest by the artist and picture dealer Lebrun against the exclusion from the new Museum at the Louvre of seventeenth-century Dutch and Flemish paintings – the sort of art in which he specialised. As well as its 'colour', he championed the moral utility of such art, especially appropriate to an egalitarian republic since it preached 'the virtues of cottages, of simple families' rather than the exalted and usually elitist messages of history painting. Another member of the society, the sculptor Espercieux, disagreed. He protested that such art did not speak to the soul, unlike that of Poussin. Lebrun compared Espercieux's approach with that of Louis XIV, who had banished Flemish paintings of labouring peasants and their families from the walls of his palaces because their subjects had been regarded as too lowly for the contemplation of a 'great monarch'. Yet, as Lebrun explained, these paintings depicted the execution of agricultural tasks, the most useful for humanity, as well as such occupations as spinning and wood felling, not to mention the care lavished by a mother on her tender infants. Such art may not have been calculated to please at court, from which its authors

48. Cited by Judith E. Schlanger, 'Le peuple au front gravé (1793)', in *Les Fêtes de la Révolution. Colloque de Clermont-Ferrand (juin 1974)*, ed. Jean Ehrard and Paul Viallaneix (Paris, 1977), p.387-95. A striking celebration of physical labour mounted in the Convention itself was the formal reception accorded to armaments workers including foundry workers on the occasion of the so-called 'fête du Salpêtre on 30 pluviôse An II/20 February 1794, commemorated in a drawing attributed to David's pupil Fulcran-Jean Harriet (Paris, Musée Carnavalet). As Valérie Mainz observes, however, the fête occurred four days before the denunciation of the Hébertistes, the Jacobins' last remaining enemies on the left, and the event may well have been staged in part to challenge the latters' monopoly of popular sectional activity. See Valerie Mainz, *L'Image du travail et la Révolution française* (Vizille, 1999), p.203-208.

had been banished as mere 'genre' painters, but its worth should be acknowledged in the enlightened atmosphere of the new republic. The label 'genre' was an irrelevancy when art portrayed the virtuous citizen or faithfully depicted the natural world – 'the only goal of art'.

Espercieux countered by pointing out that Louis XIV had indeed possessed paintings of labouring peasants, but these had been the work, not of Flemish genre painters, but of Poussin, a history painter, who had therefore depicted such activities and the persons of those engaged in them with the dignity they deserved: 'a harvester, scythe in hand, is as noble and as beautiful when tending his land as he is when defending it'. This was clearly a reference to Poussin's *Summer*, which uses a harvesting scene as a setting for the biblical story of Ruth and Boaz (fig.3, p.18). If Dutch works illustrating similar activities had been banished from Versailles, that was because they degraded their human subjects by making them appear ridiculous, 'apes, who are to the human race what Punch is to the Apollo'.[49]

In what lay the difference between the figure of a peasant in a Dutch genre painting and a similar figure depicted by a history painter? The answer is provided indirectly by another participant in this debate, identified by Udolpho van de Sandt as the painter Pierre-René Cacault. Cacault pointed out that the heroic subjects of the Revolution would be regarded as subjects for genre rather than history painting according to the traditional classification, since they were modern subjects and therefore did not admit the representation of the ideal figure.[50] Among the subjects which Cacault listed as falling into this category was, ironically enough, the death of Bara (Cacault may have been unaware that David was probably already at work on the depiction of precisely that event).

For Cacault, then, and presumably for Espercieux as well, the difference in approach between a genre and a history painter consisted in

49. *Aux armes et aux arts!*, p.267, 277, 302-306, 321-33. The debate is discussed in relation to the revaluation of the hierarchy of the genres by Udolpho van de Sandt, '"Grandissima opera del pittore sarà l'istoria". Notes sur la hiérarchie des genres sous la Révolution', *Revue de l'art* 83 (1989), p.71-76. For the context, see Udolpho van de Sandt, 'Institutions et Concours', in *Aux armes et aux arts! Les arts de la Révolution 1789-1799*, ed. Philippe Bordes and Régis Michel (Paris, 1988), p. 137-65; Jules Renouvier, *Histoire de l'art pendant la Révolution, considéré principalement dans les estampes* (Paris, 1863). The invocation of the notion of 'nobility' in relation to the work of Academic artists was by this date anachronistic but it was traditional in the context of French aesthetic debates. See Édouard Pommier, 'De l'art libéral à l'art de la Liberté: le débat sur la patente des artistes sous la Révolution et ses antécédents dans l'ancienne théorie de l'art', in *BSHAF* (1992), p.147-67 (156-58). On the representation of work and the working body in the art of this period, see Mainz, *L'Image du travail.*

50. *Aux armes et aux arts!*, p.304. See also Udolpho van de Sandt, '"Grandissima opera del pittore sarà l'istoria"'.

idealisation. Was it in that case the Flemish artist's truth to nature, the quality vaunted by Lebrun, which differentiated his depiction of the working body from that of the history painter? Was what made his work so unwelcome to Espercieux the accuracy with which he depicted bodies, if not deformed by labour, then at least stamped with particularity? If so, he was anticipating a position which would be made explicit in the following decade in the judgement which Joachim Le Breton, secretary of the Classe des Beaux-Arts of the Institut, would pass on Bouchardon's *Amour*:

> The figure has nothing of the ideal. The artist seems to have copied his model in the class of the people. The attitude is lacking in grace, as in nobility: the action is exaggerated: it is an adolescent who deploys all his strength to bend a lump of wood.[51]

In the debates in the Société populaire et républicaine des arts it was the more outspoken and committed Jacobin, Espercieux, who spoke out firmly for idealisation and against 'ignoble' particularisation. His approach appears to provide a theoretical counterpart to that taken by David in his *Bara*.

Espercieux may have preferred artists to avoid too accurate or at least deforming a depiction of the effects of work on the working body, but one unexpected episode in his exchanges with Lebrun reveals that he was far from indifferent to the effects of the division of labour on society. It also illuminates the tensions and resentments inherited from the *ancien régime* which fuelled the debate. In order to clarify the distinction he wanted to draw between the ways in which the human figure was treated by genre and history painters, Espercieux provided a detailed account of moral subjects by two representative painters, Teniers (then regarded as the greatest of Dutch artists) and Poussin. With some justice, he condemned the inexpressivity of the figures in Teniers' *Acts of charity* (Louvre) (fig.42, p.185), which depicts a man doling out bread to a group of far from obviously starving peasants.

The Poussin which he chose as a comparison was the *Testament of Eudamidas* (fig.32, p.148), presumably because this, too, depicts a scene of relatively humble life. It was also the most famous of Poussin's works – indeed, it was probably the most highly regarded painting in the world in the second half of the eighteenth century. It was particularly admired for

51. Udolpho van de Sandt ed., *Rapports à l'Empereur sur le progrès des sciences, des lettres et des arts depuis 1789. V. Beaux-arts* (Paris, 1989), p.162. In the same report, Lebrun praised Stouf's *Abel* for its role in the regeneration of French art, together with Julien's *Dying gladiator* (p.168). Commenting on the same statue in his continuation of Watelet's dictionary, Levesque considered 'le travail d'un ouvrier vigoureux' unbecoming to Love (Watelet and Levesque, *Dictionnaire*, vol.5, p.5 s.v. 'pensée').

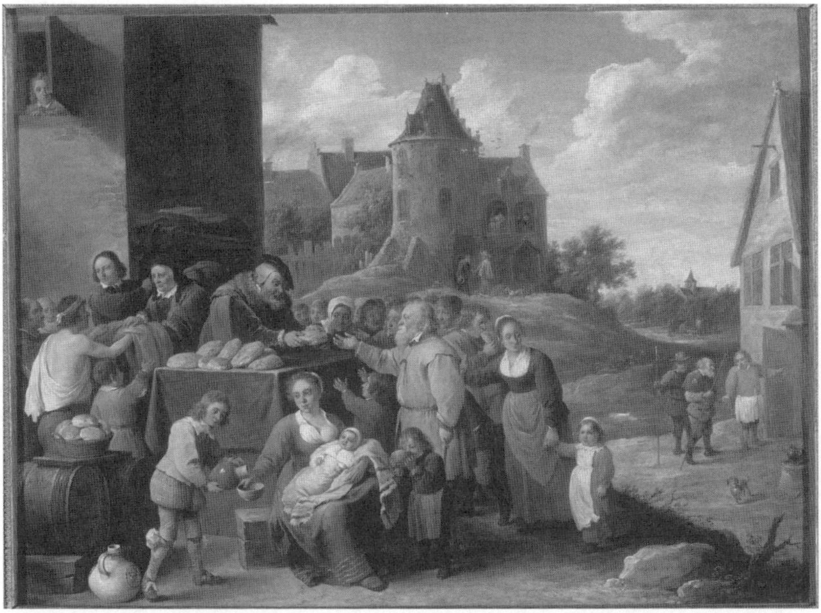

Figure 42: David II Teniers, *Acts of charity*, *c.* 1640, 57 × 77 cm, Musée du Louvre, Paris, Inv. 1879.

the expressions of its figures.[52] The *Testament of Eudamidas* illustrates an act of selflessness in the name of friendship recounted in one of Lucian's dialogues. Eudamidas, a citizen of Corinth, is dying in poverty. He has bequeathed his only property, his wife and daughter, to two rich friends, whom Poussin has depicted as a doctor and a lawyer attending the deathbed. The bequests represent a considerable financial liability. Not only are freeborn Corinthian women not expected to support themselves by work, but Eudamidas' daughter is of marriageable age, and will require a dowry. A few days after Eudamidas' death, one of his two heirs also dies, and the other takes the entire burden on himself, but does so willingly, as a tribute to friendship. The inhabitants of Corinth, who initially derided his gesture, end by admiring it. But it was not this edifying narrative which Espercieux saw when he looked at Poussin's painting. Having described the figure Eudamidas in unexceptionable terms, he turned to the other male figures, of whose friendship with the dying man he was evidently unaware:

> The doctor, like those of today, seems to want to persuade us, by his affectation of gravity, that there is some relationship between his ignorance and the great mysteries of nature. The notary is only concerned with drawing up a will which will compensate with interest the trouble which he has taken to leave his books. The sufferings of a dying man, the grief of a young girl, the deep sadness of a woman overcome by age and grief – that affects him but little; what does concern him is an écu of six francs.[53]

Espercieux's readings of the women's expressions, for which he had nothing but praise, were similar to those of other commentators. His misreading of the narrative evidently depends on his readiness to misinterpret the expressions and the motives of the two professional men.

52. Richard Verdi, 'Poussin's *Eudamidas*: eighteenth-century criticism and copies', *The Burlington magazine* 113 (1971), p.513-24, where it is noted that the confrontation of Teniers with Poussin was a standard one (p.514). It was the *Eudamidas* on which Poussin had been depicted as being at work in Julien's statue.
53. *Aux armes et aux arts!*, p.331. The history of Eudamidas was available in several forms, whether in Lucian's own narrative, both in the original and in French translations, or in those given in Montaigne's essay 'De l'Amitié' and in Pierre Charron's *De la Sagesse* (III, 7, 9), see Richard Verdi, *Nicolas Poussin 1594-1665* (London, 1995), p.259f (no.58). Eudamidas' friends are not identified as a doctor and a lawyer or notary by Lucian, and I have found no explanation of why Poussin or his patron, Michel Passart, decided to cast them as such, thereby unwittingly misleading Espercieux over a century later. By this date Poussin's painting was already in Copenhagen, and Espercieux is likely to have known it only through engravings, which may have given a distorted idea of the two friends' individual facial expressions. See Verdi, 'Poussin's *Eudamidas*'. It is noteworthy that Espercieux was prepared to interpret the narrative of a history painting set in a domestic interior in terms more appropriate to the content of a genre painting, even though he accepted that Poussin followed the conventions of history painting elsewhere in his treatment of humble subjects, as when he idealised the figures of the harvesters in *Summer*.

Under the *ancien régime* doctors and lawyers, like artists, had belonged to corporations or academies which enjoyed privileges under the Crown but whose hierarchies and jealous regard for their own privileges had fostered internal discontent and external resentment and suspicion. These institutions had been dismantled during the revolution. The abolition of the Royal Academy of Painting and Sculpture's monopoly of Salon exhibition in 1791, followed by that of the Academy itself two years later, had been undertaken in the name of liberty and equality, but had failed to defuse rivalries and resentments within the artistic community which had been growing during the previous decades.[54] The Société populaire et républicaine des arts was intended to be a radical and democratic replacement for the Academy, but its debates were frequently and acrimoniously fuelled by internal professional rivalries, especially between painters on the one hand and sculptors and architects, whose training was less expensive and thus less exclusive, on the other – a distinction similar to that which existed between doctors and surgeons.[55] Thus, for example, Lebrun was quick to question Espercieux's own competence to judge painting by observing that a mere sculptor should not be expected to appreciate the beauties of colour and chiaroscuro to be found in Flemish art.[56] In another context, Espercieux had himself openly attacked the attitude of painters who, ignoring the revolutionary principle of equality, continued to claim superiority of judgement over architects and, by implication, sculptors.[57] Espercieux's reading of narrow professional selfishness and charlatanism into the demeanour of the lawyer and the doctor in Poussin's *Testament of Eudamidas* should surely be interpreted in the light of his resentment of what he interpreted as similar behaviour by painters in the field of the fine arts. The privileges of the *ancien régime* had been abolished, but the new, regenerated society was divided by distinctions whose vitality was all the more insidious for the removal of the corporate hierarchies which had previously contained them. However vigorously the Jacobin apologist Espercieux (or for that matter, David) rejected social divisiveness in representation of the democratic body in favour of an ideal abstraction, he could not prevent preoccupations about the effects of such divisiveness in his own career from informing his own perception of

54. See Locquin, *Peinture d'histoire*, p.54-63.

55. See Nathalie Heinich, *Du Peintre à l'artiste. Artisans et académiciens à l'âge classique* (Paris, 1993), p.48-51. For Pigalle's resentment of honours bestowed on painters and not on Bouchardon in the *ci-devant* Academy (and his justification), see Jean Chatelus, *Peindre à Paris au XVIIIe siècle* (1991), p.223. The various rivalries in the medical profession reached a peak in the 1780s, with the disputes between the Paris Faculty of Medicine and the Royal Society of Medicine. See Laurence Brockliss and Colin Jones, *Medical world*, p.760-69.

56. *Aux armes et aux arts!*, p.321.

57. *Aux armes et aux arts!*, p.17.

art and the world. His point of view was symptomatic of an increasing preoccupation with social distinction, not merely in the Academy, but also in society at large. Espercieux's failure to see off the elitism of the painters in the Société populaire et républicaine des Arts merely by exposing it to the light of denunciation echoes on a small scale the impasse which the Jacobin republic had reached on the social front. It was something which Jacobin ideology sought to cover with a veil of abstraction, but which was to emerge into the light of day with increased vehemence after their fall from power at Thermidor.

7. The labels of Hercules: representing the body after Thermidor

It was at first unclear in what ways the coup of Thermidor would change French politics. Robespierre and his immediate entourage were swiftly guillotined by their colleagues in the Convention and the Reign of Terror was halted, though soon to be succeeded by its right-wing equivalent, the White Terror. But the Assembly was still composed of the men whose more or less active support for the Jacobin government had made the Reign of Terror possible. They now felt the need to distance their present from their previous actions while continuing to justify their ongoing authority as the national representation.[1] Their relationship to the *sans-culottes* remained ambiguous. A turning point came in the spring of the following year, when the Convention was twice invaded by crowds demanding bread and the immediate implementation of the Constitution of 1793 – the radical constitution which had been endorsed by the Convention itself in July 1793, as well as by national referendum. On I prairial An III/20 May 1795, the second of these attempts at direct democracy by a now leaderless crowd was brutally suppressed on the orders of the Convention. The confidence of the propertied men who had directed the Revolution returned. They had seen off the crowd, although their former complicity with it continued to haunt them. The excesses of government under Robespierre were now blamed on the 'people' rather than the Convention, and the people were demonised accordingly.[2]

The Revolution was reinterpreted as the heritage of the Enlightenment, a concept which the Conventionnels might be said to have invented.[3] Their mission henceforth would be to civilise a society which – events had proved – was not yet civilised enough to do without them.

1. See Bronislaw Baczko, translated by Michel Petheram, *Ending the terror: the French Revolution after Robespierre* (Cambridge, 1994).
2. 'The era of the property owners' unadulterated fear of the "dangerous classes" and their complete exclusion from politics by a repressive state had begun. The experience of the crowd in the Revolution had provoked the final defection of the bourgeoisie from a culture based on notions of community. In this domain, the rupture with the eighteenth century began in 1795, not in 1789', Colin Lucas, 'The crowd and politics between *ancien régime* and Revolution in France', in *The Rise and fall of the French Revolution*, ed. T. C. W. Blanning (Chicago, IL, and London, 1996), p.235.
3. See Roger Chartier, translated by Lydia G. Cochrane, *The Cultural origins of the French Revolution* (Durham and London, 1991), p.5.

What was now labelled the 'anarchy' of popular involvement in government had been an aberration which should not be allowed to recur.[4] A new constitution was drawn up by a special commission to replace the still unimplemented Constitution of 1793. The commission's proposals were presented to the Convention in messidor of the year III (June 1795) by Boissy d'Anglas. They were framed by the notion of the nation's indivisibility, evoked in the metaphor of the body politic with which he opened his speech:

> It is with a great nation as it is with a great man. The goal of the latter's labours, the principle of all his actions, of all that is most dangerous or painful, is one day to achieve a dignified and honourable repose.[5]

The aim of sustaining national unity was one which the post-Thermidorians shared with their Jacobin and other predecessors, but it was now inspired less by faith in nationhood than by fear of giving voice to dissent based on social and geographical division. The commission's proposals were geared to prevent factionalism. This meant forestalling any mechanism whereby the interests of particular social groups – above all, those of the propertyless – might coalesce and become articulate. Hence the provisions of the Constitution which were intended to prevent the revival of political clubs such as that of the Jacobins. Hence, too, the inclusiveness of the new franchise, which embraced all adult male tax payers (excluding domestic servants), irrespective of wealth:

> The poverty of the needy has as much right to protection as the wealth of the rich; the artisan's industry, as much as the farmer's harvest. Besides, would it be politic, would it assist harmony to divide a people into two portions, of which one would be clearly subject, while the other was sovereign? Would this usurpation be anything other than to arm the oppressed portion against that which oppressed it; and would it not be to plant in the state a perpetual seed of division which would end in the overthrow of your government and your laws?[6]

4. See, for example, Boissy d'Anglas, *Discours préliminaire au projet de Constitution pour la République française, prononcé par Boissy-d'Anglas, au nom de la commission des onze, dans la séance du 5 messidor, An 3*, messidor An III (1795), p.5. See also Baczko, 'L'Expérience thermidorienne', in *The Political culture of the French Revolution* (*The French Revolution and the creation of modern political culture*, vol.2), ed. Colin Lucas (Oxford, 1988), p.341-70 (366); Baczko, 'La Constitution de l'an III et la promotion culturelle du citoyen', in *L'institution de la raison*, ed. François Azouvi (Paris, 1992), p.21-37 (22).
5. Boissy d'Anglas, *Discours préliminaire*, p.1.
6. Boissy d'Anglas, *Discours préliminaire*, p.23; see also. p.55f. See also Baczko: 'The people are seen less and less as a stirring and heroic figure, more and more as emblematic and problematic, undermined from within by accusations against the 'vandals and cannibals', and yet indispensable. [...] The *people* were therefore increasingly reduced to a single function: to legitimising the Republic and, consequently, its authority' (*Ending the terror*, p.220).

There were two important restrictions in the scope of this apparently liberal provision. The first of these resulted from a two-tier election system. While all who were eligible to vote could do so at the first stage, only those who fulfilled a stringent property qualification (estimated at about 30,000 men out of an overall population of as many as 28,000,000) were allowed to take part in the second stage of the elections. It was the second-stage electors who chose the members of the two new councils which together replaced the National Assembly. Of these a lower house, the Council of the Five Hundred, had the power only to propose legislation which the other, the Council of the Ancients, could only accept or reject.[7] The executive branch consisted of a five-man Directory or *Directoire*, which subsequently gave its name to the regime as a whole. It was hoped that the checks and balances which resulted from this arrangement would prevent future dictatorship. The property requirements for members of the secondary electoral assemblies and the Councils meant that all important decisions would effectively be in the hands of the rich. The new Constitution thus helped to solve one of the most problematic issues for the rulers of the young democracy; how to maintain hereditary distinctions between individuals in a society which claimed to have abolished them – a society which recognised equality of right and opportunity, yet which was grounded in the private ownership of property and the privileged access to social resources which that entails. As Boissy d'Anglas famously explained: 'A land governed by the property owners is in the social order; that where the non-property owners govern is in the state of nature.'[8]

The other restriction imposed on the exercise of civil rights was educational. Only those who could read and write and who had learned a craft (*un art mécanique*) would be allowed to exercise the function of voters at any level. The implementation of this requirement was postponed for a decade, to allow reforms of the Republic's educational system to take effect. As the predicted benefits of liberty and the free market failed to materialise, future perfection and prosperity were increasingly invoked as a remedy for present inequalities or injustice. But since access to education was still the privilege of a propertied

7. As though to disarm the threat which bicameralism posed to organic unity in government, Boissy d'Anglas explained that the councils performed the functions of the imagination and the reason respectively (*Discours préliminaire*, p.32f.). On the Constitution, see Jacques Godechot, *Les Institutions de la France sous la Révolution et l'Empire* (Paris, 1951), p.457-67.

8. Boissy d'Anglas, *Discours préliminaire*, p.22. Several members of the Commission des Onze had been in favour of restricting the overall franchise to landowners, leading to an important press debate in the nature of citizenship. See Edgard Allix, 'La rivalité entre la propriété foncière et la fortune mobilière sous la révolution', in *Revue d'histoire économique et sociale* 6 (1913), p.297-348.

section of the population, the provision effectively reinforced the property qualification by other, social measures while appearing merely to set a premium on intellectual capacity. This aspect of Thermidorian cultural strategy was attacked by the radical journalist Gracchus Babeuf:

> [We shall demonstrate that] it is the intelligent who have given so high a price to the products of their brains, and that if it had been the strong who had ordered things, they would doubtless have decreed that the merit of the arms equalled that of the head, and that the fatigue of the whole body could receive recompense like that of the thinking part alone.
> That, without putting this equality in place, the more intelligent, the more industrious, receive a licence to accumulate, a right to despoil with impunity those who are less so.[9]

The crown of the Convention's achievements, alluded to at the end of Boissy d'Anglas' speech, would be the voting of a comprehensive new law on national education, which replaced earlier legislation projected by the Jacobins.[10]

The centrality of education to Thermidorian ideology helps to explain the outcome of a sculpture competition decided in the spring of the same year. It was part of the great national art competition of the year II, announced by the Jacobin Committee of Public Safety on 5 floréal An II/24 April 1794. The winning sculpture was to be erected in the Champs-Elysées in honour of the philosopher Jean-Jacques Rousseau. The jury's decision had been delayed by the coup of Thermidor. As a result, the twenty-five entries had been on public display in the Louvre for almost a year before the award of the prize on 28 pluviôse An III/16 February 1795. Most of the surviving submissions which have been identified represented the philosopher as a full-length figure, seated or standing, in the manner of the statues of *Grands hommes* commissioned by d'Angiviller and in one version or another of contemporary dress.[11] But the winning entry, by Moitte, represented a semi-naked figure accompanied by a naked child. It was described as 'Jean-Jacques Rousseau pondering the first steps of childhood' (fig.43, p.194). As the monument was intended for the Champs-Elysées, a popular meeting place and playground for children

9. 'Manifeste des plébéiens', *Le Tribun du peuple* no.36 (20 frimaire An IV/11 December 1795), cited in Babeuf, ed. Claude Mazauric, *Ecrits* (Paris, 1988), p.276. Writing from a different political perspective, Necker observed that the literacy qualification in the Constitution of the Year III would have excluded Charlemagne himself from full civic rights (cited by Lucien Jaume, 'Necker: examen critique de la Constitution de l'An III' in *La Constitution de l'An III[.] Boissy d'Anglas et la naissance du libéralisme constitutionnel*, ed. Gérard Conac and Jean-Pierre Machelon (Paris, 1999), p.167-82 (179)). In the present case, such faith in the future was misplaced – the Constitution of the Year III survived only until 1799.
10. See Baczko, 'L'Expérience thermidorienne'; Azouvi, *L'Institution de la raison*, *passim*.
11. See above, ch.5, p.15-18.

and their mothers, it was considered particularly appropriate that Moitte should have chosen to represent Rousseau as 'the legislator of education, the benefactor of childhood'. The outcome was reportedly an endorsement of the views of the public.[12]

The child at the philosopher's knee was identified by contemporaries with Emile, the eponymous hero of Rousseau's didactic novel on the subject of education. Moitte's representation of him as a mere toddler presumably alludes to the importance attached by the philosopher to early education. The man's evident willingness to allow the child the freedom to determine the direction of his steps reflects Rousseau's own belief in the natural goodness of childhood, corrupted only later in life by experience in society. As Gramaccini emphasised, these were also important elements in the Jacobin ethos of education, as set forth in the proposals of the Jacobin martyr Lepelletier Saint-Fargeau and in the law of 29 frimaire An II/19 December 1793, which prescribed compulsory primary education for all the Republic's children.[13]

It is not only in its vision of the educational process that Moitte's group expressed a Jacobin ideology. Unlike the figure of Cassini which Moitte had contributed to the *Grands hommes* (fig.30, p.146), the *Rousseau* monument makes no concessions to the trivially specific or modern in its dress. Instead it combines nudity with generalised classical drapery. The marks of social distinction associated with modern dress are erased by the universal language of classicism, reinforcing Jacobin commitment to primary education for all, irrespective of wealth or condition. The use of classical drapery also suggests a programme of regeneration through education – Rousseau himself had considered the cultural practices of antiquity closer to nature than those of his own time.[14] But the nudity of the older figure reveals another, more specific classical reference which explains an otherwise anomalous feature of the sculpture. The face is not unlike that given to Rousseau in his portraits, including those based on the mask which Moitte's rival, Houdon, had taken following the philos-

12. For this and other references, and for accounts of the competition, see Gisela Gramaccini, 'Sur le projet d'élever un monument en l'honneur de Rousseau', in *La Révolution française et l'Europe 1789-99*, 3 vols (Paris, 1989), vol.3, p.893-97; Guilhelm Scherf, in *L'Esprit créateur de Pigalle à Canova. Terres cuites européennes 1740-1840*, ed. James David Draper and Guilhem Scherf (Paris, 2003), p.256-58 (no.113). There had been earlier projects for a monument to Rousseau, including one which would have been financed by public subscription, like David's *Tennis court oath* (see Gramaccini).

13. Gramaccini, 'Sur le projet', p.896. See also Gramaccini, 'L'image de l'homme nouveau', p.681f; Michel Lepeletier [*sic*] Saint-Fargeau, ed. Fęlix Lepeletier, *Œuvres* (Paris, 1826), p.267-330 (314). See also Jacques Godechot, *Les institutions*, p.447.

14. See 'Lettre à M. d'Alembert sur son article Genève', in *Du Contrat social ou principes du droit politique*, (Paris, 1962), p.160, n.2. For views on the degeneracy of modern dress, see ch.5; the use of restrictive clothing for children was particularly frowned on.

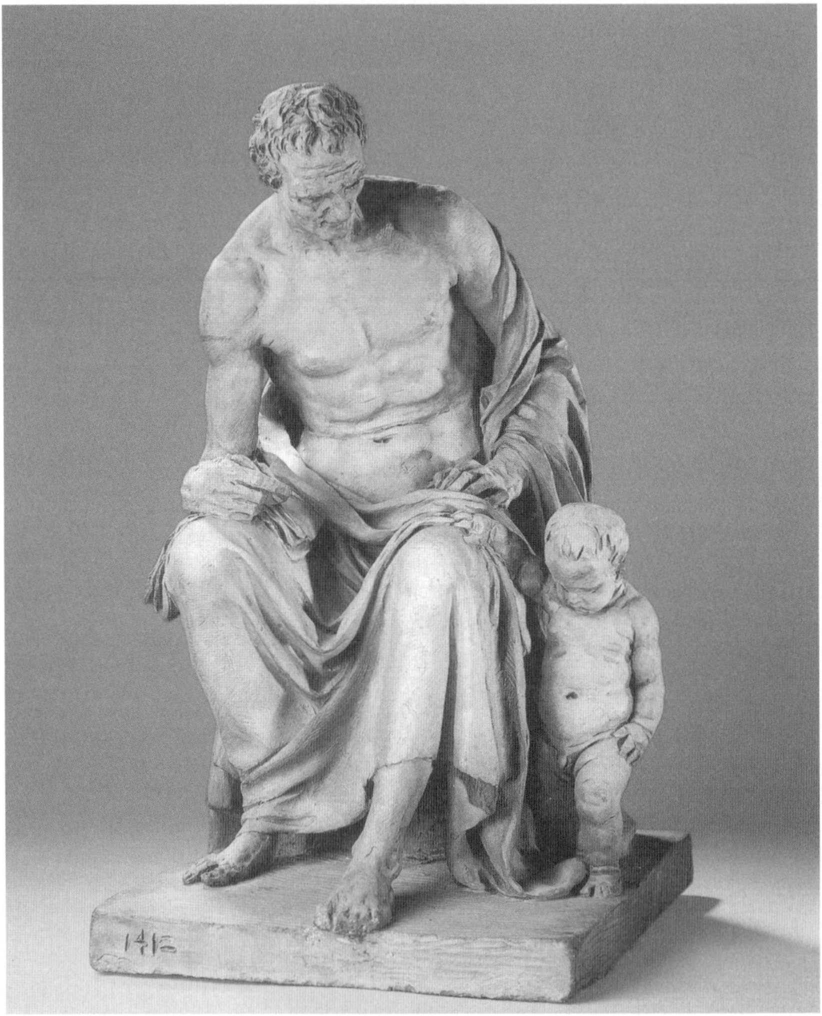

Figure 43: Jean-Guillaume Moitte, *Jean-Jacques Rousseau*, terracotta, 1790, 34 × 19 cm, Musée Carnavalet, Paris.

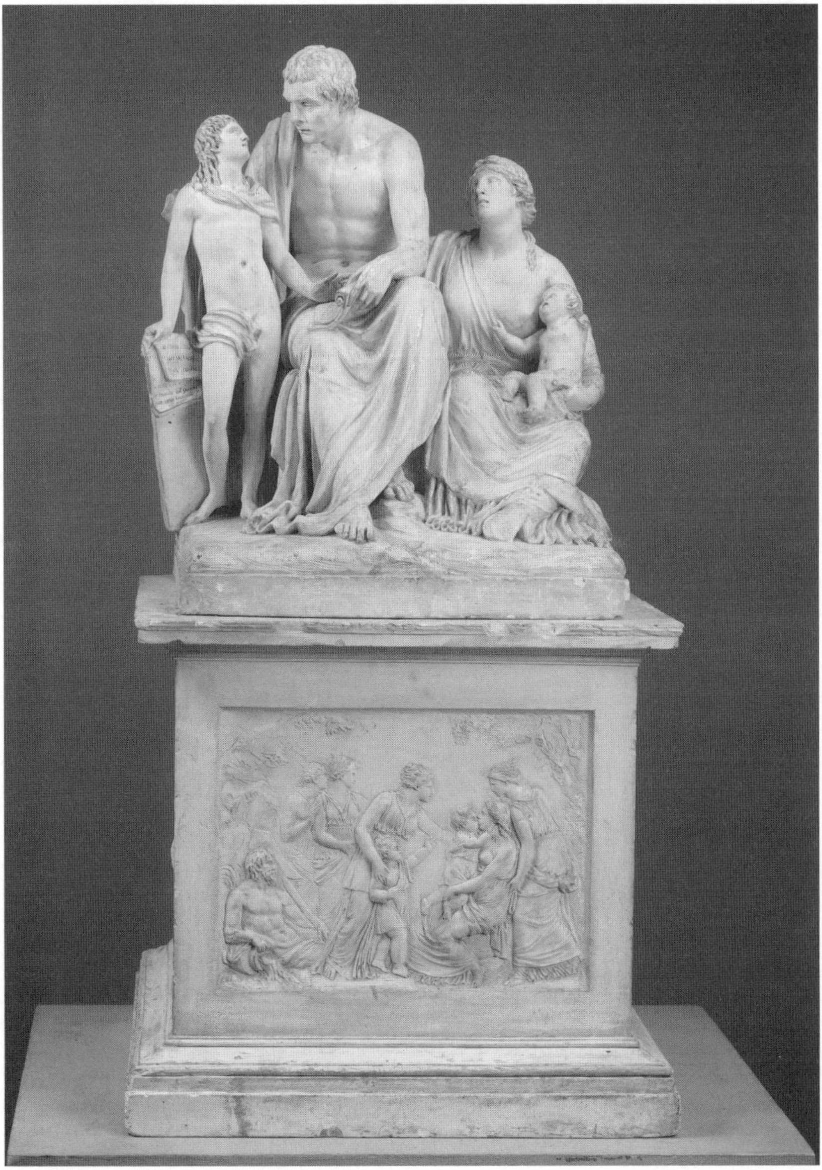

Figure 44: François Masson, *Project for monument to Jean-Jacques Rousseau*, plaster, 1798-1799, 96 × 49 cm, Musée du Louvre, Paris, RF 1984.

opher's death in 1778.[15] But the build attributed to Rousseau by Moitte seems inappropriately powerful and robust for the representation – even the idealised representation – of a man who had never laid claim to good health.[16] This is because his anatomy did not originally belong to Rousseau at all. As Gramaccini recognised, Moitte's composition is built around a copy of the fragmentary *Belvedere torso* (fig.20, p.109). At this date, the *Torso* was universally regarded as a representation of Hercules. According to Winckelmann, it represented Hercules in his divine form, at rest after his labours.[17] Moitte was not the only sculptor of his age who tried to 'complete' the *Torso* in such a way.[18] But in a sculpture designed for a Jacobin competition, the identification with Hercules had a specific resonance. Moitte's *Rousseau* stands for the French people, like the figures of Hercules in David's projects for the Opéra curtain and the colossal statue on the Pont Neuf, produced at the same time as that at which Moitte was at work on his submission to the Rousseau competition. Beside the Herculean Rousseau, Emile stands for the regenerated citizen of the future. The representation of the people as a child in need of re-education had become a distinctive feature of Jacobin discourse.

At first, internal opposition to the Revolution in the royalist west and the federalist south-east had been viewed as the effect of counter-revolutionary propaganda. But the persistence and intensification of armed resistance had impelled the Jacobins to adopt another explanation – like a child unused to freedom, the young nation had made mistakes, but these could and would be corrected by a programme of re-education.[19] But if Moitte's group personifies the people under two

15. Houdon produced busts of Rousseau in classical as well as contemporary dress. See Anne L. Poulet and Guilhem Scherf, *Houdon sculpteur des Lumières 1741-1828* (Paris, 2003), p.173-77 (no.27), who illustrate the surviving death mask (fig.1, p.175).
16. A life-long hypochondriac, Rousseau was, for example, ranked among the typically skinny geniuses of his age by the medical writer J. G. Zimmermann, together with Voltaire and Wieland ('Wieland's legs are like a pair of flutes'). [J. G. Zimmermann], *A Treatise on experience in physic*, 2 vols (London, 1778), vol.2, p.299 (originally published in German as *Von der Erfahrung in der Arzneykunst* in 1763).
17. Winckelmann, *History*, vol.1, p.374, 382f, vol.2, p.341-43.
18. For more about the group of Hercules and Hebe by Moitte's English contemporary, John Flaxman (now London, Victoria & Albert Museum), see Margaret Whinney, *Sculpture in Britain 1530-1830* (London, 1964), p.188). Auguste-Louis-Marie Ottin chose to execute a marble copy of the Torso as an *envoi* from Rome in 1838 (Paris, Ecole des Beaux-Arts) because he had already decided that his final *envoi* would be a statue of Hercules presenting the golden apples of the Hesperides to Eurystheus (formerly Luxembourg gardens) (Antoinette Le Normand, *La Tradition classique et l'esprit romantique. Les sculpteurs de l'Académie de France à Rome de 1824 à 1840* (Rome, 1981), p.117). The latter's pose, however, appears to have been based on that of the *Farnese Hercules* (p.264) rather than the *Torso*. I owe this example to Philip Ward-Jackson. For further instances see Haskell and Penny, *Taste and the antique*, p.313.
19. See Christian Alain Muller, 'Du "peuple égaré" au "peuple enfant" [.] Le discours

aspects, like David's *Triumph of the French people*, there are not the same grounds for potential conflict between the two roles assigned to the people in Moitte's project as there were in David's project. Instead, the two are united in their devotion to a single goal – regeneration through education. Moitte's incorporation of the figure of Hercules into that of Rousseau was not yet as incongruous in 1795 as it would soon become. Representations of the French Hercules – more usually in the pose of the *Farnese Hercules* than in that of the *Torso* – continued in official use.[20] The pose of Hercules gave resonance to representations of the citizen in other contexts as well. Thus, for example, when the miniaturist J.-B. Augustin took advantage of Academic deregulation to exhibit for the first time at the Salon in 1796, he made his debut with a self-portrait miniature described as being *en grande miniature* – a miniature of Herculean dimensions. It represented the artist's ample figure swathed in quasi-classical drapery of the sort used in Moitte's *Cassini* and in the pose of the *Farnese Hercules* – though with the latter's club replaced by a portfolio of male nude *académies*, thereby implying that a grasp of life drawing was the strength on which the citizen artist relied.[21]

Superficially, the educational aspirations proclaimed by Moitte's Jacobin sculpture were equally in tune with the aspirations of government following Thermidor. A fundamental shift, however, was already taking place in the official approach which was in line with the new model of ideal citizenship. For the Jacobins, the education of the citizen had been designed to foster virtue and commitment to the Revolution. For the Thermidorians, its aim was to teach competence of judgement. This is clear from the debates on the literacy provisions of the new Constitution.[22] This perspective was most fully expressed in the creation of an *Institut national*, proposed by Boissy d'Anglas himself in February 1794 and again invoked at the end of his report on the Constitution. The Institut superseded the academies of the *ancien régime*, but without their old, corporate functions. To some extent it functioned as an instrument whereby government sought to regain control of a cultural field which

politique révolutionnaire à l'épreuve de la révolte populaire en 1793', *Revue d'histoire moderne et contemporaine*, 47 (2000), p.93-112.

20. Particularly on coins, see Jean-Charles Benzaken, 'Hercule dans la Révolution française (1789-1799) ou les "nouveaux travaux d'Hercule"', in *Les Images de la Révolution française. Actes du colloque 25-27 octobre 1985*, ed. Michel Vovelle (Paris, 1988), p.203-14; Lynn Hunt, *Politics, culture, & class in the French Revolution* (Los Angeles and London, 1984), p.113.

21. See Halliday, *Facing the public*, p.125-27, fig. 21.

22. See Baczko,'La Constitution de l'An III et la promotion culturelle du citoyen', especially p.31, n.1. Boissy d'Anglas' report already signalled the abandonment of the commitment to universal education with the responsibility for primary education passed to local authorities instead of the state (*Discours préliminaire*, p.57). See also Godechot, *Institutions*, p.448.

was fragmenting following the removal of older privileges and regulations. Only the elite from each of the arts or sciences were admitted. The second of the three classes into which the Institut was originally divided, that of the moral and political sciences, constituted its ideological keystone, bringing together scientists, historians, geographers and men of letters, many of them active in politics, in the service of the Republic. One of the most active members of the class, the medical writer P. G. J. Cabanis, described the Institut as 'a living encyclopedia'. It could be seen as giving practical application to the values and achievements of the *Encyclopédie* of Diderot and d'Alembert, at once the symbol and the embodiment of the Enlightenment.[23]

There was no more effective or energetic spokesman than Cabanis for the values associated with the Institut. He was perhaps the most immediately influential and certainly the most ambitious of the *médecins philosophes* active in late eighteenth-century French culture. Between 1796 and 1800, he delivered a series of memoirs at the Institut. These were published from 1798 onwards by the Class of Moral and Political Sciences, eventually appearing as an independent publication in 1802 and frequently thereafter with the collective title *Rapports du physique et du moral de l'homme*. For Cabanis, 'physiology, the analysis of ideas and morality are merely three branches of a single science, which can justly be called *the science of man*'.[24] Temperament occupied a position on the confines of the physical and the moral. It therefore constituted one of the central elements in Cabanis' vision of the science of man, together with sex and age. The *Rapports* helped to inaugurate a period of renewed interest in temperament theory in a medical world preoccupied with the question of hygiene in the broadest sense. For a time, temperament appeared to offer the basis for new ways of regarding and ultimately regulating the human species.[25] Cabanis' view of temperament and its

23. See François Azouvi, 'L'Institut national: une "encyclopédie vivante"?', in Azouvi, *Institution de la raison*, p.51-61. For accounts of the theories and aims of the men associated with the foundation of the Institut, usually grouped together under the label 'Idéologues', see Sergio Moravia, *Il Tramonto dell'illuminismo: filosofia e politica nella società francese (1770-1810)* (Bari, 1968); Moravia, *Il Pensiero degli idéologues: scienza e filosofia in Francia (1780-1815)* (Florence, 1974); Martin S. Staum, *Minerva's message. Stabilizing the French Revolution* (Montreal, 1996). These earlier accounts should be read in the light of Jean-Luc Chappey, *La Société des observateurs de l'homme (1799-1804)[.] Des anthropologues aux temps de Bonaparte* (Paris, 2002), especially p.68-73, 116.
24. Cabanis, *Œuvres philosophiques*, ed. Claude Lehec and Jean Cazeneuve, 2 vols (Paris, 1956), vol.1, p.126. For accounts of Cabanis in English see Martin S. Staum, *Cabanis: Enlightenment and medical philosophy in the French Revolution* (Princeton, NJ, 1980); Elizabeth A. Williams, *The Physical and the moral: anthropology, physiology, and philosophical medicine in France, 1750-1850* (Cambridge, 1994), p.85-93. See also Chappey, *Société des observateurs de l'homme*, p.56-67.
25. See Roselyne Rey, 'La transmission du savoir médical', in Azouvi, *L'Institution de la raison*, p.29-49; Staum, *Minerva's message*, p.95-117.

relationship to the physiology of sensation were ultimately based on Haller's. But Cabanis' approach differed in one very important respect. French physicians associated with the medical school at Montpellier had modified Haller's physiology by questioning the dual operations of irritability and sensibility. They favoured a monistic model in which these functions were attributed to sensibility alone. Sensibility thus came to be seen as 'the connecting principle for all vital processes [...] the communicative and coordinating force that allowed the body to function as an integrated whole'.[26] This approach was followed by Cabanis, who understood the action of sensibility in a sense which extended well beyond older definitions. In addition to the accepted role of the nervous system in receiving and transmitting sensation, Cabanis' model of sensibility accorded important roles to the brain, which he thought of as an active rather than as a merely passive organ, 'secreting' and transmitting ideas on the basis of the perceptions which it received, but also to impressions originating in the internal organs and operating at a subconscious level. This extended model of sensibility underlay his claim that 'the difference of the temperaments depends above all on that of the centres of sensibility, on the relations of strength or weakness and the sympathetic communications of the different organs'.[27]

The whole of the sixth and twelfth of the twelve memoirs which composed the *Rapports du physique et du moral de l'homme* were devoted to the temperaments, as was a substantial section of the first. (The first three memoirs dealt with general issues including sensation; the fourth, with the influence of age; the fifth, with that of sex; the seventh, eighth, ninth, tenth and eleventh with the influence of sickness, regime, climate, instinct and related issues and the moral.) The most extended treatment of the temperaments is found in the sixth memoir, 'De l'influence des tempéraments sur la formation des idées et des affections morales',

26. Anne C. Vila, *Enlightenment and pathology: sensibility in the literature and medicine of eighteenth-century France* (Baltimore, MD, and London, 1998), p.46. Haller had by his own account been tempted to make similar claims for irritability: 'It is well-known that man likes to give importance to his own discoveries. He would naturally want to conquer the world by means of his opinions, and establish a universal monarchy for the hypothesis of which he believes himself the creator.' More modest in this than Descartes or Newton, as he himself observed, he had resisted the temptation. When experiments failed to uncover irritability in the arteries, Haller was, to use his own majestic metaphor, thrown back from that province onto the empire which he had already made his own, that of the muscles (*Mémoires sur la nature sensible et irritable des parties du corps animal*, 4 vols (Lausanne, 1756-1760), vol.4, p.34f.). Entertaining no such qualms, his French translator, Tissot, looked to irritability to explain almost everything, including the temperaments (vol.1, p.xxxf.). On the relationship of Cabanis' model of sensibility to Haller's theories, see Moravia, *Il Pensiero degli Idéologues*, p.201-16.
27. Cabanis, *Œuvres*, vol.1, p.152. For Cabanis' theory of internal sensations, see Staum, *Cabanis*, p.191-99.

which was read at a sitting of the Institut on 22 ventôse An V/12 March 1797 (according to the Institut minutes) and was first published in the memoirs of the Institut in fructidor An VII/August or September 1799. According to the information given at the end of the first memoir as published by the Institut in thermidor an VI/July-August 1798, Cabanis initially planned to place the memoir on the temperaments next, ahead of those on the sexes and on age (in that order). This agreed with the order in which these topics were treated in the first memoir, as Cabanis noted. The same source also dates the first reading of both the memoir on the sexes and that on the temperaments to the same day (22 fructidor An IV/8 September 1796), followed twenty six days later by that on the ages.[28] The intended order of publication presumably accounts for the structure of the memoir on the temperaments, where a lengthy exordium discusses the relationship of medicine to philosophy and the whole question of difference between human beings. This contrasts with the brief opening paragraphs of the memoirs on age and the sexes which now precede that on the temperaments. Much of this material is as relevant to the memoirs on age and the sexes as to that on the temperaments and was presumably designed to provide an introduction to all three.[29]

In the first memoir Cabanis presented an introduction to the question of temperament. He gave a summary of the four traditional temperament 'types', while explicitly rejecting a humoral aetiology. In this, his approach agreed with that of other followers of Haller, such as William Cullen, whom he cited. According to Cullen, the ancients had at first 'distinguished [the temperaments] by actual observation; but very soon they formed a theory with regard to them, from whence they formed appellations which have continued to be applied to them ever since'.[30] Cabanis explicitly rejected the idea of a '*tempérament tempéré* par excellence' the perfect *temperamentum ad punctum* of the Galenists. In real life there was no single, perfect balance. He reported that the moderns had rejected the traditional fourfold classification, instancing Haller's addition of a fifth *temperamentum baeoticum, quadratum, rusticum,* which he referred to as the *temperamentum musculosum torosum.* His discussion of the humours echoed Haller's. In line with his general views on sensibility,

28. Cabanis, *Œuvres*, vol.2, p.548f; vol.1, p.161. The reason for the changes of order in the publication of the memoirs is not recorded.

29. *Œuvres philosophiques*, vol.1, p.316-34, p.235, p.272. The first memoir originally began with a 'history of the temperaments'. See Rey, 'La transmission du savoir médical', p.133, n.12.

30. William Cullen, M.D., *A Treatise of the materia medica*, 2 vols (Edinburgh, 1789), vol.1, p.61f. See also Cullen's *Traité de matière médicale, traduit de l'anglois par la seule edition donée [sic] par l'auteur à Edimbourg en 1789; par M. Bosquillon*, 2 vols (1789-1790), vol.1, p.59-63; Cabanis, *Œuvres*, vol.1, p.149f.

Cabanis suggested that difference of temperament depended on the relative strength or weakness of specific organs and systems of organs and, in particular, on that of the sensitive and motor functions of the organisation as a whole.

In the introduction to his sixth memoir – that which was devoted exclusively to the temperaments – Cabanis claimed that he was following the ancients in seeking to unite medicine with philosophy. For Cabanis, the doctrine of the temperaments had been 'perhaps the principal fruit' of the 'great endeavour to achieve an all-embracing view of man', which was how he viewed ancient medicine. The authority of the ancients was to be revered, but when it came to such matters of everyday experience as the temperaments, we should 'interrogate nature, and not books', trusting in the first place to our own observations, without too much regard for the views of earlier observers:

> One can in the present subject, more perhaps than in any other, address nature directly and with confidence. All the elements of the question are before our eyes; and the laws which we seek to determine are eternal.[31]

He proceeded to expand his discussion to embrace the question of human difference in general. For Cabanis, what chiefly distinguished the human from other animals was the degree of difference between individual human beings – 'differences analogous and in a sense correspondent to those to be observed between the species'.[32] Such differences were evident in external signs – height, build, manner of movement and expression of the passions. They were complemented by a similar variety in the conformation of the body's interior organs. Such differences involved the nature of the individual's nervous system as a whole, whether considered under the aspect of its active or its passive properties – that is, whether as activating the organs or as receiving 'the impressions by virtue of which it then acts on the motor organs, to make them produce their movements and execute their functions'. 'Physical sensibility' was to be equated with life itself. Various causes, chemical and other, might be suggested for differences in the active workings of the nervous system in different individuals. A presentation of the four traditional temperament types follows which is dependent on accounts in Hippocrates and Galen, but is linked in each case to differences in sensibility which are accounted for in terms of the physiology of the organs.[33]

31. Cabanis, *Œuvres*, vol.1, p.317f.
32. Cabanis, *Œuvres*, vol.1, p.318f.
33. Cabanis, *Œuvres*, vol.1, p.321-41. Cabanis summarised the differences between his own aetiology of the temperaments and the humoral accounts of the ancients in a footnote (p.345 (n.1), p.352f).

The four traditional temperaments are dealt with fairly briefly. The remainder of the memoir is largely devoted to a discussion of two temperaments unremarked by the ancients. The first of these is Haller's muscular temperament; the other, its complementary opposite, the 'cerebral' temperament. The latter appears to have originated in the writings of another German-speaking medical writer, J. G. Zimmermann. Although Zimmermann did not classify the cerebral and muscular dispositions as temperaments, he related them to each other, as Cabanis was to do:

> Violent and long continued exertions of the mind fatigue the body, as much as excessive bodily labour enervates the mind; much study, without exercise, weakens the body; and a laborious life, in which the mind is unemployed, gradually weakens the mind. This is the reason why the most trifling meditation fatigues the vulgar, and why literary men are unable to support the least degree of bodily labour. The vulgar, whose ideas do not extend beyond instinct, can have no abstracted knowledge, because to abstract there is required both knowledge and genius. Hard labour is what they call working; and reading, and thinking, and writing, are in their opinion, a life of idleness.[34]

Although among other things a physician, Zimmermann took his cue here, not from medicine, but from a letter by the Roman philosopher Seneca, which gives advice on the comportment proper to the studious life.[35] When it came to physiology, Zimmermann was rather vague:

> We confessedly are not able to say in what manner a violent effort of the mind acts upon the medullary substance of the brain, and through it over the rest of the system [...]. It may be presumed, that a certain motion takes place in the parts, through the medium of which the soul thinks, and by which it executes its functions. It is impossible indeed to say what this motion is, but we need only observe the difference between a penetrating and a stupid brain, to be convinced of the probability of some such motion. In a penetrating head, every thing is apparently in agitation. [....] On the other hand, the little stock of ideas of a stupid head seems to form one indistinct mass; if I may be allowed the expression.

Zimmermann suggested that these phenomena were related to the extent of 'mobility in the brain':

> This mobility would seem to be founded on the greater or less degree of sensibility in the brain: stupid people having but little or no sensibility, except in matters of interest; in all other things they seem to be without conception.[36]

34. [J. G. Zimmermann], *A Treatise on experience in physic*, 2 vols (London, 1778), vol.2, p.296.
35. Seneca, *Epist.*, 15. Zimmermann enjoyed an international reputation as the author of *Solitude*, almost as famous in its day as Gessner's *Death of Abel*.
36. Zimmerman, *Treatise*, vol.2, p.296f.

Cabanis was able to provide the physiological explanation which had been beyond Zimmermann. He reclassified the cerebral and the muscular dispositions as temperaments and attributed the difference between them to the relative preponderance of the nervous or sensitive system and of the motor system in the physical organisation of the individual. The 'nervous and cerebral system' predominated in those of a cerebral temperament; the muscular system, which informed the 'organs of movement', in those who were temperamentally muscular. The characteristics of the two new temperaments were built on this distinction. A cerebral temperament might be encountered in people with strong or weak muscles. In conjunction with strong muscles, it tended to occur in men; with weak, in women. The muscular temperament might depend on the original strength of the fibres or on the 'extraordinary' influence of the nervous on the muscular system, the second eventuality being pathological rather than healthy.[37]

The only sure external sign of difference between the two temperaments was the presence or absence of well-developed muscles.[38] Yet on this basis Cabanis divided the human race into two groups who had almost nothing in common. The second half of the sixth memoir is devoted to an exposition of the characteristics of the cerebral and the muscular temperaments. The four temperaments of traditional doctrine are quietly dropped. Cabanis regarded the division of humanity into the cerebral and the muscular as self-evident and all-pervasive. Even a discussion of the balanced temperament found in Galen (the *temperamentum ad punctum*) took only these two into account, ignoring the temperaments known to Galen himself. But it was above all the characteristics of the muscular temperament which preoccupied Cabanis. Implicit in the contrast which he set up between the two temperaments was a polarity between the normal and the pathological, even though his discussion of a putative ideal temperament suggested that some sort of balance between the muscular and the cerebral was desirable.[39] Just as in his memoir on the sexes it was woman, not man, whose identity was conditional on her sex,[40] so it was the muscular and

37. Cabanis, *Œuvres*, vol.1, p.347f.; Cf. vol.1, p.352.

38. See also Hallé, 'Mémoire sur les observations fondamentales d'après lesquelles peut être établie la distinction des tempéramens', in *Mémoires de la société médicale d'émulation, séante à l'Ecole de Médecine de Paris.* Pour l'An VII de la République française, troisième Année, An VIII, p.342-94 (367).

39. Cabanis, *Œuvres*, vol.1, p.352-54. On the bipolarity of the normal and the pathological in late eighteenth-century medical thought, see Michel Foucault, *Birth of the clinic: an archaeology of medical perception*, translated by A. M. Sheridan Smith (London, 1988), p.35f.

40. 'Cabanis united sex and gender, in our sense, when he considered women. A female body, mind and social role were all one. Male tasks and lives are not similarly dependent on their special natural properties' (Ludmilla Jordanova, 'Sex and gender', in *Inventing human*

not the cerebral temperament which imprisoned its possessor in a particular consciousness and an existence circumscribed by ultimately physiological considerations. An over-developed cerebral temperament might affect the subject's health adversely (a condition particularly observable in artists and men of science), but this was as nothing compared with the baneful consequences of a pronounced muscular temperament. According to Cabanis, those cursed with the latter were morally and intellectually inferior to the cerebral. Perhaps surprisingly, their inferiority was also physical:

> Those bodies, so vigorous in executing movements, seem somehow to possess no more than mechanical strength: true energy, the radical energy of the nervous system, is much more frequently met with in bodies which appear weak and thin. The slightest indisposition is often enough to lay porters and labourers low. [...] Robust bleedings or inconsiderately employed purges rapidly enervate and prostrate them.[41]

It is here that the reader realises the full import of Cabanis' own observation that the degree of difference encountered among humans was of an order which elsewhere occurred only between animals of different species:

> The slightest observation suffices to demonstrate that the circumstance which distinguishes this temperament must necessarily give a distinct stamp to all the habits; that between the man of deep and lively feelings and he who lives only through exercise or the awareness of his external strength, there are fundamental differences; that their *mores* must sometimes seem scarcely to belong to the same system of existence; that finally time and the practice of life, in developing and strengthening their different characters, can only make more apparent this dividing line.[42]

Increasing muscular strength made people 'more apt to attack than to observe; to overthrow and destroy, than to subdue gently, by resorting to the laws of nature'. Worse still, violent exercise operated like a drug. It became more and more necessary to people who practised it, like strong liquor to those who developed an appetite for it (most inordinate drinkers in fact shared this temperament, according to Cabanis). The muscular man had less feeling – less sensitivity to outward impression or inner emotion – than the cerebral. Preoccupied as he was by movement

---

science: eighteenth-century domains, ed. Christopher Fox, Roy Porter and Robert Wokler (Berkley, CA, and London, 1995), p.172).

41. Cabanis, *Œuvres*, vol.1, p.349. This was based on Cabanis' observation from his work in public hospitals. The idea that heavy bleeding was good for muscular subjects may derive from Galen, according to whom those of athletic build possessed too much blood (*De bono habitu*, in Galen, *Medicorum Graecorum opera quæ extant. Editionem curavit C. G. K. Gr. and Lat.*, ed. C. G. Kühn, 26 vols (Leipzig, 1821-1833), vol.4, p.754).

42. Cabanis, *Œuvres*, vol.1, p.350.

and action, 'his existence is necessarily circumscribed by a few narrow views and his brutal impulses'.[43] The ultimate dependence of both these temperaments on modifications of sensibility as well as their mutually inverse relationship were evident from the behaviour of epileptics, convulsionaries and the raving mad, all of whom displayed increased physical strength accompanied by a corresponding diminution of mental awareness during an attack.

In some respects Cabanis' descriptions of the two temperaments fit the character sketches of the dove and the woodpecker which Bewick's *British birds* provided at about the same date (see Chapter 1 above). Like Bewick, Cabanis related physiological difference to differences of *habitus*. The conclusion of the sixth memoir and the whole of the final, twelfth memoir were given over to the questions of acquired temperament and selective breeding (Cabanis accepted the inheritance of acquired characteristics). Cabanis expressed surprise that men had already successfully intervened to create improved breeds of dogs, horses, cattle and tulips, yet had neglected the possibilities of similarly developing the human race itself. At first, he gave the impression of being concerned with the perfectibility of the human race as a whole, like his brother-in-law the philosopher Condorcet. But further on it emerges that this was not quite the goal of his inquiries. The example of selective breeding chosen by Cabanis – that of a stud in which horses are bred to perform different tasks – makes it evident that he looked forward to the production of a race of human beings specifically bred to labour. Perhaps aware that such a suggestion might provoke unease, he sought to reassure his auditors that such an arrangement would be in the order of things. Returning to the comparison with which he had opened his reflexions on human difference, he observed:

> On this point, as on many others, there exists a great difference between man and the rest of the animals. Man, by the singular extent and delicacy of his sensibility, is subject to the action of an infinite number of causes: consequently, nothing would be more chimerical than to want to bring all the individuals of the species to an exactly common and uniform type. Men, as we envisage them here, would thus be equally suited to social life; they would not be equally so to all the employments of society.[44]

43. Cabanis, *Œuvres*, vol.1, p.350f.
44. Cabanis, *Œuvres*, vol.1, p.358. The last distinction answers to that made by Sieyès between civil and political rights. On the relinquishment by later medical writers of the goal of universal perfectibility envisaged by Condorcet, see Vila, *Enlightenment and pathology*, p.256f. For more charitable interpretations of Cabanis' eugenicist speculations, see Daniel Teysseire, 'Lien social et ordre politique chez Cabanis', *Studies on Voltaire and the eighteenth century* 267 (1989), p.353-400; Teysseire, 'Eugénisme et euthanasie chez Cabanis', in *Transactions of the eighth international congress on the Enlightenment* 1992, p.272-75, and Staum, *Minerva's message*, p.95-117.

It was thus not merely the observation, but the manipulation and even the manufacture of human difference which preoccupied Cabanis. This was a topic which he returned to in the twelfth memoir, on 'acquired temperaments'. There, the baneful moral sensibility associated with the muscular temperament in the sixth memoir was presented as the necessary consequence of strenuous labour – independently, it would appear, of any temperamental predisposition. The moral randomness of this consequence of the division of labour in society had troubled Diderot when he observed the effects of heavy labour on the children of the faubourg Saint-Marcel.[45] But Cabanis, like Adam Smith, expressed no qualms about the arbitrariness of the conditions under which some people and not others were condemned to the moral brutalisation associated with the muscular temperament. It may be true that by using eugenic and other means 'Cabanis' goal was in the long term to eliminate temperamental obstacles to good citizenship'.[46] He certainly shared Smith's faith in the benefits which would accrue to all from the unrestricted operations of a free market, with which he thought that even charity should not be allowed to interfere.[47] But he also maintained the 'natural' inequality of human faculties (which Smith did not) whereby nature had 'rejected in advance' equality of fortunes.[48] The civil disqualification of the temperamentally muscular was grounded by Cabanis in physiology, not, as in the writings of most of his contemporaries, in property ownership. For him, the division of labour was determined by nature, not society. All human society depends for its survival on human labour. Nowhere did Cabanis suggest that members of the property-owning and therefore non-labouring class to which he himself belonged should share the burden – and the temperament – of their labouring fellow citizens. It must be presumed therefore that in Cabanis' view of society the muscular temperament would necessarily remain the condition of the unpropertied – a perpetual barrier to their moral and intellectual development and to their participation in political self-determination.

His speculations on selective human breeding indicate that Cabanis was at least as interested in the accentuation of human inequalities as in their amelioration. If so, his views accorded with those of Sieyès, who had already privately speculated on selective breeding as the means to the

45. Cabanis, *Œuvres*, vol.1, p.630.

46. Staum, *Minerva's message*, p.99. See also Chappey, 'Les idéologues face au coup d'état du 18 brumaire an VIII[.] Des illusions aux désillusions', *Politix*, 14 (n.56) (2001), p.55-75 (69).

47. See *Quelques principes et quelques vues sur les secours publics*, in Cabanis, *Œuvres*, vol.2, p.1-63, and the analysis of J. F. Spitz, *L'Amour de l'égalite. Essai sur la critique de l'égalitarisme républicain en France 1770-1830* (Paris, 2000), p.153-56.

48. Cabanis, *Œuvres*, vol.2, p.18.

creation of a human race more readily adapted to the requirements of economic progress. Sieyès' proposal had been predicated on the 'necessary' division of the nation into:

> Two peoples, the producers and the human instruments of production, intelligent people and workers [*ouvriers*] who possess only passive strength, educated citizens and auxiliaries to whom are allowed neither the time nor the means to receive education; would it not be desirable, especially in very hot or very cold countries, that there should be a species intermediate between men and animals, a species capable of serving man for consumption and production?[49]

In attributing a difference of sensibility to those of cerebral and muscular temperaments, Cabanis defined a fundamental difference in their nervous systems as a whole. In this respect his approach to temperament resembled that which he took to the issue of sexual difference. For Cabanis, difference of sex, like difference of temperament, was ultimately to be accounted for in terms of sensibility:

> The principal concern of moral anthropology was [...] not sex but sensibility, the vital principle that these theorists deemed responsible for determining all aspects of human life and all variations thereon.[50]

The case made by Cabanis in the fifth memoir for the necessary subservience of women to men and for their exclusion from public life was vigorously argued, but it was no more so than that which he made for the necessary inferiority of the muscular to the cerebral in the memoir on the temperaments. Like Kant, Cabanis appears to have seen difference defined by temperament and difference defined by gender as equally valid – although of course Cabanis was able to explain each in physiological terms. The only indication that one type of difference took precedence over the other in his thought appears to be the order in which the memoirs were eventually published – an order which, as has been seen, was fixed at a relatively late stage, and only after Cabanis' delivery of both memoirs at the Institut.[51]

49. *Notes et fragments inédits*, in *Écrits politiques*, p.75. Sieyès thought that such a race might be produced by interbreeding varieties of great apes with human beings, both white and black. For the rapprochement of Cabanis and his allies in the Institut with Sieyès at this period, see Chappey, 'Les idéologues face au coup d'état', p.63. See also *Conseil des cinq-cents. Discours prononcé par Cabanis, sur le message du Conseil des Anciens, relatif aux journaux calomniateurs des premières autorités. Séance du premier fructidor An* 7 (An VII/1799), p.3f.
50. Vila, *Enlightenment and pathology*, p.241.
51. See above, n.28. Cabanis does not appear to have addressed the issue of whether one form of difference – temperament or sex – should be given priority over the other. His discussion of the male and female nervous system in the memoir on the sexes recalls his distinction between two types of cerebral temperament, those allied to strong and weak muscular systems (see above, p.12), which he explicitly divided along sexual lines (a

Cabanis' memoir on the sexes has been widely cited in discussions of the changing ways in which sexual difference was accounted for in late eighteenth-century thought. The old Galenic model of sexual identity depended on degrees of vital heat, arranged hierarchically between male and female terms. It was replaced by a model of 'biological divergence' between the sexes: 'An anatomy and physiology of incommensurability replaced a metaphysics of hierarchy in the representation of woman in relation to man'.[52]

Insofar as this description fits Cabanis' memoir on the sexes,[53] is it not equally applicable to his polarisation of the cerebral and muscular temperaments? Are not the developments of sensibility in the two temperaments – the one attuned to feeling, the other to violent action, so that they 'seem scarcely to belong to the same system of existence' – equally incommensurable? The Galenic model of temperamental identity, like that of sexual identity, depended on gradations in the distribution of heat and moisture. Haller himself had acknowledged his own break with the fluidity of that model when he had located the workings of the muscular temperament in the inherent texture of the fibres, their *congenitum stamen*.[54] For Cabanis, too, it was through the fibres that sensibility operated and acquired its distinctive qualities in individuals, whether those qualities related to temperament, to sex or to both.

---

discussion which could be taken to imply that the cerebral is the 'normal' temperament and the muscular merely a deviation, since there is no equivalent differentiation of types of muscular temperament) (*Œuvres*, vol.1, p.277, 280-83; see also vol.1, p.348). Earlier, he accorded a prominent if not a determining role to the organs of generation in his account of the formation of the types of bilious and melancholic temperaments, but he did not differentiate that role according to sex. Thus, for example, he blamed a religious disposition on the inordinate activities of the organs of generation in those of a melancholy temperament, but appears to have regarded this reaction as operating similarly in both sexes, since he explicitly referred to both male and female melancholics (*Œuvres*, vol.1, p.345f.).

52. Thomas Laqueur, *Making sex: body and gender from the Greeks to Freud* (Cambridge, MA, 1990), p.5f. See also Knibiehler, 'Les Médecins et la "nature feminine" au temps du Code Civil', *Annales ESC* 31 (1976), p.824-45. This development is particularly associated with Roussel's *Système physique et moral de la femme*, published in 1775. Cabanis is significant in this context 'both because he synthesised the various strands of the medicine and philosophy of sensibility and because he established the Rousselian model of women as canonical for the next generation of moral anthropologists' (Vila, *Enlightenment and pathology*, p.229).

53. The extent to which the label 'incommensurability' fits that model has been questioned by Vila, *Enlightenment and pathology*, p.242. Her criticism would also apply to the dichotomy of the cerebral and muscular temperaments insofar as Cabanis accepted a sliding scale of difference there as well (*Œuvres*, vol.1, p.354). On the construction of 'these dichotomies, where two opposed terms mutually define each other' such as male/female and town/country, as a feature of Enlightenment discourse, see L. J. Jordanova, 'Natural facts: a historical perspective on science and sexuality' in *Nature, culture and gender*, ed. Carol MacCormack and Marilyn Strathern (Cambridge, 1980), p.42-69.

54. *Elementa physiologiae*, vol.2, p.147.

Such an outlook represented a significant break with the way in which the whole question of difference between human beings had been approached by writers earlier in the century. Then the emphasis had been on similarity and equality rather than the discrepancies to which Cabanis was drawing attention:

> The very posing of the question by the Dijon Academy in 1753 – 'What is the origin of inequality among men, and is it authorized by natural law?' – which Rousseau answered with his thunderous discourse, implied that inequality was a phenomenon in the history of man which had to justify itself and had to be explained.[55]

Frank Manuel accorded Cabanis a significant role in the evolution away from this perception of collective human identity – 'the reversal from the eighteenth-century view of men as more or less equal, or at least similar, in nature [...] to the early nineteenth-century emphasis upon human uniqueness, diversity, dissimilarity, culminating in theories of inequality and organicism'.[56] Eighteenth-century theories of perception and sensibility owed at least as much to the philosophers Locke and Condillac as to medical writers. There was therefore a presumption that everyone experienced the world in more or less the same way.[57] It was precisely this presumption which Cabanis' more sophisticated, physiological model of the operations of human sensibility enabled him to challenge in his account of the cerebral and the muscular temperaments.

Laqueur and others have linked the ideological shift in the discourse on gender to changes in the condition of women in revolutionary and post-revolutionary France. Anne Vila is critical of this position, pointing to chronological discrepancies and attributing the change instead to exigencies imposed by transformations of the discourse on sensibility itself.[58] As I have argued elsewhere, however, the removal of barriers to women's involvement in professional life and their subsequent achievements led to an intensification of the rhetoric of incommensurability deployed by their male rivals, at least in the fine arts.[59] Cabanis' theory of

55. Frank E. Manuel, 'From equality to organicism', in *Freedom from history, and other untimely essays* (London, 1972), p.222.
56. Manuel, 'From equality', p.221-22.
57. See K. M. Figlio, 'Theories of perception and the physiology of mind in the late eighteenth century', *History of science* 13 (1975), p.177-212. Cabanis reproved his more philosophically minded predecessors, Helvétius and Condillac, for their lack of physiological awareness (*Œuvres*, vol.1, p.141).
58. Roussel's *Système physique et moral de la femme*, a key text, was published well before the Revolution, in 1775. See Vila, *Enlightenment and pathology*, p.227, with references.
59. *Facing the public*, p.191-97, with references. See also Knibiehler, 'Les médecins et la "nature feminine" au temps du Code Civil', *Annales ESC* 31 (1976), p.824-45, for women in the medical profession and Carla Hesse, *The other Enlightenment: how French women became modern* (Princeton, NJ, and Oxford, 2001), p.42 and *passim*, for the situation of women

the temperaments can also be related to a political context. The doctrine of the temperaments was already being transformed into a tool of differentiation, whether of class, gender or race, during the third quarter of the eighteenth century (see Chapter 3 above). But there are significant differences between Cabanis' treatment of the muscular temperament and earlier accounts of temperament difference which can only be accounted for in terms of the social and political context in which he was operating. This was an aspect of his views to which Cabanis was evidently sensitive, and which he sought to gloss over by invoking earlier authorities for his theory. He claimed, for example, that his version of the muscular temperament was 'absolutely the same' as Haller's and that he had merely defined it with greater precision and accuracy,[60] but this was scarcely the case. What made Cabanis' characterisation of the muscular temperament fundamentally different from Haller's was its social referent. For Haller, the muscular individual – weak in irritability though strong in fibre – had been close in some respects to the phlegmatic. He had been described by Haller as *boeoticus* and *rusticus* ('Boeotian' and 'rustic').[61] Both these socially coloured adjectives were dropped by Cabanis (who also suppressed them in his account of Haller's doctrine), and replaced by the more neutral physical descriptors *musculosus* and *torosus* (i.e., 'muscular' and 'knotty' – equivalents, in a general sense, to Haller's *quadratus* or 'square-built'). But it was not merely greater niceness of observation which informed this change. Haller's muscular subject was defined as *boeoticus* and *rusticus* because he displayed what were regarded as typical peasant qualities (as defined by non-peasants, at least).[62] Cabanis' did not. Addicted to mindless violence and to alcohol, destructive of life and property, sickly in body in spite of appearance, Cabanis' muscular subject was an urban brute, not a country yokel. He was insensitive, but in a dynamic, not a passive way. His was an active and efficacious brutality, not the passively bovine brutality traditionally attributed to those who toiled in the fields. This was the temperament proper to the *turba forensis*, the *peuple* according to André Chénier.[63] It was the temperament of the *sans-culotte*, or at least the *sans-*

writers, who, like women artists, experienced the consequences of revolutionary deregulation.

60. Cabanis, *Œuvres*, vol.1, p.349f.

61. See above, ch.3.

62. On the insensitivity of the peasant, see, for example, the observations of Tissot, cited by Vila, *Enlightenment and pathology*, p.194. Zimmermann's account of the stupid man, with its emphasis on lack of 'mobility' in the brain and on the capacity to retain only a few simple ideas (*A Treatise on experience in physic*, vol.2, p.296) resembles Haller's rather than Cabanis' version of the muscular temperament.

63. See above, ch.5.

culotte of Thermidorian mythology. If there were any physiological considerations which impelled Cabanis to depart from Haller's characterisation of the muscular temperament in this way, he failed to present them. By suppressing Haller's own description he took care to preclude speculation on his reasons for the change.

The other indicator of the political preoccupations underlying Cabanis' memoir comes in a passage in which he attempted to relate his characterisation of the muscular temperament to classical examples. The ancients may have failed to identify the muscular as a separate temperament, but according to Cabanis, they at least knew how to connect muscular strength with moral and psychological defects. Their athletes reputedly lacked discernment:

> Hercules, their prototype, though a god, was himself more famous for his courage than for his wits; and the comic poets allowed themselves more than once to attribute what is vulgarly called uncouth behaviour [*ce qu'on appelle vulgairement des balourdises*] to him, and to make the people laugh at his expense.[64]

This was a questionable example, as Cabanis must have recognised. It is true that Hercules appears as a figure of fun in Greek plays such as the *Frogs* of Aristophanes and the *Alcestis* of Euripides, but he was accorded divine authority in the same works. The burlesque treatment of deities was a comic convention and did not involve any judgement on the moral character attributed to them. The unsatisfactoriness of this example points to a more fundamental weakness in Cabanis' case for the muscular temperament. As has been seen, an important element in Cabanis' argument for the importance of temperament was the ease with which the marks of the temperaments could be recognised. This demonstrated that there could be no doubt about the objective existence of temperament types even if the humoural explanations offered by Hippocrates and Galen had been shown to be invalid. There was of course abundant evidence for the identification of the four original temperaments in antiquity. But ancient literary sources were less helpful in providing even indirect evidence for Cabanis' two new temperaments. In particular, the ancients appear to have been largely unaware of the drawbacks of the

64. Cabanis, *Œuvres*, vol.1, p.349f. Anthelme Richerand, a follower of Cabanis, gave a different reason for doubting the intelligence of the mythological Hercules – the ease with which he was taken in by 'all the kings he served and by all the women he loved' (Richerand, *Nouveaux élémens de physiologie*, 4th edn, 2 vols (Paris, 1807), vol.2, p.465). While this has nothing to do with the sort of *balourdises* attributed to Hercules by the dramatists, it has clear affinities with the character attributed to the 'people' by their representatives from December 1793 onwards (see Christian Alain Muller, 'Du "peuple égaré" au "peuple enfant" [.] Le discours politique révolutionnaire à l'épreuve de la révolte populaire en 1793', in *Revue d'histoire moderne et contemporaine* 47 (2000), p.93-112).

muscular temperament, so glaringly obvious to Cabanis. Worse still, they admired and actively promoted the cultivation of muscle. Ancient educational and cultural practices were geared to the development and celebration of physical strength through strenuous exercise, whether in the gymnasium or in sacred games such as the Olympics.[65] Cabanis cited a famous aphorism of Hippocrates on the instability of perfect health in athletes in support of his position. But there Hippocrates had merely presented the physical problems which according to him resulted from too intensive training. States of peak form were inherently slippery in that change by definition could only be for the worse. It was therefore prudent to reduce the state swiftly by controlled medical means. Hippocrates said nothing of the moral consequences of athletic development, as Cabanis was forced to admit.[66]

Cabanis' observations on Hercules would have suggested a specific visual prototype to his original auditors, the *Farnese Hercules* (fig.5, p.24). It was usual for medical writers to instance famous examples of ancient sculpture as archetypes of the qualities commonly associated with the god or hero they represented. The statues most frequently used in this way were those of the *Apollo Belvedere* and the *Medici Venus*.[67] Medical writers who adopted Cabanis' account of the muscular temperament explicitly linked their descriptions to the *Farnese Hercules*.[68] But Cabanis'

65. 'The idea of effort is the very essence of athletics as the Greeks understood the term' (E. Norman Gardiner, *Athletics of the ancient world* (Oxford, 1980), p.1).
66. Cabanis, *Œuvres*, vol.1, p.349f. See also Hipp, *Aph.*, 1, 3. Hallé took a similar position in his entry on *hygiène* in the *Encyclopédie méthodique*, citing the same passage and claiming that 'all the ancients condemn this excessive state' *(Encyclopédie méthodique, ou par ordre de matières; par une Société de gens de lettres, de savans et d'artistes. Médecine. Par une société de médecins*, 13 vols, 1792-1830, vol.7 (1798 / An VI), p.373-437 (382). Galen dealt with the same issue in what is effectively an extended commentary on Hippocrates' aphorism (*De Bono habitu*, ed. Kühn, 4:750-54) and again in *Galeni ad Thrasybulum liber, utrum medicinae sit an gymnastices hygiene* (*ed. cit.*, 5: 820-78), where he cited a passage in Book 3 c.18 of Plato's *Republic* which would have answered Cabanis' purposes very well, since it specifically connects athletic training with a disposition to anger and a deafness to argument (Plato 411 D, E. See also Galen, *Medicorum Graecorum opera quæ extant. Editionem curavit C. G. K. Gr. and Lat.*, ed. C. G. Kühn, 26 vols (Leipzig, 1821-1833), vol.5, p.824f.). That Cabanis was apparently unaware of this passage confirms the well-known neglect of Plato in eighteenth-century European culture. There were other, often political critiques of athletes and their lifestyle in antiquity, but these would have been less useful to Cabanis (the ancient athlete was a relatively privileged citizen). See Bronislaw Bilinski, 'L'agonistica sportiva nella Grecia antica. Aspetti sociali e ispirazioni letterarie' in *Accademia polacca di scienze e lettere*: Conferenze: fascicolo 12 (Rome, 1960); Bilinski, *Agoni ginnici. Componenti artistiche ed intellettuali nell'antica agonistica greca*, in *Conferenze dell'Accademia polacca delle scienze* (Rome, 1979), p.75.
67. See above, ch.4, where it was suggested that this practice may have owed something to Galen's citation of the *Canon* of Polyclilytus in his *De Temperamentis*.
68. Such as Husson (*Essai sur une nouvelle doctrine des tempéramens; Présenté et soutenu à l'École de Médecine de Paris, le 18 nivôse, An VII de la République* (An VII), p.50f.); Hallé (Mémoire sur les observations fondamentales d'après lesquelles peut être établie la distinction des

own choice of the figure of Hercules was presumably dictated less by a consideration for the wisdom of the ancients than by the connotations of popular power which ancient statues of Hercules had acquired when they had been adapted to represent the modern, French Hercules during the Revolution – connotations which persisted after Thermidor in coins, medals and statues such as Moitte's *Rousseau*.

Many French republican institutions had been self-consciously modelled on those of antiquity. By the later 1790s, however, the changing political situation was leading to a more selective application of classical precedents in contemporary life. Popular participation in government as practised in what Cabanis would later call 'the anarchical democracies of antiquity'[69] was discouraged, generally with success, both in the aftermath of the *journées* of germinal and prairial in 1795 and in the period following the coup of 18 fructidor an V/4 September 1797, when the Directoire introduced a more authoritarian style of government. But the identification of the cultural institutions of the new republic with those of the republics of antiquity was still encouraged in what were seen as appropriate contexts. Among the practices of ancient civic life revived by the French were athletic competitions. Games based on those of ancient Greece were staged at the festivals of the Republic, but they elicited increasingly unfavourable responses, at least from the educated classes. It was not merely that the games set a premium on physical strength. They also provided no guarantee that the winners would be socially acceptable in any other respect. When foot and horse races were held on the Champ de Mars to celebrate the second anniversary of the fall of the Jacobins on 10 thermidor an IV/28 July 1796, the victor in the equestrian event turned out to be not some modern Hiero of Syracuse, but the son of a horse dealer, as the deputy and journalist Sébastien Mercier noted with dismay.[70] Chaussard, an ex-Jacobin and a friend of David, published a long and vigorous denunciation of what he saw as the

Tempéramens' in *Mémoires de la société médicale d'émulation, séante à l'Ecole de Médecine de Paris*. Pour l'An VII de la République Française. Troisième Année, An VIII, p.342-94 (367); Richerand (*Nouveaux élémens de physiologie*, vol.2, p.465), Cabuchet (*Essai sur l'expression de la face dans l'état de santé et de maladie, présenté à l'École de Médecine de Paris, le 2 frimaire an 10* (Paris, an X), p.30).

69. In his 'Quelques considérations sur l'organisation sociale en général et particulièrement sur la nouvelle constitution par Cabanis imprimées par l'ordre de la commission[.] Séance du 25 frimaire An VIII', reprinted in Cabanis, *Œuvres*, vol.2, p.474. See below.

70. Louis Sébastien Mercier, *Le Nouveau Paris*, ed. Jean-Claude Bonnet (Paris, 1994), p.714. Mercier may have been consoled by the result of the foot race, won by the son of a leading banker. See A. Aulard, *Paris pendant la réaction thermidorienne et sous le Directoire: recueil de documents pour l'histoire de l'esprit public à Paris*, 5 vols (Paris, 1898-1902), vol.3 (1898), p.52 (citing a report in the *Rédacteur* of 11 thermidor An IV / 29 July 1796).

excessive preoccupation of the ancients with athletics in a book dealing with the festivals of ancient Greece.[71]

Witnessing such games at festivals under the Consulate, Helen Maria Williams attributed her own disappointment and that of other spectators to changes in cultural values, for which she gave a variety of explanations. In particular, she suggested that 'the machinery of war consisting more in personal valour than it does in modern times, corporeal powers were held in higher estimation' in antiquity than in her own day.[72] Williams' observation was increasingly true in post-Revolutionary France. The *virtus* or valour of the ancient citizen warrior had provided an apt enough universal model in earlier stages of the Revolution, when France faced the immediate threat of invasion by foreign armies, but this was no longer the case in the later 1790s, by which time the army was becoming increasingly professionalised.[73] The identification of the institutions of the new republic with those of the republics of antiquity persisted, but was viewed as problematic, particularly by those who, like Cabanis, wanted to move towards a more élite republican model.[74]

Two hundred years later, Cabanis' crudely ideological approach to ostensibly scientific material would embarrass his more sympathetic

71. [Chaussard], *Fêtes et courtisanes de la Grèce: supplément aux voyages d'Anacharsis et d'Antenor*, 4 vols (Paris, An XI/1801), vol.2, p.116-22. On Chaussard, see below, ch.8, p.1. Much of Chaussard's text derived from a recent edition of Cornelius de Pauw's *Recherches philosophiques sur les grecs* (Part 1: 2, 5) in De Pauw, *Œuvres philosophiques*, 7 vols (Paris, An III/1794-1795), vol.6, p.135-45. But Chaussard's comment in a later discussion that 'physical force [...], far from being a sure indicator is, on the contrary, often in inverse proportion to moral force' ((Chaussard), *Fêtes*, p.183) is his own, and may point to an awareness of Cabanis' or Hallé's views).
72. Helen Maria Williams, *Sketches of the state of manners and opinions in the French Republic, towards the close of the eighteenth century. In a series of letters*, 2 vols (London, 1801), vol.2, p.287. Writing in the *Journal de Paris*, Roederer was merely relieved at the evident lack of enthusiasm displayed by a crowd of more than 100,000 spectators: 'In 1790, everyone was an actor in public affairs; a constitution, a revolution were being made. Today, the revolution, the Constitution have been achieved. It is for the government to attend to our business, and public spirit can express itself no better than in enjoying confidently and in security the pleasures it is offered and those which each can obtain for himself' (P. L. Roederer, ed. Baron A. M. Roederer, *Œuvres*, 8 vols (Paris, 1853-1859), vol.6, p.154 (12 thermidor An IV). For a proposal made in 1800 for a national games or *Franciade* based on the Olympics, see Staum, *Minerva's message*, p.129.
73. See Martyn Lyons, *France under the Directory* (Cambridge, 1975), p.146-58.
74. For a comprehensive attempt to distance contemporary republicanism from its classical prototypes, see the sixth of the lectures delivered by Volney at the École Normale in 1795 in C. F. Volney, *Œuvres complètes* (Paris, 1837), p.592. Significantly, Volney also discouraged the teaching of history to those destined merely for the mechanical trades ('What does it matter to the farmer, the artisan, the merchant or the businessman that there once existed an Alexander, an Attila, [...] a republic of Carthage, Sparta or Rome?' (p.581); see also p.577). For Theremin, see n.85 below.

commentators.[75] But Cabanis himself was as significant a figure in contemporary politics as he was in medicine. He played a series of important roles in dismantling the democracy of the first French Republic and he did not hesitate to invoke his own authority as an expert on the physical and the moral when it came to persuading his colleagues of the advisability of ditching the democratic process. The coup of 18 fructidor An V/4 September 1797, when the Directoire moved against right-wing opponents suspected of royalist sympathies (including two of the Directors) and abolished freedom of the press, was a turning point in the history of the Directoire. In the short term this was because it demonstrated that the democratic safeguards of the constitution could be violated with relative impunity in the interests of maintaining firm, centrist government. Cabanis and other members of the Institut were enthusiastic supporters of the coup and of the policies which followed it, which included the wholesale manipulation of election results. It was as a result of one particularly shameless instance of such manipulation that Cabanis himself was 'elected' to the Council of the Five Hundred in 1798.[76] On 21 germinal An VI/10 April 1798 the 680 electors of the Seine (Paris) electoral assembly met to begin the lengthy electoral process. In spite of opposition, a left-leaning majority (led, not by some irresponsible *sans-culotte*, but by the respected lawyer Cambacérès, future second Consul of the Republic and Archchancellor of Napoleon's Empire) had made considerable progress by the morning of 26 germinal, when they arrived to discover that between one and two hundred government supporters or *directoriaux* had absconded with the official record of the proceedings to an unknown location. This turned out to be the headquarters of the Institut. There, the *directoriaux* constituted themselves as a rival assembly which proceeded to its own elections, subsequently validated by the government which overturned the activities of the original, larger assembly. Cabanis was a member of the breakaway group. The choice of the Institut as the site for its deliberations suggests that his personal involvement in this subversion of the electoral process was not peripheral. He was rewarded with election to the Five Hundred.

75. See, for example, the accounts given by Teysseire and Staum (see n.44 above) and in Staum, *Cabanis*, p.218. In none of these accounts are the social implications of the muscular temperament, on which Cabanis' own text placed such emphasis, reported. Staum explains the involvement of Cabanis and his Idéologue colleagues in the Brumaire coup as part of their 'search for stability' (*Minerva's message*, p.179).

76. See J.-R. Suratteau, *Les Elections de l'An VI et le "coup d'état du 22 floréal" (11 mai 1798): étude documentaire, statistique et analytique. Essai d'interprétation* (Paris, 1971), p.244-47. On Cabanis' political career, see Sergio Moravia, *Il Tramonto dell'illuminismo: filosofia e politica nella società francese (1770-1810)* (Bari, 1968), p.303-12 and, specifically on the period from Fructidor to Brumaire, Chappey, 'Les Idéologues face au coup d'état'.

Cabanis became an important figure in the search for a new constitutional solution, one in which a strengthened executive and a reduction in the role of popular representation would obviate the need to subvert election results. He already appears to have favoured a radically reduced public sphere based on intellectual rather than property qualifications whose principal mouthpiece would be the Institut.[77] The choice of Sieyès, known to be unhappy with the Constitution of the Year III, as one of the directors in 1799 was seen as a sign for action by those including Cabanis who wanted to limit the operations of democracy. The by now predominately left-wing Councils were turning the Directoire's tactics on itself. The first indications of parties of government and opposition appeared in French republican politics, with a resurgence of political associations and an independent press.[78] Sieyès and his followers represented such developments as threats to the future of civilisation itself, views to which Cabanis, as a member of the Five Hundred, lent eloquent support.[79]

Together with other colleagues from the Institut, Cabanis was involved in the conspiracy which brought the Directoire to an end in the coup of 18 brumaire An VIII/9 November 1799, a move designed to 'resolve once and for all the nagging problem of popular participation'.[80] The conspirators' strong man was a fellow member of the Institut, Napoleon Bonaparte. Cabanis was among twenty conspirators picked from the two Councils who met on 16 brumaire to prepare the coup, planned for two days later, following the transfer of the Councils from Paris to Saint-Cloud on the pretext that another coup was being planned by the left.[81] The coup did not go smoothly. Bonaparte panicked when confronted by the unexpected resistance of the Councils. The presence of mind of his brother, Lucien, president of the Council of the Ancients, and the military intervention of Murat saved the day for the conspirators. Members of the Councils fled in panic, and it was with difficulty that Lucien managed to round up a hundred or so of them on the following

77. Suratteau, *Elections.*

78. Bernard Gainot, *1799, un nouveau Jacobinisme?: la démocratie représentative, une alternative à brumaire* (Paris, 2001); Isser Woloch, *Jacobin legacy. The democratic movement under the Directory* (Princeton, NJ, 1970).

79. See Cabanis, *Opinion sur les réunions s'occupant d'objets politiques. le 6 fructidor An 7* (An VII/ 1799); *Discours prononcé par Cabanis, sur le message du Conseil des Anciens, relatif aux journaux calomniateurs des premières autorités.*

80. Lynn Hunt, David Lansky and Paul Hanson, 'The Failure of the Liberal Republic in France, 1795-1799: the road to Brumaire', *Journal of modern history* 51 (1979), p.734-59 (754).

81. [V. Lombard de Langres] *Le Dix-huit brumaire, ou tableau des événemens qui ont amené cette journée; des moyens secrets par lesquels elle a été préparée; des faits qui l'ont accompagnée, et des résultats qu'elle doit avoir; auquel on a ajouté des anecdotes sur les principaux personnages qui étaient en place; et les pièces justicatives, etc.*, An VIII de la République (1799), p.129.

evening to vote for what was to be their own demise.[82] In what was effectively the official announcement of the coup, Cabanis urged his colleagues to accept the situation. He addressed them as an expert on the mechanisms of the physical and moral, employing a succession of organicist metaphors. He and his colleagues were, he claimed, ready to die for 'Equality, Liberty, Republic', but these were vain words without stable social institutions to support them. How could a people enjoy true liberty when annual elections insured that they would be 'in a fever' for six months out of every twelve? But it was when reporting the views of the people that Cabanis revealed the true extent of his expertise. Other members of the Council had claimed to speak on their behalf. Only Cabanis, by virtue of his profession, could do so with real authority. He encountered 'the penniless labouring class' '*la classe indigente et manouvrière*' on a daily basis. He explained on their behalf that they held in horror 'the pretended popular laws' 'of the neo-Jacobins'. None was more enthusiastic than they for 'a prompt return to a system of justice and security', since they understood that this was their own best guarantee of (future) wealth and comfort. Such would be the despair of the people if denied these benefits that, strange to say, they would rise up and bring the whole social edifice crashing down in ruin.[83]

Cabanis continued to play an influential role. He was appointed to the commission set up to advise on yet another new constitution, that of the Year VIII. He emerged as perhaps the most effective and authoritative apologist of the new government's ideology in the Councils. It was not merely his vaunted familiarity with the ways of the labouring classes which gave his views such authority. The insights which he claimed into the medical underpinnings of social activity in general were calculated to make his prescription for a healthy political constitution all the more persuasive. He managed to present the Constitution of the Year VIII as an extension of the democratic process rather than the restriction, which it in fact was. The new constitution would provide representative government after a fashion, as Cabanis explained, and it would have a salutary effect on the people at the same time:

> The principal object, the great advantage of this form of government is that the people [...] make no laws, they do not administer, they do not judge, as they did in the anarchical democracies of antiquity; but that their legislators,

82. Jean Tulard, *Le 18 brumaire: comment terminer une Révolution* (Mesnil-sur-l'Estrée, 1999), p.146.

83. During debates earlier in the day rumours had been spread of an uprising in the fauxbourgs of Paris and an impending march on Saint-Cloud [Lombard de Langres], Tulard, *18 brumaire*, p.218; for Cabanis' speech, see p.313-33; Cabanis, 'Discours prononcé par Cabanis à la suite du rapport de la commission des sept. Séance extraordinaire du 19 brumaire An VIII', An VIII, in Cabanis, *Œuvres*, vol.2, p.451-56.

> their administrators and their judges be always selected from those designated by them. [....] In the true representative system, everything is thus done in the name of the people and for the people; nothing is done directly by them: they are the sacred fount of all the powers, but they do not exercise any [...]: in a word, they are free, but they are calm.[84]

Seen from the perspective of Cabanis' views on the democratic process, his earlier division of the muscular from the cerebral temperament had clear political implications. Muscular development or lack of it was an indication of how people made their living. In social terms, Cabanis' distinction differentiated those who gained their livelihood by physical labour from those who did not. (The gym had yet to be invented as a forum for bourgeois recreation and display.) Cabanis provided a physiological explanation of why propertied people like him were so different from their labouring fellow-citizens, even though he preferred to emphasise intellectual qualifications or the lack of them. It was disregard for this distinction which had doomed the 'anarchic' democracies of antiquity, and which made the curtailment of the democratic process so desirable in the new French republic. For those who attended to the lessons of science, the new theory of the temperaments provided an unanswerable argument for excluding the unpropertied – those forced to work manually for a living – from the political process. The muscular were unfit to vote because they were temperamentally less able to take things in. By defining cultural prejudices as precultural patterns, Cabanis' theory of the temperaments provided a physiological justification for a reduction in participatory democracy.

A pamphlet by Theremin, Sieyès' confidant and his regular mouthpiece, provided sound economic arguments which complement Cabanis' physiological justification for the abolition of democracy. He revived the familiar argument that the type of democracy practised by the ancients had been based on slavery. Freed by their slaves from the need to bother about how they made their livelihood, citizens of the ancient democracies had been free to devote themselves more or less exclusively to public life. The Jacobins had given political power to those who had to work for a living, with disastrous results. Their attempt to extend democracy in 1793 had been an untimely 'irruption of antiquity' into contemporary life, producing 'disparity between ideas and things'. A modern republic was 'necessarily subordinated to the system of public economy in which we live'. Democracy was clearly incompatible with modern economic and social needs. What the modern citizen feared was

84. 'Quelques considérations sur l'organisation sociale en général et particulièrement sur la nouvelle Constitution par Cabanis imprimées par l'ordre de la commission [.] Séance du 25 frimaire An VIII', reprinted in Cabanis, *Œuvres*, vol.2, p.473, 481. On the medicalisation of the discourse of the body politic in this speech, see A. de Baecque, *Body politic*, p.314-20.

not slavery, but poverty. He was therefore more interested in the pursuit of wealth than in that of liberty, and valued the latter chiefly as a means to the former. Politics only got in the way of profits. What was needed was civil, not political liberty.[85] These were essentially the arguments which Sieyès had deployed in 1789 as a basis for the distinction between active and passive citizens.[86] But in Theremin's hands, they were used to question the feasibility of representative democracy itself. If government required such expertise, was it not best left in the hands of experts, those properly qualified to do everything 'in the name of the people and for the people'? This is what initially appeared to be happening at Brumaire. Members of the Institut were admitted to the new political institutions, including the three bodies created to replace the Councils of the Directoire – the Legislative Body, the Tribunate and the Senate. Under the Constitution of the Year VIII, the membership of these bodies was to be chosen either by the executive consuls (effectively, Bonaparte) or by each other.

It is unlikely that Cabanis' pathologisation of Hercules' sculpted anatomy contributed directly to the eventual rejection of Moitte's *Rousseau* project for the Champs-Elysées. Hercules still personified the people in the late 1790s, but chiefly for those on the left, as in a painting of the *Triumph of the French people* by the unrepentant Jacobin Philippe-Auguste Hennequin, a pupil of David, exhibited at the Salon of 1799.[87] By 1798, the Jacobin ambition of universal primary education had gone, even in the diluted form proposed by the Thermidorians. Moitte had completed the life-size plaster version of his monument in preparation for executing it in marble by 1798, when it was quietly dropped, in spite of his protests. It was replaced by another project, by Masson, the result of a direct commission, not a competition (fig.44, p.195).

The commitment of government to public commissions decided by public competition was also a thing of the past. Masson's *Rousseau* preserves the classical drapery of Moitte's project, but without the Herculean build or pose.[88] The infant learning to tread the paths of freedom has been replaced by a dutifully attentive adolescent who displays no inclination to stray from the sage's side. The figure of a

85. *De l'incompatibilité du systême démagogique avec le systême d'économie politique des peuples modernes* (An VIII). Theremin, who was also Chef de bureau at the Committee of Public Safety, attempted to act as a go-between between Sieyès and Kant (Luc Ferry, 'Kant', in *Dictionnaire critique de la Révolution française*, p.1008).

86. In *Observations sur le rapport du comité de Constitution, concernant la nouvelle organisation de la France* (1789). See also Rosanvallon, *Le sacre du citoyen*, p.85-88.

87. See Stefan Germer, 'In search of a beholder: on the relation of art, audiences and social spheres in post-Thermidor France', *Art bulletin* 74 (1992), p.19-28 (25).

88. On Masson's project, see Gramaccini, 'Sur le projet d'élever un monument en l'honneur de Rousseau'.

woman with another child to Rousseau's left alludes to the vogue for breastfeeding, another cause promoted by the philosopher and one fashionable in the Directoire among those who campaigned to restrict women to the biological role of mother.[89] The woman's presence helps to promote a fantasy (particularly inappropriate in Rousseau's case) of patriarchal family values. With the progressive if stealthy withdrawal of the State from its earlier commitment to universal schooling, education had once more become a private rather than a civic responsibility.[90] The civic purpose of education was itself in question following Brumaire. The reference to the *Belvedere torso* – the French Hercules – has disappeared, together with the mute *gravitas* and momentousness of Moitte's group. No longer an allusion to the social institutions of antiquity, classical drapery has become merely the badge of good taste. But, as we will see in the next chapter, there was one work of art which incarnated the ideals of the Brumaire moment in more triumphal fashion.

89. See Elisabeth Badinter, *L'amour en plus[.] Histoire de l'amour maternel (XVIIe-XXe siècle)* (Paris, 1980), p.195-98 and *passim*.

90. Rousseau had forced their mother to abandon each of his children to the care of the Paris foundling hospital, the *Enfants-trouvés*. On the representation of education as a family activity in portraiture of this date, see Halliday, *Facing the public*, p.172, n.30.

8. The trouble with Tatius: David's *Sabines* and the end of public art

As a Jacobin conspicuous for his personal loyalty to Robespierre, David was lucky to escape with his life at Thermidor. Had he attended the Convention on 9 Thermidor (he stayed away in order to take medication) he would probably have accompanied the other Jacobins to the scaffold on the following day. As it was, he was imprisoned for nearly a year, released, then briefly re-imprisoned during the government fear of a popular uprising which accompanied the *journée* of I prairial An III/20 May 1795. He reappeared at the Salon (at which he had not exhibited during the period of his service in the Convention) later in the same year with a pair of portraits. But he was already at work on what was to be his most substantial undertaking hitherto, a vast history painting of *The Intervention of the Sabine women* (fig.45, p.222).

Finished in 1799, the *Sabines* was a turning point in French history painting. Under the *ancien régime*, major history paintings had usually been undertaken in response to specific demand, often as the result of a public commission on behalf of Church or State. Uncommissioned and without destination, the *Sabines* was painted to be exhibited for money, a purpose which it fulfilled so successfully that David was able to buy a modest estate with the proceeds.[1] The success of the *Sabines* exhibition served both as a lesson and as a warning to later history painters. It fuelled fantasies about the potency of art and the independence of the artist, but it warned of their increasing social marginalisation at the same time.

The *Sabines* was calculated to attract critical reactions and commentary. The painting's exhibition was accompanied by the publication of pamphlets by David himself and by his friend Jean-Baptiste (Publicola) Chaussard, a civil servant during the Reign of Terror, a 'classic' Jacobin,[2]

1. For background and bibliography, see Antoine Schnapper and Arlette Sérullaz, p.323-53. Discussions of the painting published since have included those by Stefan Germer, 'In search of a beholder: on the relation between art, audiences, and social spheres in post-Thermidor France', *Art bulletin* 74 (1992), p.19-36; Dorothy Johnson, *Jacques-Louis David: art in metamorphosis* (Princeton, NJ, 1993), p.121-36; and Ewa Lajer-Burcharth, *Necklines: the art of Jacques-Louis David after the Terror* (New Haven, CT, and London, 1999), p.130-235.
2. See Bernard Gainot, *1799, un nouveau Jacobinisme?* (Paris, 2001), p.469. On Chaussard's career, see Marc Régaldo, 'Profil perdu: l'idéologue Chaussard', in *Approches des lumières. Mélanges offerts à Jean Fabre* (Paris, 1974), p.381-401.

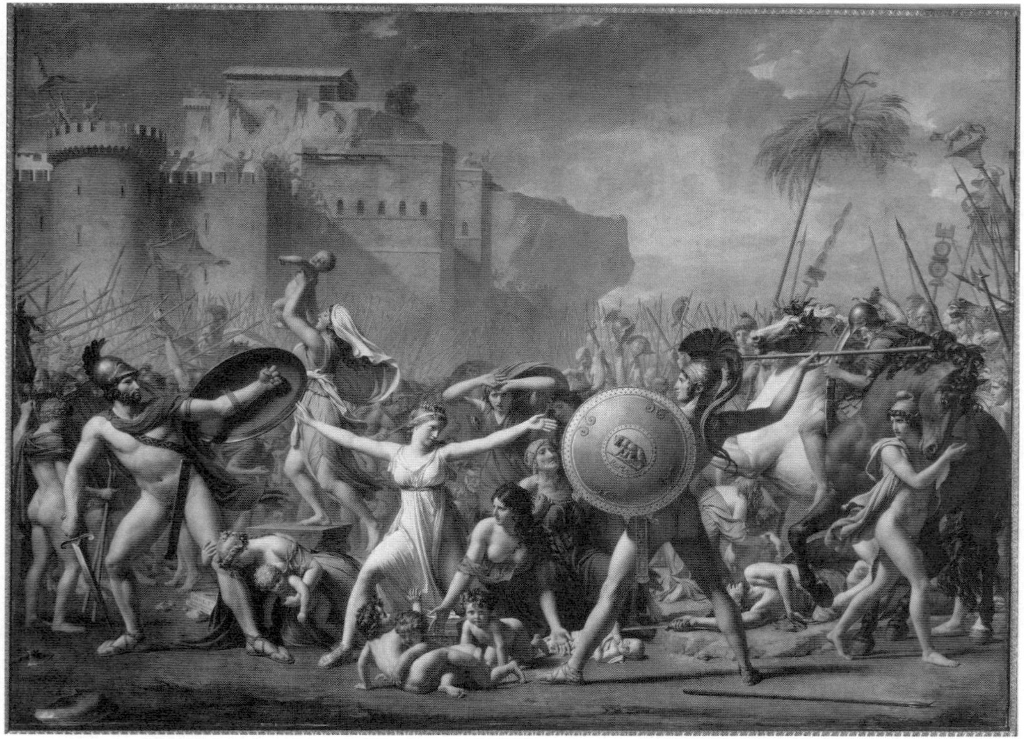

Figure 45: Jacques-Louis David, *Intervention of the Sabine women*, oil on canvas, 1795-1799, 385 × 522 cm, Musée du Louvre, Paris, RF 3691.

and an art critic.[3] The painting received considerable press coverage both at its first exhibition, which lasted from 1799 until 1805, and later. It was shown again in 1808 and in 1810, in which year it was shortlisted for Napoleon's Prix décennaux. Following the Restoration the *Sabines* was purchased for the Crown. It went on public display at the Luxembourg in 1820 and at the Louvre from 1826. There it came to be seen as epitomising the achievements and failures, the strengths and the shortcomings of the sort of classical history painting associated with the school of David. The painter had helped to insure that this would be the case by publishing a pamphlet to accompany the initial exhibition in which he claimed to have realised afresh the peculiar qualities of ancient art. Such emphasis on the aesthetic rather than the moral aspects of history painting was a novelty on the part of David, consonant with the circumstances of the *Sabines* exhibition.[4] At the same time, the political implications of the painting's subject, the reconciliation of hostile political factions by the intervention of a group of women, were intended to attract comment and reflection.[5] They have continued to do so. Recent accounts of the painting have concentrated on the role of the women – particularly that of the central figure, Hersilia, who stands at the crux of the composition.[6] But early spectators were at least as concerned with the artist's characterisation of the principal male figures to either side of her as with that of Hersilia. Where later commentators have seen a polarity based on gender roles, David's contemporaries were struck by a hierarchical distinction of social and physical types among both the women *and* the men, but chiefly between the two male protagonists. What this difference signified and why it mattered is the subject of this chapter. In particular, the *Sabines* and its early critiques will be looked at in the light of Cabanis' doctrine of the cerebral and muscular temperaments. In the light of this evidence, the original purpose of the painting's exhibition will be re-examined.

The narrative illustrated in the painting is well known. It derives from the Roman historian Livy and from a later account in Plutarch's *Life of Romulus*, and is conveniently set forth in David's pamphlet.[7] The first Romans, a largely male group, seized the womenfolk of a neighbouring

3. [J.L. David], *Le Tableau des Sabines, exposé publiquement au palais national des sciences et des arts, salle de la ci-devant académie d'architecture. Par le c^{en} David, membre de l'Institut national*, 1799; P. Chaussard, *Sur le tableau des Sabines, par David*, An VIII/1800.
4. Philippe Bordes, *David*, p.80. See also [J.L. David], *Tableau des Sabines*, p.16. On the significance of the mode of the painting's exhibition, see Annie Becq, 'Expositions, peintres et critiques: vers l'image moderne de l'artiste', *Dix-huitième siècle* 14 (1982), p.131-48.
5. Chaussard, *Sur le tableau des Sabines*, p.4. See also Valerie Mainz, 'David's *Les Sabines* and the colouring of history painting post Thermidor', *Interfaces* 10 (1996), p.47-59 (50-54).
6. See, in particular, Lajer-Burcharth, *Necklines*, p.30-235.
7. [J. L. David], *Tableau de Sabines*, p.9-14.

tribe, the Sabines, in order to provide themselves with wives and mothers for their children. Three years later, the Sabine men, under their leader, Tatius, captured the city of Rome (depicted in the background of the painting). They defended it against a counterattack by the Romans themselves, led by their own king, Romulus. At this point the women, by now Roman wives and mothers as well as Sabine sisters and daughters, intervened to demand reconciliation. Softened by their pleas, the Sabine men made peace with the Romans.

David chose to depict the moment of the women's intervention, with the battle well under way. Tatius, on the left, has already attacked Romulus with a spear. Deflected by the Roman's shield, it lies in the foreground. As Tatius recoils to gather momentum for an onslaught with his sword, Romulus steadies his own spear for release.[8] There is an obvious contrast in the pose of the two men, but also in their physique – the heavier, more muscled – perhaps more mature – Tatius is pitted against the smooth and slender figure of Romulus. Contemporary writers identified this as a contrast in types of male beauty – that of ordinary humanity in the case of Tatius as against ideal beauty, exemplified by the body of the demi-god Romulus.[9]

The status and definition of ideal beauty was itself a live issue at this date, but this was not the aspect of the contrast which interested commentators. They sought the significance of this difference, not in aesthetics, but in the characters of the two leaders as depicted by David. The difference in pose and physique between Romulus and Tatius points to two different attitudes to combat – reliance on brute strength in the case of Tatius; skill and calculation in that of Romulus. The impetuous Tatius has already used half his weaponry (his spear) in vain, and has expended considerable energy in doing so – note how the tip of his spear has buckled under the force of its impact against his opponent's shield. Heated and furious, he now has to rely on the power of his arm and sword alone. Romulus may appear a weaker specimen physically, but he clearly holds the upper hand by this point in the fight. Calm and collected, he is still in a position to time and direct his own first strike. His sword remains as yet in its scabbard. Critics compared his attitude, like his physique, with that of Apollo – an allusion to the *Apollo Belvedere*, a representation of that god which, it was generally agreed, depicted him at the moment of victory, having just launched the arrow (from a now vanished bow) which struck and killed the Python. The same critics

8. Ch. P. Landon, *Journal des arts, de littérature et de commerce* (10 nivôse An VIII/30 December 1799), p.3.

9. See especially Ch. P. Landon, *Journal des arts, de littérature et de commerce* (10 nivôse An VIII/30 December 1799), p.3 and (20 nivôse An VIII/10 January 1800), p.6; [Amaury Duval], 'Beaux-Arts. Examen du tableau des *Sabines*, *La Décade*, (10 pluviôse An VIII/30 January 1800),

likened the figure of Tatius to Hercules or Ajax, heroes famous for strenuous feats of physical strength.[10]

The situation of the two men in the painting implies an underlying difference in their attitude to conflict and ultimately to life in general – a difference of *temperament*. The wrath of the laddish Tatius is set against the cooler, more rational approach of Romulus, who also knows something about the laws of dynamics, to judge by the poise with which he handles his spear. The passion of the engaged partisan confronts the serenity of the born commander. Brawn as opposed to brain. That surely is how the difference of these two bodies was intended to be read, literally down to the fingertips.

As David and his friends indicated, the *Sabines* alluded to the revolutionary conflict and its aftermath. It did this by illustrating the power of private affections to end conflict in the public sphere – a commonplace of republican ideology during the Directory.[11] But it also provided a framework which might encourage reflection on the nature of the antecedent conflict and its outcome in the context of recent French history. On this interpretation, the Herculean figure of Tatius, leader of the city's usurpers, could hark back to an earlier, more violent phase of the Revolution in which the inhabitants of the Parisian sections had on occasion played a direct and often bloody role in government. Tatius exemplifies some salient disadvantages of the muscular temperament as characterised by Cabanis – lack of forethought, which has led him to make his rash initial attack with the spear, and a propensity to ungovernable rage. This was in any case how pro-government apologists tended to represent the behaviour of the revolutionary crowd during this period, whether or not they were in a position, like Cabanis, to offer a scientific explanation.[12] Romulus' more placid and calculating approach to slaughter, on the other hand, might suggest the imperturb-

---

p.226-30; P. Chaussard, *Sur le tableau des Sabines*, p.7-8; [Dupont], *Critique du tableau des Sabines du citoyen DAVID*, An VIII (Paris, Bibliothèque nationale (Cabinet des Estampes), Collection Deloynes, vol.21, no.599); Chaussard, 'Notice historique et inédite sur M. Louis David', in *Le Pausanias français: état des arts du dessin en France à l'ouverture du XIXe siècle: Salon de 1806* (1808), p.159-61; [Alexandre Lenoir], *Concours pour les prix décennaux. Peinture. Examen du tableau des Sabines et de l'école de M. David, Premier Peintre de sa Majesté l'Empéreur et Roi, Chevalier de l'Empire, Officier de la Légion d'Honneur, Membre de l'Institut de France* (1810), p.11 and 15; *Rapports et discussions de toutes les classes de l'Institut de France, sur les ouvrages admis au concours pour les Prix décennaux* (1810), p.19; F. P. [Fabien Pillet] in *Journal de Paris*, 23 September 1810, p.1878f. For a full bibliography of critical reactions, see Schnapper and Sérullaz, *Jacques-Louis David*, p.338-39.

10. Chaussard, *Sur le tableau des Sabines*, p.7; [Amaury Duval], p.227; [Alexandre Lenoir], p.11. The interpretation of the pose of the Apollo and the stress on the effortlessness of his pose both derive from Winckelmann. See above, ch.4.

11. See Halliday, *Facing the public*, p.88-91.

12. See, for example, Mercier, *Le Nouveau Paris*, p.713.

ability of the temperamentally cerebral – the men of Brumaire, like Bonaparte and Cabanis himself. Romulus' apparent advantage over his opponent at the moment of the women's intervention could be read as an indication that it was the cerebral, not the muscular temperament which had the best chance of success in the long run. This is not to suggest that Tatius or Romulus should be identified as overt symbols of the parties to the revolutionary conflict in any direct sense. The painting, like Cabanis' theory of the temperaments, would have lost much of its authority to convince if it had been so easily reducible to mere commentary on contemporary events. Rather, it provoked a general reflection on the likely outcome of a particular type of conflict – a conflict between apparently ill-matched adversaries, where brawn was pitted against brain. It gained any authority and resonance it possessed in that respect from the objectivity which is commonly held to attach to the correct formulation and application of scientific theory, irrespective of the immediate social context. Whether the parties concerned were interpreted as representatives of two ancient tribes or two contemporary social groups, the nature and course of their conflict were governed by the laws of temperament.

A significant parallel between David's approach and that of Cabanis lies in the fidelity with which both claimed to have followed the theories and practices of the ancients. Cabanis' views, political and medical, involved the rejection of aspects of the classical tradition dear to earlier French republicans. Yet he was no less concerned to provide classical precedents for his medical views – hence his attempt to argue that the Greeks had been aware of the drawbacks of the muscular temperament in spite of an utter lack of supporting evidence. David's approach in the *Sabines* reveals a similar preoccupation with ancient precedent and a similar underlying ambivalence. The painting was presented by the artist as heralding a return to principles of classical art forgotten or at least neglected in modern times. As already indicated, however, such a view scarcely holds true of the painting's ideological content. The judgements that spectators were invited to make about the temperament, moral character and intelligence of the two protagonists, and any conclusion that they were expected to draw about where power should lie in society, related to the social and political outlook of French republicans under the Directory – men such as David and Cabanis – not to views held by the Romans or the Greeks. Yet, paradoxically, the visual means employed by David to emphasise the role of temperament involved departures from contemporary artistic practice which were apparently sanctioned by the art of antiquity. In spite of the painting's vast scale, David rejected the traditional compositional formulae of history painting in favour of an arrangement designed to recall classical sculptural reliefs. The flatness and lack of chiaroscuro which resulted displeased his more conservative critics,[13] but they enabled him to enhance the contrast of attitude and physique of his two male protagonists by displaying them in a balanced manner, for all the world like two specimens facing each other across a double-page spread in a medical textbook.

David's other innovation, notoriously, was to make the figures of Tatius and Romulus naked. This was a more controversial issue for the inhabitants of Paris, where the nudity of statues in what were now public spaces (formally royal) had recently given rise to debate, and David's decision provoked adverse comment (he was eventually compelled to change the position of Tatius' scabbard in order to hide his genitals).[14] The artist claimed that he had decided to divest the figures of their clothing in accordance with conventions of nudity in classical art, whereby gods and heroes were so portrayed. This justification holds good for Romulus, who was a demi-god, and whose figure is appropriately idealised, but it is more problematic in the case of Tatius. This is not because Tatius as an ordinary mortal was not entitled to such treatment, as was wrongly asserted by one hostile critic.[15] Public figures were portrayed in the nude in the late republican and imperial periods. But the nudity of their statues involved idealisation as well, as was well known to David's contemporaries and presumably to David himself.[16] Had David followed classical convention in this as in other respects, he would have been forced to give Tatius a similar physique to that of the idealised Romulus, thus erasing the difference of build between the two figures. The contrast of temperament between the two would thereby have been lost.

David's original scheme had involved clothed figures. It survives in two pen and wash drawings of the whole composition now in the Louvre, as well as in other drawings.[17] The later of these drawings (fig.46, p.231) presents a composition close to that of the finished painting – an indication that the decision to divest the male protagonists of their clothing was taken relatively late in the day. A comparison between drawing and painting reveals at once how much the legibility of the difference between the two men's physical and moral characters depended on the removal of their clothes.

13. See Johnson, *Jacques-Louis David*, p.131-32.
14. Johnson, *Jacques-Louis David*, p.128-29.
15. [Dupont], *Critique du tableau des Sabines*, p.2. See also [J. L. David], *Tableau des Sabines*, p.15-16.
16. Winckelmann, *Histoire de l'art chez les anciens*, 2 vols (Paris: H. J. Jansen, An II/1794-An XI/1803), vol.2, p.383; Antoine Chrysostome Quatremère de Quincy, *Essai sur la nature, le but et les moyens de l'initation dans les beaux-arts* (1825), p.417.
17. See Schnapper and Sérullaz, *Jacques-Louis David*, nos.147, 152 and 153, p.340 and 347-48. See Pierre Rosenberg and Louis-Antoine Prat, *Jacques-Louis David 1748–1825: catalogue raisonné des dessins* (Milan, 2002), nos.146 and 158.

The decision to represent the two figures as nudes thus entailed a more fundamental shift of emphasis in the painting's message. The earlier project, in which differences in the men's physique were largely hidden beneath their armour, was evidently intended to foreground the painting's message of reconciliation rather than difference. This is consonant with the political situation during 1798 and the first half of 1799 and what we know to have been David's and especially Chaussard's sympathies. Although he too was a member of the Institut, David's political antecedents and affiliations were closer to those of the men stigmatised as 'anarchists' in Cabanis' speeches than to Cabanis' own. He was, for example, a subscriber to the newspaper published by the radical Gracchus Babeuf.[18] He remained on good terms with other ex-Jacobins and was evidently sympathetic with the Jacobin cause. A distinctive feature of the Jacobin revival of 1799 was the emphasis placed on cultural activity, promoted by organisations such as the Portique républicain, which was dedicated to the promotion of a spirit of civic engagement in the Jacobin tradition, even though it was organised separately from its more overtly political counterpart, the Club de Manège. Chaussard was an active member of both organisations. The Portique's mission was the promotion of art committed to the Republic. Many of its members, including Chaussard, were active in the cult of Théophilanthropie, the alternative republican religion promoted initially by one of the directors, Laréveillère-Lépaux. Like the Théophilanthropes, the Portique's members aimed to enlist the persuasive power of artistic expression in its campaign to convert the public to the cause of Reason.[19] Members of the Portique were preoccupied with the dissemination of republican art to as wide a public as possible while at the same time distancing themselves from the Institut and related institutions. David's decision to exhibit the *Sabines* for an indefinite period to a paying audience and outside the institutional confines of the Salon and the Beaux-arts section of the Institut is often interpreted as the consequence of personal rather than political differences between David and his colleagues. But it was clearly a project which would have made good sense in terms of the aspirations of the Portique républicain. The painting's original message, too – the efficacy of private feelings in healing divisions bred in public life – was in harmony with the principles preached by the Portique's members, notably Chaussard.[20]

18. See above ch.7.
19. On the Portique républicain, see J.-L. Chappey, 'Le Portique républicain et les enjeux de la mobilisation des arts autour de Brumaire An VIII', in *Les Arts de la scène et la Révolution française*, ed. Philippe Bourdin and Gérard Loubinoux (Clermont-Ferrand, 2004), p.487-507.
20. David was not a member of the Portique (its regulations denied membership to members

It is easy enough to propose a cultural and political context in which the exhibition of a version of *Sabines* based on the Louvre drawing might have been appropriate from a neo-Jacobin point of view – some time before the closure of the Manège and the defeat of the Jacobins in the summer of 1799. But the decision to divest Romulus and Tatius of their clothes changes the painting's intended impact. It isolates the two men from the other figures and invites comparison between them. There is a corresponding shift in the spectator's response to the composition – away from the theme of reconciliation and towards the physical differences between the painting's two protagonists. The consequences of David's decision were well expressed by the critic Amaury Duval:

> Would I be able to discern beneath a tunic those admirable outlines offered by the nude? The clothed man is a man in disguise: he is only himself when naked; it is men who should be painted, not their simulacra.[21]

David had enlisted what he claimed was the true language of classical art – nudity – to encourage a reading which had nothing classical about it at all, but which related instead to contemporary physiology and the readings of anatomical difference which it promoted. By undressing his male protagonists, he appeared to have unveiled the truth about their identity. Beneath the socially imposed sameness of more or less uniform military dress lurked the 'real' men, harbouring apparently innate and irreconcilable differences of temperament and moral character expressed in their physique and their actions. The two figures are examples of two different approaches to the nude. Heroic or ideal nudity is contrasted with something more akin to everyday nakedness. David's own apologia for the nudity of his figures was restricted to the question of precedents in ancient art, avoiding the issue of heroic versus unheroic nudity. But Chaussard's pamphlet addressed both aspects. He first called for the employment of nudity on the grounds that physical beauty was the principal means whereby the painter could illustrate moral beauty – a justification for the depiction of idealised nudes – but went on to argue, like Amaury Duval, that more could be learned about moral identity from representations of the naked than from those of the clothed figure:

> the painter and the sculptor can only express moral beauty by means of physical beauty [...]. Voltaire's observation, a mere pleasantry in its original context, *To judge a man properly, you must see him naked,* becomes a deep truth

---

of the Institut). For Chaussard's views on the social mission of art, see his *Essai philosphique sur la dignité des arts* (An VI/1798). See also Édouard Pommier, *L'Art de la liberté*, p.344-49; Halliday, *Facing the public*, p.85-91.

21. [Amaury Duval], 'Beaux-Arts. Examen du tableau des *Sabines*', *La Décade*, p.229.

> for the artist. There is one man who must fear to see himself naked; it is modern man, it is the being as morally as he is physically degraded.[22]

The rhetoric of this passage is recognisably neo-Jacobin, close to that of a pamphlet by Chaussard published by the Club de Manège a few months earlier, before the closure of the clubs and before Brumaire, in which he had called for the subjection of citizens and their property to a moral censorship on the ancient Roman model.[23]

If David's painting is compared with the Louvre drawing in which the two protagonists were represented in armour (fig.46, p.231), it is evident that David has been concerned to accentuate difference of class between the two figures.

This is equally true of his treatment of the group of women between them. As the critics approvingly noted, the artist managed to distinguish the rank of the genteel Hersilia from that of her less refined sisters, thereby locating social distinction in the private as well as the public sphere. Here, too, a comparison with the drawing shows that most of the indicators of difference among the women were introduced or given fresh emphasis at a relatively late stage – between the drawing and the painting itself. The woman baring her breast to the left of Romulus, for example, was transformed from a woman of similar age to Hersilia in the drawing into an aged grandmother in the painting. The woman on the ground to Hersilia's right, the woman in red behind her, and the woman to the left of Hersilia raising her child as she confronts the Sabine soldiers were all given more emphatically anguished, open-mouthed expressions in the final painting, creating a contrast with the more restrained and decorous facial expression of Hersilia which was not present in the drawing, and whose significance was seized on by critics as an indicator of relative gentility or lack of it:

> Each of these women has her own expression which indicates her rank in society. Hersilia's grief is noble: she is visibly not sobbing; all her expression is in her eyes. She looks tenderly at her husband, in the belief that that will be sufficient to disarm him. But others rend the air with their screams: their traits are distorted. One in particular gives way to the most violent despair.[24]

22. Chaussard, *Sur le tableau des Sabines*, p.37-38. For further contemporary expressions of concern with the representation of physical types in conformity with social character, see François Benoît, *L'Art français sous la Révolution et l'Empire. Les doctrines, les idées, les genres* (Paris, 1897), p.69.
23. ([P.-J.-B. Chaussard], *Coup d'œil sur l'intérieur de la République française, ou esquisse des principes d'une révolution morale*, An VII/1799). See also [J. L. David], *Tableau des Sabines*, p.15f.
24. [Amaury Duval], 'Beaux-Arts', p.228. See also Chaussard *Sur le tableau des Sabines*: 'Hersilia dominates the centre of this group, as does Romulus among the warriors [...] especially by the dignity of her grief, the final trait which stamps a being and a soul above the common sort' (p.8); [Alexandre Lenoir], *Concours pour les prix décennaux*, p.11.

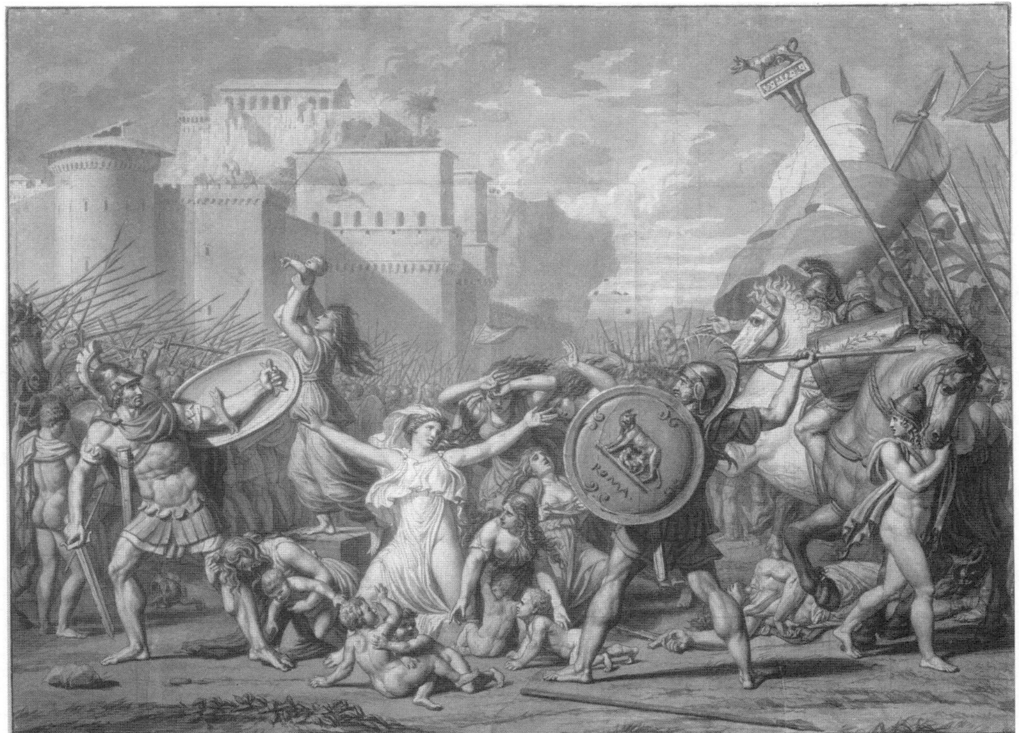

Figure 46: Jacques-Louis David, *Intervention of the Sabine women*, pen, brown and black ink, pencil, grey wash and heightening, 47.6 × 63.6 cm, Musée du Louvre, Paris, Inv. 26.183.

As the critic Landon explained, Hersilia's pale complexion, which contrasts so strikingly with the swarthiness of the other women, and which evidently provoked adverse comments, was also calculated to indicate social distinction.[25] Like degrees of muscular development in the men, shades of skin colour indicated the nature and location of a woman's habitual occupations. Whereas Hersilia's paleness derives from a secluded indoor existence, the darker complexions of her companions suggest exposure to the sun and thus outdoor work. This is a more discrete, but no less precise indicator of temperamental difference than bulging biceps.

Unlike the men, the women are clothed, but their dress, though different in colour, is of uniform type. What differentiates both the dress and the hair of the women is the manner in which they are worn – that is, the degree of disarray to which they have been subjected under pressure of events. Predictably, it is the well-bred Hersilia who has best maintained neatness of dress and hair on the battlefield. Her braids are still in place and her breasts remain covered. She has let nothing slip, unlike the woman on her knees in the right foreground. Status is thus conveyed, not by distinctions of dress, but by the different ways that it is worn, and what they imply about the habitus of the individual women. As with the men's nudity, the effect is to suggest that such indicators of class difference are inevitable consequences of individual character, not social constructions.

The characterisation of the women according to class by means of complexion and comportment complements and ultimately reinforces the contrast of temperament between the principal men. The difference between Hersilia's self-control and the unbridled anguish of the other Sabine women corresponds with that between the sang-froid of Romulus and Tatius' rage. Differentiation of character also enables the spectator to perceive how personal interaction is governed by temperament. Indeed, Hersilia demonstrates her own awareness that her husband reacts to sensations in a fundamentally different way to his more muscular opponent. As Amaury Duval perceived, she knew that a winning look was enough to sway the sensitive Romulus. The woman hanging grimly onto Tatius' left leg has evidently understood that a more physically forceful mode of persuasion was needed in order to get through to the temperamentally muscular.

As with the nudity of the two principal male figures, this differentiation was given its final form relatively late in the day, and without introducing any external marks of status. Nudity and classical dress had found favour as modes of representation in French Revolutionary cul-

25. Landon, *Journal des arts* (20 nivôse An VIII/10 January 1800), p.9.

ture. As Lynn Hunt has stated, 'both had the effect of erasing the reference to contemporary social distinctions and enforcing the sense of consensus that stood above social differentiation'.[26] All the more remarkable, then, was David's imaginative leap in employing the classical bodies of both the women and the men in the *Sabines* to reassert and redefine the visual expression of social distinction as a property of the unadorned human body and its gestural language. But this was only part of a more ambitious project, one which he shared with Cabanis and other post-revolutionary liberals, that of making the operations of human society explicable in their own terms. As Lynn Hunt has also argued, the search for secular principles of social legitimation which 'made the workings of the social both more visible and more problematic' encouraged closer scrutiny of the human body.[27] Like Cabanis' medical writings, David's *Sabines* in its definitive form contains an attempt to interpret historical events in terms of social interaction and, ultimately, human physiology. Implied in both projects was the hope that such knowledge would make possible a better and more efficient organisation of social life in the future. David's success was attested by the enthusiastic response of Chaussard, Landon, Amaury Duval and Alexandre Lenoir, all of whom gladly took up and elaborated the indications offered by David in their own accounts of the painting.

The *Sabines* appeared to offer a new way of treating historical subjects, as much by its attention to the social and the physiological as by its adoption of what the artist claimed to be a truly classical approach. Yet it retained this significance only briefly. By the autumn of 1800, Chaussard was explaining the significance of the figures' nudity in a different light. Introducing the first issue of a newly founded and short-lived newspaper of which he appears to have been the editor, the *Bulletin universel des sciences, des lettres et des arts*, he played on the insecurities of prospective readers by describing the pitfalls which attended the attempts of the insufficiently equipped to appreciate art with discernment – pitfalls, needless to say, from which a reading of the *Bulletin universel* would help to protect them:

> The multitude – and this is a truth confirmed throughout history – applauds only trivial and easy imitation. In the Museum, it is not the *Transfiguration* [of Raphaël, seized as booty by the French from the pope] which attracts the crowd, but the *Judge flayed on the orders of Cambyses* [by Gerard David, Bruges]; in the Salon, the image of broken glass [a *trompe-l'œil* by the genre painter

26. Lynn Hunt, 'Freedom of dress in revolutionary France', in *From the royal to the republican body: incorporating the political in seventeenth- and eighteenth-century France*, ed. Sara E. Melzer and Kathryn Norberg (Berkeley, CA, 1998), p.224-49 (235).
27. Hunt, 'Freedom', p.231-32. Cf. Brian C. J. Singer, *Society, theory and the French Revolution* (London, 1986).

> Boilly on show at the Salon] has made more people run to it than the drama of Orestes [*Les Remords d'Oreste*, a classical history painting by David's pupil, Hennequin, at the same Salon]. In this respect the journalists themselves are part of the crowd. How many have fallen into the trap of a bright, stagey composition! How many have preferred Tatius to Romulus in David's painting![28]

The right viewing of the *Sabines* has here become a question of aesthetic rather than moral discernment. The aesthetic capacity to which it provides a touchstone is defined in terms of social distinction – the ability to distinguish the ideal from the merely real. This was indeed an ability which the new post-revolutionary public of amateurs and Salon visitors conspicuously lacked[29]. Chaussard's new interpretation provided an indication of how the painting would subsequently be assessed, as well as of the social value which would attach to high art more generally in the new, bourgeois culture of the nineteenth century. When the Decennial Competition of 1810 pitted the *Sabines* against a painting by one of David's pupils, Girodet, *Une Scène de déluge* (Salon of 1806, Paris, Louvre) (fig.47, p.235), it was Girodet's painting which critics – and the members of the Institut itself – preferred to the *Sabines*, in spite of the protests of Montalivet, the Minister of the Interior.[30]

Why did the *Sabines*' popularity fade so quickly? In part, because the preoccupations and ambitions of both David and Cabanis at the time of Brumaire were soon overtaken by events. The course of history, not merely that of history painting, was about to take a very different direction from that anticipated by Bonaparte's early supporters. A dictatorship was swiftly established. Cultural achievements distinctive of the Revolutionary decade were as far as possible obliterated. Christianity and slavery were reintroduced. The republican calendar and democracy were abolished. By 1810 it must have become painfully obvious that the concerns addressed in both Cabanis' medico-political theorising and in David's painting – issues which had appeared of such vital importance in the autumn of 1799 – had in fact been contingent on political circumstances which had now been swept away, apparently forever.

But there are indications, too, of broader reasons for dissatisfaction with the didactic function of art in post-revolutionary culture. Girodet's *Déluge* depicts a totally imaginary scene in which a hapless father tries to

28. [Chaussard], 'Exposition des ouvrages de peinture' in *Bulletin universel des sciences, des lettres et des arts* no.1 (20 brumaire An IX/11 November 1800), p.6.
29. See Martial Guédron, *De Chair et de marbre: imiter et exprimer le nu en France, 1745-1815* (Paris, 2003), p.19f.
30. F. Boyer, 'Napoléon et l'attribution des grands Prix décennaux (1810-1811)', *Bulletin de la société de l'histoire de l'art français* (1947-1948), p.66-72.

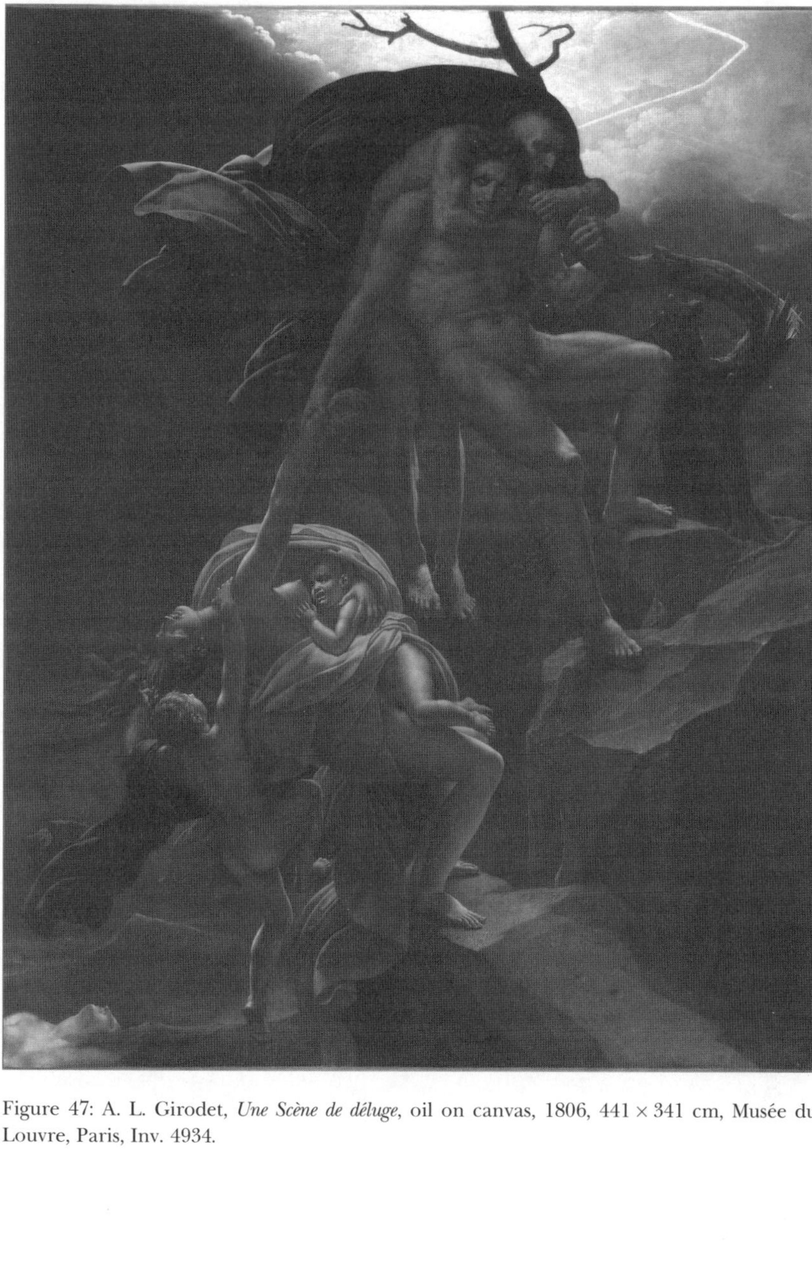

Figure 47: A. L. Girodet, *Une Scène de déluge*, oil on canvas, 1806, 441 × 341 cm, Musée du Louvre, Paris, Inv. 4934.

prevent his family from being swept away by the flood swirling round the rock on which they have taken refuge. Half-throttled by his aged father, he grasps with one hand his fainting wife, herself burdened by two children, and with the other the branch, already breaking, of a puny tree. At first sight, the *Déluge* looks like some sort of anti-*Sabines*. It certainly paints a different picture of family life. But the point of the painting is not to be sought in any lesson which it might impart. The *Déluge* is not about choice, but feeling. Its success was a victory for what Stefan Germer called the 'spectacularisation' of history painting.[31]

There is plenty of nudity in the *Déluge*, but it does not further our understanding of the individual characters in Girodet's drama. Nor in any case would such knowledge enable us to forestall what is evidently a hopeless outcome. Here nudity stands, as critics realised, as a form of cultural allusion – in this case, to Michelangelo. In other words, nudity signifies that this is a work of art, and that that is how it is to be consumed. The artist is all artist – an expert in the concoction and transmission of feeling – and the freedom of the spectator is the freedom to interpret, not political freedom. As judges and critics in 1810 conceded, the *Sabines* was incontestably superior in terms of genre – even of taste and style, but Girodet's painting won on the counts of imagination, energy, boldness and appeal.[32] David had embodied reason in Romulus and passion in Tatius, confident that his spectators would regard themselves as sufficiently cerebral to identify with Romulus. From that perspective, the success of the Girodet was a triumph for base instinct. The era of enlightened history painting, like the era of enlightened democracy, appeared to be over, almost as soon as it had begun. In what it reveals about the problematic relationship between history painting and social purpose, the fate of the *Sabines* was indeed a lesson for the artists of the succeeding century.

31. 'The mass viewership of the Salon exhibitions no longer judged a picture on the basis of its moral message, but rather according to the sensational value of its subject matter' (Germer, p.31). Germer was writing about the Salon of 1799.

32. *Rapports et discussions de toutes les classes de l'Institut de France*, p.14; [Alexandre Lenoir], *Concours pour les prix décennaux* p.28; [Fabien Pillet] *Journal de Paris* (23 September 1810), p.1878f.

Bibliography

i. Texts first published before 1800

[Amaury Duval], 'Beaux-Arts. Examen du tableau des *Sabines*', *La Décade*, 10 (pluviôse An VIII/30 January 1800), p.226-30.

Audran, Girard, *Les Proportions du corps humain mesurées sur les plus belles figures de l'antiquité* (Paris, 1683).

Boerhaave, Hermannus, *Praelectiones academicae in proprias institutiones rei medicae, edidit et notas addidit Albertus Haller*, 5 vols (Turin, 1742-1745).

Boissy d'Anglas, *Discours préliminaire au projet de Constitution pour la République française, prononcé par Boissy-d'Anglas, au nom de la commission des onze, dans la séance du 5 messidor, An 3* (messidor An III/ 1795).

Buffon, Georges Louis LeClerc comte de, *The Natural history of birds. From the French of the Count de Buffon*, translated by W. Smellie, 9 vols (London, W. Strahan and T. Cadell, 1793).

Cabanis, Pierre Jean Georges, *Conseil des cinq-cents. Discours prononcé par Cabanis, sur le message du Conseil des Anciens, relatif aux journaux calomniateurs des premières autorités. Séance du premier fructidor An 7* (An VII/1799).

–, *Opinion sur les réunions s'occupant d'objets politiques. Le 6 fructidor An 7* (An VII/1799).

Camper, Pierre, *Dissertation sur les variétés naturelles qui caractérisent la physionomie des hommes des divers climats et des différens ages* (Utrecht, 1792).

Caylus, Anne-Claude-Phillipe Comte de, *Vie d'Edmé Bouchardon, sculpteur du roi* (Paris, 1762).

Chaussard, P. J. B., *Essai philosphique sur la dignité des arts* (Paris, an VI/ 1798).

–, *Sur le tableau des Sabines, par David* (Paris, An VIII/1800).

[Chaussard, P. J. B.], *Coup d'œil sur l'intérieur de la République française, ou esquisse des principes d'une révolution morale* (Paris, An VII/ 1799).

[Chaussard, P. J. B.], 'Exposition des ouvrages de peinture', in *Bulletin universel des sciences, des lettres et des arts*, no.1 (20 brumaire An IX/11 November 1800), p.6.

Cullen, William, M. D., *A Treatise of the materia medica*, 2 vols (Edinburgh, Charles Eliot, 1789).

–, *Traité de matière médicale, traduit de l'anglois par la seule edition donée [sic?] par l'auteur à Edimbourg en 1789; par M. Bosquillon*, 2 vols (1789-1790).

Dandré-Bardon, François-Michel, *Le Monument de la ville de Reims* (1765).

[David, J. L.], *Le tableau des Sabines, exposé publiquement au palais national des sciences et des arts, salle de la ci-devant académie d'architecture. Par le citoyen David, membre de l'Institut national* (Paris, 1799).

Détournelle, Athanasius, *Aux Armes et aux arts! Peinture, sculpture, architecture, gravure. Journal de la Société républicaine des arts, séante au Louvre, Salle du Laocoon, Rédigé par Détournelle, Architecte. Première partie* (An II/1794).

Dumas, Charles-Louis, *Principes de physiologie, ou introduction à la science expérimentale, philosophique et médicale de l'homme vivant* (Paris, An VIII/1800).

[Dupont], *Critique du Tableau des Sabines Du Citoyen DAVID* (Paris, An VIII) Bibliothèque Nationale (Cabinet des Estampes), Collection Deloynes, vol.21, no.599.

Falconet, Etienne, *Œuvres d'Etienne Falconet, statuaire, contenant plusieurs écrits relatifs aux beaux-arts*, 6 vols (Lausanne, Société typographique, 1781).

Ferry, Luc, 'Kant', in F. Furet, M. Ozouf and B. Baczko, *Dictionnaire critique de la Révolution française* (Paris, 1988).

Gessner, Salomon, *The Death of Abel. In five books from the German of Mr. Gessner of Zurich, in Switzerland. A new translation* (London, Dodsley, 1764).

Hallé, [Jean-Noël] 'Mémoire sur les observations fondamentales d'après lesquelles peut être établie la distinction des Tempéramens', in *Mémoires de la Société Médicale d'Emulation, séante à l'Ecole de Médecine de Paris.* Pour l'An VII de la République française. Troisième année (An VIII), p.342-94.

Haller, Albrecht von, *Mémoires sur la nature sensible et irritable des parties du corps animal*, 4 vols (Lausanne, 1756-1760).

–, *Elementa physiologiae corporis humanae*, 8 vols (Lausanne and Berne, 1757-1766).

–, *Elementa physiologiae corpus humani*, 8 vols (Lausanne, 1760-1769).

–, translated by William Cullen, M. D., *First lines of physiology, printed under the inspection of William Cullen, to which are added* [...] *all the notes and illustrations of Prof. Wrisberg*, 2 vols (Edinburgh, G. G. J. and J. Robinson, 1786).

Husson, Henri-Marie, *Essai sur une nouvelle doctrine des tempéramens; Présenté et soutenu à l'École de Médecine de Paris, le 18 Nivôse, An VII de la République* (An VII/1799).

Lavater, J. G. [*sic*], *Essai sur la physiognomie, destiné à faire connoître l'homme et à le faire aimer*, 4 vols (The Hague, 1781-1803).

Leclerc, Daniel, *Histoire de la médecine, où l'on voit l'origine & les progrès de cet art, de siècle en siècle; les sectes, qui s'y sont formées; les noms des médecins, leurs découvertes, leurs opinions, & les circonstances les plus remarquables de leur vie* (Amsterdam, 1723).

Le Gendre, *Description de la Place de Louis XV que l'on construit à Reims; des ouvrages à continuer aux environs de cette place, et de ceux à faire dans la suite pour l'utilité et l'embellissement de cette ville* (Paris, 1765).

[Lombard de Langres, Vincent] *Le Dix-huit brumaire, ou tableau des événemens qui ont amené cette journée; des moyens secrets par lesquels elle a été préparée; des faits qui l'ont accompagnée, et des résultats qu'elle doit avoir; auquel on a ajouté des anecdotes sur les principaux personnages qui étaient en place; et les pièces justicatives, etc.* (An VIII de la République/1799).

Pauw, Cornelius de, *Œuvres philosophiques*, 7 vols (Paris, An III/ 1794-1795).

Pliny the Elder *Caii Plinii Secuni Historiae Naturalis libri XXXVII, quos recensuit et notis illustravit* G. Brotier 6 vols (Paris, Barbou, 1779).

Quatremère de Quincy, *Considérations sur les arts du dessin en France* (Paris, 1791).

Reale Accademia Ercolanese di Archeologia, *Le Antichità di*

Ercolano esposte, 8 vols (Naples, 1757-1792).
Roussel, Pierre, *Système physique et moral de la femme, ou table philosophique de la constitution, de l'état organique, du tempérament, des moeurs, et des fonctions propres au Sexe* (Paris, 1775).

Sieyès, Emmanuel Joseph, *Observations sur le rapport du comité de Constitution, concernant la nouvelle organisation de la France* (Versailles, 1789).

Watelet, C.-H., *L'Art de peindre. Poëme, avec des réflexions sur les différentes parties de la peinture* (Paris, 1761).
Watelet, C.-H., and Claude-Henri Levesque, *Dictionnaire des arts de peinture, sculpture et gravure*, 5 vols (Paris, 1792).
Winkelmann [*sic*], Giovanni, *Storia delle arti del disegno presso gli antichi, tradotta dal tedesco e in questa edizione corretta e aumentata dall'abate Carlo Fea giureconsulto* (Rome, 1783).
Winkelmann [J. J. Winckelmann], *Histoire de l'art chez les anciens*, 2 vols (Paris, H. J. Jansen, An II/1794-An XI/1803).
Winckelmann, Johann Joachim, *Johann Joachim's Geschichte der Kunst des Alterthums* (Dresden, 1764).

[Zimmermann, J. G.], *A Treatise on experience in physic*, 2 vols (London, 1778).

ii. Texts published after 1800

Allix, Edgard, 'La rivalité entre la propriété foncière et la fortune mobilière sous la Révolution', *Revue d'histoire économique et sociale* 6 (1913), p.297-348.
Allport, G. W., *Pattern and growth in personality* (New York, 1961).
Andress, David, *The French Revolution and the people* (London, 2004).
Arias, Paolo Enrico, *Policleto* (Florence, 1964).
Aulard, A., *Paris pendant la réaction thermidorienne et sous le Directoire: recueil de documents pour l'histoire de l'esprit public à Paris*, 5 vols (Paris, 1898-1902).

Babeuf, *Ecrits, introduction and annotated by Claude Mazauric* (Paris, 1988).
Baczko, Bronislaw, 'La Constitution de l'An III et la promotion culturelle du citoyen', in *L'Institution de la raison*, ed. François Azouvi (Paris, 1992), p.21-37.
–, 'L'expérience thermidorienne', in *The French Revolution and the creation of modern political culture: the political culture of the French Revolution*, ed. Colin Lucas (Oxford, 1988), p.341-70.
–, *Ending the Terror: the French Revolution after Robespierre*, translated by Michel Petheram (Cambridge, 1994).
Badinter, Elisabeth, *L'Amour en plus[.] Histoire de l'amour maternel (XVIIe-XXe siècle)* (Paris,1980).
Baecque, Antoine de, *Le Corps de l'histoire: métaphores et politique (1770-1800)* (Paris, 1993).
–, 'L'homme nouveau est arrivé. La 'régénération' du Français', *Dix-huitième siècle* 20 (1988), p.193-208.
–, *The Body politic. Corporeal metaphor in revolutionary France, 1770-1800*, translated by Charlotte Mandell (Stanford, CA, 1997).
Baldensperger, Fernand, 'Gessner en France', *Revue d'histoire littéraire de la France* 10 (1903), p.437-56.
Barthes, Roland, 'Les planches de l'"Encyclopédie"', in *Le Degré zéro*

de l'écriture suivi de nouveaux essais critiques (Paris, 1972), p.89-105.
Barton, Tamsyn, *Ancient astrology* (London and New York, 1994).
Becq, Annie, 'Expositions, peintres et critiques: vers l'image moderne de l'artiste', *Dix-huitième siècle* 14 (1982), p.131-48.
–, *Genèse de l'esthétique française moderne 1680-1814* (1984; Paris, 1994).
Benoît, François, *L'Art français sous la Révolution et l'Empire. Les doctrines, les idées, les genres* (Paris, 1897).
Benzaken, Jean-Charles, 'Hercule dans la Révolution française (1789-1799) ou les "nouveaux travaux d'Hercule"', in *Les Images de la Révolution française. Actes du colloque 25-27 octobre 1985*, ed. Michel Vovelle (Paris, 1988), p.203-14.
Bewick, Thomas, *History of British birds* (Newcastle, 1797; 1804).
Bilinski, Bronislaw, 'L'agonistica sportiva nella Grecia antica. Aspetti sociali e ispirazioni letterarie', *Accademia Polacca di Scienze e Lettere*: Conferenze: fascicolo 12 (Rome, 1960).
–, *Agoni ginnici. Componenti artistiche ed intellettuali nell'antica agonistica greca*, in *Conferenze dell'Accademia Polacca delle Scienze* (Rome, 1979).
Bindman, David, *Ape to Apollo: aesthetics and the idea of race in the eighteenth century* (London, 2003).
Blanckaert, Claude, 'La valeur de l'homme: l'idée de nature humaine chez Buffon', in *Buffon 88: actes du colloque international Paris-Montbard-Dijon*, ed. J. Gayon et al. (Paris, 1992), p.583-600.
Bleyl, Mathias, review of Philippe Bordes, *Le Serment du Jeu de Paume* (1983), *Kunstchronik* 38 (1985), p.384-88.
Bordes, Philippe, '"Brissotin enragé, ennemi de Robespierre": David, conventionnel et terroriste', in *David contre David [.] Actes du colloque organisé par le service culturel au musée du Louvre du 6 au 10 décembre 1989*, ed. Régis Michel (Paris, 1993), p.321-47.
–, *David* (Paris, 1988).
–, 'Le recours à l'allégorie dans l'art de la Révolution française', in *Les Images de la Révolution française*, ed. Michel Vovelle (Paris, 1988), p.243-49.
–, *Le Serment du Jeu de Paume de Jacques-Louis David* (Paris, 1983).
Bourdieu, Pierre, translated by Richard Nice, *Distinction: a social critique of the judgement of taste* (Cambridge, MA, 1984).
Boyer, F., 'Napoléon et l'attribution des grands prix décennaux (1810-1811)', *Bulletin de la société de l'histoire de l'art français* (1947-1948), p.66-72.
Brewer, John, *The Pleasures of the imagination: English culture in the eighteenth century* (London, 1997).
Brewer, John and Stella Tillyard, 'The moral vision of Thomas Bewick', in *The Medical world of early modern France*, ed. Laurence Brockliss and Colin Jones (Oxford, 1997), p. 375-408.
Bukdahl, Else-Marie, *Diderot critique d'art. II. Diderot, les salonniers et les esthéticiens de son temps*, translated by Jacques Piloz (Copenhagen, 1982).

Cabanis, Pierre Jean Georges, *Œuvres philosophiques de Cabanis*, ed. Claude Lehec and Jean Cazeneuve, 2 vols (Paris, 1956).
Cabuchet, François, *Essai sur l'expression de la face dans l'état de santé et de maladie, présenté à l'Ecole de Médecine de Paris, le 2 frimaire An 10* (Paris, An X-1801).
Chappey, Jean-Luc, 'Les idéologues face au coup d'état du 18 brumaire An VIII [.] Des illusions aux désillusions', *Politix* 14 (2001), p.55-75.
–, 'Le Portique républicain et les

enjeux de la mobilisation des arts autour de Brumaire An VIII', in *Les Arts de la scène et la Révolution française*, ed. Philippe Bourdin and Gérard Loubinoux (Clermont-Ferrand, 2004), p.487-507.

–, *La Société des observateurs de l'homme (1799-1804)[.] Des anthropologues aux temps de Bonaparte* (Paris, 2002).

Charlton, D. G., *New images of the natural in France: a study in European cultural history 1750-1800. The Gifford Lectures in the University of St Andrews 1982-83* (Cambridge, 1984).

Chartier, Roger, translated by Lydia G. Cochrane, *The Cultural origins of the French Revolution* (Durham and London, 1991).

Chatelus, Jean, *Peindre à Paris au XVIIIe siècle* (Paris, 1991).

Chaussard, P. J. B., *Le Pausanias français: état des arts du dessin en France à l'ouverture du XIXe siècle: Salon de 1806* (Paris, 1808).

[Chaussard, Publicola], *Fêtes et courtisanes de la Grèce: supplément aux voyages d'Anacharsis et d'Antenor*, 4 vols (Paris, An XI/1801).

Childs, Gilbert, *Understanding your temperament* (London, 1995).

Chouillet, Jacques, *La Formation des idées esthétiques de Diderot 1745-1763* (Paris, 1973).

Coleman, William, 'Health and hygiene in the *Encyclopédie*: a medical doctrine for the bourgeoisie', *Journal of the history of medicine and allied sciences* 29 (1974), p.399-421.

Correspondance littéraire, philosophique et critique, adressée à un souverain d'Allemagne, depuis 1753 jusqu'en 1769, par le baron Grimm et par Diderot. Première partie (1813).

Crow, Thomas E., *Painters and public life in eighteenth-century Paris* (New Haven, CT, and London, 1985).

Cuno, James (ed.), *French caricature and the French Revolution, 1789-1799* (Chicago, IL, 1988).

Davis, P., and J. Holmes, 'Thomas Bewick (1753-1828), engraver and ornithologist', *Archives of natural history* 20 (1993), p.167-84.

Delamétherie, J. C., *De l'Homme considéré moralement; de ses mœurs, et de celles des animaux*, 2 vols (Paris, an IX-1802).

Delpierre, Madeleine, 'A propos d'un manteau de représentant du peuple de 1798 récemment offert au Musée du Costume', *Bulletin du Musée Carnavalet* (1972), p.13-23.

Démoris, René, 'Les Passions en peinture au dix-huitième siècle', in *Le Siècle de Voltaire. Hommage à René Pomeau*, ed. C. Mervaud and S. Menant, 2 vols (Oxford, 1987), vol.1, p.381-92.

Dérodé-Géruzez. P. A., *Observations sur les monuments et établissements publics de la ville de Reims, sur les embellissements projétés et les améliorations dont ils sont susceptibles* (Reims, 1827).

Diderot, Denis, *Correspondance*, ed. Roth and Varloot (Paris, 1955-1970).

–, *Diderot on art*, translated by John Goodman, 2 vols (New Haven, CT, and London, 1995).

–, *Eléments de physiologie*, ed. Jean Mayer (Paris, 1964).

–, *Lettre sur les aveugles*, ed. R. Niklaus (Geneva, 1951).

–, *Œuvres completes*, ed. J. Assézat and M. Tourneux, 20 vols (Paris, 1875-1877).

–, *Œuvres esthétiques*, ed. P. Vernière (Paris, 1965).

Diderot & l'art de Boucher à David. Les Salons: 1759-1781 (Paris, 1984).

Dionysius Halicarnassensis, *De Isocrate Iudicium, in Dionysius of Halicarnassus. The critical essays*, ed. Stephen Usher (Cambridge MA and London, 1974).

Dowley, Francis H., 'D'Angiviller's *Grands hommes* and the significant moment', *Art bulletin* 39 (1957), p.259-77.

Doyle, William, *The Oxford history of the French Revolution* (Oxford, 1989).

Draper, James David and Guilhem Scherf, *Augustin Pajou royal sculptor 1730-1809* (New York, 1998).

Draper, James David and Guilhem Scherf, (ed.), *L'Esprit créateur de Pigalle à Canova. Terres cuites européennes 1740-1840* (Paris, 2003).

Duchesneau, François, 'Diderot et la physiologie de la sensibilité', *Dix-huitième siècle* 31 (1999), p.195-216.

Elias, Norbert, translated by Edmund Jephcott, *The Court society* (Oxford, 1983).

Eméric-David, T. B., *Recherches sur l'art statuaire considéré chez les anciens et chez les modernes* (1805; Paris, 1863).

Encyclopédie méthodique, ou par ordre de matières; par une société de gens de lettres, de savans et d'artistes. Médecine. Par une société de médecins, 13 vols (1792-1830).

Explication des ouvrages de peinture, sculpture, architecture et gravure, des Artistes vivans, exposés au Musée Napoléon, le 1er jour Complémentaire, An XII de la République française (an XII de la République/1804).

Fabre, Jean, *André Chénier. L'homme et l'œuvre* (Paris, 1955).

Fabre, Jean, 'L'article "Peuple" de l'"Encyclopédie" et le couple Coyer-Jaucourt', in Centre Aixois d'Études et de recherches sur le dix-huitième siècle, *Images du peuple au dix-huitième siècle (Colloque d'Aix-en-Provence 25 et 26 octobre 1969)* (1973), p.11-24.

Febvre, Lucien, 'Travail: évolution d'un mot et d'une idée', *Journal de psychologie* 21 (1948), p.19-29.

Feist, Peter H., 'Chodowieckis Calas', in *Ars Auro Prior, Studia Joanni Bialostocki Sexa genario dicata*, ed. Alijca Dyczek-Gwizdz (Warszawa, 1981), p.575-83.

Figlio, K. M., 'Theories of perception and the physiology of mind in the late eighteenth century', *History of science* 13 (1975), p.177-212.

Foissy-Aufrère, M.-P. and J. Cl. Martin, R. Michel, E. Pommier and M. Vovelle, *La Mort de Bara* (Avignon, 1989).

Foucault, Michel, *Birth of the clinic: an archaeology of medical perception*, translated by A. M. Sheridan Smith (London, 1988).

–, *Les Mots et les choses. Une archéologie des sciences humaines* (Paris, 1966).

Friederichs, C., *Amor mit dem Bogen des Herkules, Marmorstatue im Museum zu Berlin. Siebenundzwanzigstes Programm zum Winckelmannsfest der Archäologischen Gesellschaft zu Berlin* (Berlin, 1867).

Friedmann, Georges, 'L'*Encyclopédie* et le travail humain', *Annales economies sociétés civilisations* 8 (1953), p.53-61.

Fritz, Gérard, *L'Idée de peuple en France du XVII au XIXe siècles* (Strasbourg, 1988).

Furcy-Raynaud, Marc (ed.), 'Correspondance de M. d'Angiviller avec Pierre', *Nouvelles archives de l'art français*, 3e série, 21 (1905), 22 (1906).

–, 'Inventaire des sculptures exécutées au XVIIIe siècle pour la direction des bâtiments du Roi', *Archives de l'art français*, nouvelle série, 14 (1927).

Furet, François, *Interpreting the French Revolution* (Cambridge, 1981).

–, *Penser la Révolution française* (Paris, 1977).

Gaehtgens, Thomas W., 'La statue de Louis XIV et son programme iconographique', in *Place des Victoires: histoire, architecture, société*, ed. Isabelle Dubois, Alexandre Gady and Hendrik Ziegler (Paris, 2003), p.9-35.

Gagnebin, Bernard, 'La gravure de

"la malheureuse famille Calas"', *Gazette des Beaux-Arts* 1319 (1978), p.197-202.

Gainot, Bernard, *1799, un nouveau Jacobinisme?: la démocratie représentative, une alternative à brumaire* (Paris, 2001).

Galen, *Medicorum Graecorum opera quæ extant. Editionem curavit C. G. K. Gr. and Lat.*,ed. C. G. Kühn, 26 vols (Leipzig, 1821-1833).

Galen, Margaret Tallmadge May, ed. and translated by, *Galen on the usefulness of the parts of the body Peri chreias moríon De Usu partium*, 2 vols (Ithaca, NY, 1968).

Gardiner, E. Norman, *Athletics of the ancient world* (Oxford, 1980).

Garrioch, David, *Neighbourhood and community in Paris, 1740-1790* (Cambridge, 1986).

–, *The Formation of the Parisian Bourgeoisie 1690-1830* (Cambridge, MA, 1996).

Geffroy, Annie, 'Le peuple selon Robespierre', in *Peuple, plèbe, populace. Idées, représentations, quotidien de l'ancien régime au temps des Girondins*, Actes du colloque de Bordeaux, *Revue française d'histoire du livre* 66-67 (1990), p.213-26.

Gelbart, Nina R., 'The French Revolution as medical event: the journalistic gaze', *History of European ideas* 10 (1989), p.417-27.

Germer, Stefan, 'In search of a beholder: on the relation of art, audiences and social spheres in post-Thermidor France', *Art bulletin* 74 (1992), p.19-28.

Gilman, Sander L., *Seeing the insane* (1982; Lincoln and London, 1996).

Godechot, Jacques, *Les institutions de la France sous la Révolution et l'Empire* (Paris, 1951).

Goodden, Angelica, *Diderot and the body* (Oxford, 2001).

Gouhier, Henri, 'Le Refus du symbolisme dans l'humanisme cartésien', in *Umanesimo e simbolismo*, ed. E. Castelli (Padua, 1958), p.65-74.

Gramaccini, Gisela, 'L'image de l'homme nouveau [.] Exemples de la sculpture publique à la fin de l'*ancien régime* et à l'époque révolutionnaire', in *La Révolution française et les processus de socialisation de l'homme moderne* (Rouen and Paris, 1989), p.675-89.

–, 'Sur le projet d'élever un monument en l'honneur de Rousseau', in *La Révolution française et l'Europe 1789-99*, 3 vols (Paris, 1989), vol.3, p.893-97.

Guédron, Martial, *De Chair et de marbre: imiter et exprimer le nu en France, 1745-1815* (Paris, 2003).

Guilhaumou, Jacques, 'Le peuple est-il divisible en classes? A propos du débat sur "la division des intérêts de classe" (1789-1793)', in *Peuple, plèbe, populace: idées, représentations, quotidien de l'ancien régime au temps des Girondins : actes du colloque organisé du 12 au 14 mai 1989, Centre interdisciplinaire bordelais d'étude des Lumières*, ed. Anne-Marie Cocula and Jean Mondot (Bordeaux, 1993), p.161-71.

Halliday, Tony, *Facing the public: portraiture in the aftermath of the French Revolution* (Manchester and New York, 2000).

Halperin, David M., 'Forgetting Foucault: acts, identities and the history of sexuality', *Representations* 63 (1998), p.93-120.

Hargrove, June (ed.), *The French Academy: classicism and its antagonists* (Newark and London, 1990).

Haskell, Francis and Nicholas Penny, *Taste and the antique: the lure of classical sculpture 1500-1900* (New Haven, CT, and London, 1983).

Heinich, Nathalie, *Du Peintre à l'artiste. Artisans et académiciens à l'âge classique* (Paris, 1993).

Helman, Cecil G., 'Feed a cold, starve a fever – folk models of infection in an English suburban community, and their relation to medical treatment', *Culture, medicine and psychiatry* 2 (1978), p.107-37.

Hellmuth, Eckhard (ed.), *The Transformation of political culture: England and Germany in the late eighteenth century* (Oxford, 1990), p.375-408.

Henry, C., *Mémoires inédits de Charles-Nicolas Cochin sur le Comte de Caylus, Bouchardon, les Slodtz* (Paris, 1880).

Hesse, Carla, *The Other Enlightenment: how French women became modern* (Princeton, NJ, and Oxford, 2001).

Hibberd, John, *Salomon Gessner. His creative achievement and influence* (Cambridge, 1976).

Higonnet, Patrice, 'Sans-culottes', in *Dictionnaire critique de la Révolution française*, ed. François Furet and Mona Ozouf (Paris, 1988), p.418-24.

Hippocrates, *Aphorisms* (Hippocratic Writings) (London, 1983), p.206-36.

–, *De Natura Hominis* (Hippocratic Writings) (London, 1983), p.260-71.

Hogarth, William, *Works* (London, 1838).

Hould, Claudette, (ed.), *L'Image de la Révolution française* (Quebec, 1989).

Hunt, Lynn, 'Freedom of dress in revolutionary France', in *From the Royal to the republican body: incorporating the political in seventeenth- and eighteenth-century France*, ed. Sara E. Melzer and Kathryn Norberg (Los Angeles, 1998), p.224-49.

–, *Politics, culture, & class in the French Revolution* (Los Angeles and London, 1984).

Hunt, Lynn, David Lansky, and Paul Hanson, 'The failure of the liberal republic in France, 1795-1799: the road to Brumaire', *Journal of modern history* 51 (1979), p.734-59.

Janson, Horst W., 'Observations on nudity in neoclassical art', in *Stil und Überlieferung in der Kunst des Abendlandes. Akten des 21 Internationalen Kongresses für Kunstgeschichte in Bonn 1964* (Berlin, 1967), vol.1, p.198-207.

Jaume, Lucien, 'Necker: examen critique de la Constitution de l'An III' in *La Constitution de l'An III [.] Boissy d'Anglas et la naissance du libéralisme constitutionnel*, ed. Gérard Conac and Jean-Pierre Machelon (Paris, 1999), p.167-82.

Jobert, Berthélemy, 'The "Travaux d'encouragement": an aspect of official arts policy in France under Louis XVI', *Oxford art journal* 10 (1987), p.3-14.

Johnson, Dorothy, *Jacques-Louis David: art in metamorphosis* (Princeton, NJ, 1993).

Jones, Colin, 'Bourgeois revolution revivified: 1789 and social change', in *Rewriting the French Revolution*, ed. Colin Lucas (Oxford, 1991), p.69-118.

–, *The Great nation: France from Louis XV to Napoleon* (London, 2002).

Jones, H. Stuart (ed.), *A Catalogue of the ancient sculptures preserved in the municipal collections of Rome. The sculptures of the Museo Capitolino* (Oxford, 1912).

Jordanova, Ludmilla (ed.), *Languages of nature: critical essays on science and literature* (London, 1986).

–, 'Natural facts: a historical perspective on science and sexuality', in *Nature, culture and gender*, ed. Carol MacCormack and Marilyn Strathern (Cambridge, 1980).

–, 'Sex and gender', in *Inventing human science: eighteenth-century domains*, ed. Christopher Fox, Roy Porter and Robert Wokler

(Berkley, CA, and London, 1995), p.166-69.

Junius, Franciscus, *The Literature of classical art, 2: A lexicon of artists & their works*, ed. and translated by Keith Aldrich, Philipp Fehl and Raina Fehl (Berkeley, CA, 1991).

Kaitaro, T., *Diderot's holism. Philosophical anti-reductionism and its medical background* (Frankfurt, 1997).

Kant, Immanuel, translated by Werner S. Pluhar, *Critique of pure judgement* (Indianapolis, IN, and Cambridge, 1987).

–, translated by John T. Goldthwait, *Observations on the feeling of the beautiful and sublime* (1959; Berkeley, CA, Los Angeles and London, 2003).

Klibansky, Raymond, Erwin Panofsky and Fritz Saxl, *Saturn and melancholy. Studies in the history of natural philosophy, religion, and art* (London, 1964).

Knibiehler, Yvonne, 'Les médecins et la "nature feminine" au temps du Code Civil', *Annales economies sociétés civilisations* 31 (1976), p.824-45.

Koepp, Cynthia J., 'The alphabetical order: work in Diderot's *Encyclopédie*', in *Work in France: representation, meaning, organisation and practice*, ed. Stephen Kaplan and Cynthia Koepp (Ithaca, NY, and London, 1986), p.229-57.

Kunzle, David, 'Plagiaries-by-memory of the *Rake's progress* and the genesis of Hogarth's second picture story', *The Journal of the Warburg and Courtauld Institutes* 29 (1966), p.311-48.

Lajer-Burcharth, Ewa, *Necklines: the art of Jacques-Louis David after the Terror* (New Haven, CT, and London, 1999).

Laqueur, Thomas, *Making sex: body and gender from the Greeks to Freud* (Cambridge, MA, 1990).

Laveissière, Sylvain, *Prud'hon. La justice et la vengeance divine poursuivant le crime* (Paris, 1986).

Lefebvre, Georges, translated by Elizabeth Moss Evanson, *The French Revolution from its origins to 1793* (London, 1962; 2001).

Leftwich, Gregory V., 'Polykleitos and Hippocratic medicine', in *Polykleitos, the Doryphorus and tradition*, ed. Warren G. Moon (Madison, WI, 1995), p.38-51.

Leith, J. A., 'Allégorie et symbole dans la Révolution française', in *L'Image de la Révolution française*, ed. Claudette Hould (Montreal, 1989), p.95-113.

Lenoir, Alexandre, *Concours pour les prix décennaux. Peinture. Examen du tableau des Sabines et de l'école de M. David, Premier Peintre de sa Majesté l'Empéreur et Roi, Chevalier de l'Empire, Officier de la Légion d'Honneur, Membre de l'Institut de France* (1810).

Le Normand, Antoinette, *La Tradition classique et l'esprit romantique. Les sculpteurs de l'Académie de France à Rome de 1824 à 1840* (Rome, 1981).

Lucian, *Hercules gallicus*, in *Works*, translated by A.M. Harmon, 8 vols (London, 1927), vol.2.

LeMay, Edna Hindie, '"Peuple" dans le discours des Constituants 1789/91' in *Peuple, plèbe, populace. Idées, représentations, quotidien de l'ancien régime au temps des Girondins, Actes du colloque de Bordeaux, Revue française d'histoire du livre*, 66-67 (1990), p.203-12.

Lepeletier [*sic*] Saint-Fargeau, Michel, ed. Félix Lepeletier, *Œuvres* (Paris, 1826).

Locquin, Jean, *La Peinture d'histoire en France de 1747 à 1785* (Paris, 1912; 1978).

Lordat, Jacques, *Exposition de la doctrine médicale de P.-J. Barthez, et mémoires sur la vie de ce médecin* (Paris, 1818).

Lucas, Colin, 'The crowd and politics between *ancien régime* and revolution in France', in *The Rise and fall of the French Revolution*, ed. T. C. W. Blanning (Chicago, IL, and London, 1996), p.199-235 (originally published in *The Political culture of the French Revolution* (Oxford, 1988), p.259-85).

–, 'Nobles, bourgeois and the origins of the French Revolution', *Past and present* 60 (1973), p.84-126.

Lyons, Martyn, *France under the Directory* (Cambridge, 1975).

Mainz, Valerie, *L'Image du travail et la Révolution française* (Vizille, 1999), p.203-208.

–, 'David's *Les Sabines* and the colouring of history painting post Thermidor', *Interfaces* 10 (1996), p.47-59 (50-54).

Manuel, Frank E., 'From equality to organicism', in *Freedom from history, and other untimely essays* (London, 1972).

Marion de Procé, P. M., *Quelques Vues générales sur les doctrines des tempéraments, et sur le tempérament lymphatique en particulier; thèse présentée et soutenue à la Faculté de Médecine de Paris; le 11 août 1812* (Paris, 1812).

–, 'Sur plusieurs espèces nouvelles de poissons et de crustacés observées dans un voyage de France à Manille', *Bulletin de la société philomathique de Paris*, 1822, sér. 3, vol.9, p.129-34.

Mattick, Paul, *Art in its time: theories and practices of modern aesthetics* (London and New York, 2003).

Mayer, Jean, *Diderot, homme de science* (Rennes, 1959).

Maza, Sarah, *Private lives and public affairs: the causes célèbres of pre-revolutionary France* (Berkeley, CA, Los Angeles and London, 1993).

Mazauric, Claude, *La Révolution française et les processus de socialisation de l'homme* (Rouen and Paris, 1989).

McClellan, Andrew, 'D'Angiviller's great men and the politics of the Parlement', *Art history* 13 (1990), p.175-92.

Melot, Michel, 'Caricature and the Revolution', in *French caricature and the French Revolution*, ed. James Cuno (Chicago, IL, 1988) p.25-32.

Mercier, Louis Sébastien, *Le Nouveau Paris*, ed. Jean-Claude Bonnet (Paris, 1994).

Merrick, Jeffrey, 'Politics on pedestals: royal monuments in eighteenth-century France', *French history* 5 (1991), p.234-65.

Merrick, Jeffrey and Bryant T. Ragan, Jr (ed.), *Homosexuality in early modern France: a documentary collection* (Oxford, 2001).

Métraux, Guy P. R., *Sculptors and physicians in fifth-century Greece. A preliminary study* (Montreal and Kingston, 1995).

Michaelis, Adolf, 'Tre Statue Policletee', *Annali dell'Instituto di Correspondenza Archeologica* 50 (1878), p.7.

Michel, Régis, *Le Beau idéal* (Paris, 1989).

–, 'Diderot and modernity', *Oxford art journal* 7 (1985), p.36-51.

–, 'Diderot et la modernité', in *Diderot et l'art de Boucher à David* (Paris, 1984), p. 110-21.

Michel, Régis, Arlette Sérullaz, Udolpho van de Sandt, *David e Roma* (Rome, 1981).

Mitchell, Harvey, 'Rationality and control in French eighteenth-century medical views of the peasantry', *Comparative studies in society and history* 21 (1979), p.81-112.

Montagu, Jennifer, *The Expression of the passions: the origin and influence of Charles Lebrun's Conférence sur l'expression générale et particulière* (New Haven, CT, and London, 1994).

Montesquieu, Charles-Louis de Secondat, baron de La Brède et de, *Œuvres complètes* (Paris, 1949).

Moravia, Sergio, *Filosofia e scienze umane nell'età dei lumi* (1982; Florence, 2000).

–, *Il Pensiero degli Idéologues: scienza e filosofia in Francia (1780-1815)* (Florence, 1974).

–, *Il tramonto dell'illuminismo: filosofia e politica nella società francese (1770-1810)* (Bari, 1968).

Moreau (de la Sarthe), J. L., *Histoire naturelle de la femme, suivie d'un traité d'hygiène appliqué à son régime physique et moral aux différentes époques de la vie* (Paris, 1803).

Mortier, Roland, 'Diderot et la notion de peuple', *Europe* 1 (1963), p.78-88.

Mouilleseaux, Jean-Pierre, 'David: a classical painter against the Academy and a teacher of the French school', in *The French Academy: classicism and its antagonists*, ed. June Hargrove (Newark, NJ, and London, 1990), p.131-39.

Muller, Christian Alain, 'Du "peuple égaré" au "peuple enfant" [.] Le discours politique révolutionnaire à l'épreuve de la révolte populaire en 1793', *Revue d'histoire moderne et contemporaine* 47 (2000), p.93-112.

Nutton, Vivian, 'Humoralism', in *Companion encyclopedia of the history of medicine*, 2 vols, ed. W. F. Bynum and Roy Porter (London, 1993), vol.1, p.281-91.

Ozouf, Mona, translated by Alan Sheridan, *Festivals and the French Revolution* (Cambridge, MA, and London, 1988) (French edition, 1976).

Panofsky, Erwin, 'The history of the theory of human proportions as a reflection of the history of styles', in *Meaning in the visual arts* (New York, 1955).

–, *Idea: a concept in art theory* (New York and London, 1968).

Paulson, Ronald, *Hogarth's graphic works* 3rd revised edn (London, 1989).

Percival, Melissa, *The Appearance of character: physiognomy and facial expression in eighteenth-century France* (Leeds, 1999).

Pertué, Michel, 'La représentation des citoyens dans les institutions révolutionnaires', in *La Révolution française et le processus de socialisation de l'homme moderne (Colloque international de Rouen 13, 14 et 15 Octobre 1988)*, ed. Claude Mazauric (Rouen, 1989), p.85-93.

Pigeaud, Jackie, *L'Art et le vivant* (Paris, 1995).

–, 'Cabanis et les rapports du physique et du moral', *Revue médicale de la Suisse Romande* 106 (1986), p.47-59.

–, 'L'esthétique de Galien', *Métis* 6 (1991), p.7-42.

–, 'Homo quadratus. Variations sur la beauté et la santé dans la médecine antique', *Gesnerus* 42 (1985), p.337-52.

Piguet, Marie-France, *Classe, histoire du mot et genèse du concept des physiocrates aux historiens de la Restauration* (Lyons, 1996).

Pindar, *Nemean odes, isthian ode, fragments*, translated by William H. Race (Harvard, 1997).

Plato, *The Republic*, translated by Desmond Lee (London, 2007).

Pliny the Elder, *The Elder Pliny's chapters on the history of art, translated by K. Jex-Blake with commentary and historical introduction by E. Sellers* (Oxford, 1896).

Pollitt, J. J., *The Ancient view of Greek art: criticism, history and terminology* (New Haven, CT, and London, 1974).

Pommier, Edouard, *L'art de la liberté:*

doctrines et débats de la Révolution française (Paris, 1991).
–, 'De l'art libéral à l'art de la liberté: le débat sur la patente des artistes sous la Révolution et ses antécédents dans l'ancienne théorie de l'art', *Bulletin de la société de l'histoire de l'art français* 1992, p.147-67.
–, 'Rêver devant l'antique un Winckelmann à la main', in *La Mort de Bara* (Avignon, 1989), p.78-81.
–, 'Winckelmann et la vision de l'antiquité classique dans la France des Lumières et de la Révolution', *Revue de l'art* 83 (1989), p.9-20.
Potts, Alex, *Flesh and the ideal: Winckelmann and the origins of art history* (New Haven, CT, and London, 1994).
–, 'Natural order and the call of the wild: the politics of animal picturing', *Oxford art journal* 13 (1990), p.12-33.
–, 'De Winckelmann à David: l'incarnation des idéaux politiques', in *David contre David*, ed. R. Michel, p.647-69.
Poulet, Anne L. and Guilhem Scherf, *Clodion 1738-1814* (Paris, 1992).
–, *Houdon sculpteur des Lumières 1741-1828* (Paris, 2003).
Pressly, Nancy L., *The Fuseli circle in Rome* (London, 1979).
Proust, Jacques, *Diderot et l'Encyclopédie* (Paris, 1962).
–, 'L'image du peuple au travail dans les planches de l'"*Encyclopédie*"' in Centre Aixois d'Études et de Recherches sur le dix-huitième siècle, *Images du peuple au dix-huitième siècle (Colloque d'Aix-en-Provence 25 et 26 octobre 1969* (Paris, 1973), p.65-86.
Pupil, François, *Le Style troubadour ou la nostalgie du bon vieux temps* (Nancy, 1985).

Quatremère de Quincy, Antoine Chrysostome, *Essai sur la nature, le but et les moyens de l'initation dans les beaux-arts* (Paris, 1825).
Quintilian, translated by Donald A. Russell, *The Orator's education* (Cambridge, MA, and London, 2001).

Ragan Jr, Bryant T., 'The Enlightenment confronts homosexuality', in *Homosexuality in modern France*, ed. Jeffrey Merrick and Bryant T. Ragan Jr (New York and Oxford, 1996), p.8-29.
Rapports et discussions de toutes les classes de l'Institut de France, sur les ouvrages admis au concours pour les Prix décennaux (1810).
Régaldo, Marc, 'Profil perdu: l'idéologue Chaussard', in *Approches des lumières. Mélanges offerts à Jean Fabre* (Paris, 1974), p.381-401.
Renouvier, Jules, *Histoire de l'art pendant la Révolution, considéré principalement dans les estampes* (Paris, 1863).
Rey, Roselyne, 'La transmission du savoir médical', in François Azouvi, *L'Institution de la raison: la révolution culturelle des idéologues* (Paris, 1992), p.129-49.
Rey, Roselyne, 'Diderot et les sciences de la vie dans l'Encyclopédie', *Recherches sur Diderot et sur l'Encyclopédie* 18-19 (1995), p.47-53.
Ribeiro, Aileen, *Fashion in the French Revolution* (London, 1988).
Richerand, Balthasar Anthelme, *Nouveaux élémens de physiologie*, 4th edn (Paris, 1807).
Rippere, Vicky, 'The survival of traditional medicine in lay medical views: an empirical approach to the history of medicine', *Medical history* 25 (1981), p.411-14.
Robespierre, Maximilien, *Œuvres complètes de Maximilien Robespierre*, 10 vols (Paris, 1910-1967).

Robespierre, Claude Mazauric, (ed.), *Robespierre. Ecrits* (Paris, 1989).
Roche, Daniel, translated by Marie Evans in association with Gwynne Lewis, *The People of Paris. An essay in popular culture in the 18th century* (Leamington Spa, 1987), p.36-63.
Rocheblave, S., *Jean-Baptiste Pigalle* (Paris, 1919).
Roederer, P. L., *Œuvres*, ed. Baron A. M., 8 vols (Paris, 1853-1859).
Roger, Jacques, *Les Sciences de la vie dans la pensée française du XVIIIe siècle. La génération des animaux de Descartes à l'Encyclopédie* (Paris, 1963).
Rosanvallon, Pierre, *Le Sacre du citoyen. Histoire du suffrage universel en France* (Paris, 1992).
Roscher, Wilhelm, *Ausführliches Lexikon der griechischen und römischen Mythologie* (Leipzig, 1886-1890).
Rosen, Charles and Henri Zerner, *Romanticism and realism: the mythology of nineteenth-century art* (New York and London, 1984).
Rosenberg, Pierre, and Louis-Antoine Prat, *Jacques-Louis David 1748-1825: catalogue raisonné des dessins* (Milan, 2002).
Rousseau, G. S., and R. Porter (ed.), *The Ferment of knowledge* (Cambridge, 1980).
Rousseau, Jean-Jacques, *Du Contrat social ou principes du droit politique* (Paris, 1962).
Rudolph, Gerhard, 'La méthode Hallérienne en physiologie', *Dix-huitième siècle* 23 (1991), p.75-84.

Sabatier, Gérard, *Versailles ou la figure du roi* (Paris, 1999).
Sarazin, Charles, 'La Place Royale de Reims', in *Travaux de l'Académie Nationale de Reims*, 128, année 1909-10 (Rheims, 1911), p.1-162.
Scherf, Guilhem, 'La galerie des "Grands hommes" au cœur des salles consacrées à la sculpture française du XVIIIe siècle', *Revue du Louvre* 5-6 (1993), p.58-67.
Scherf, Guilhem, and Gilles Grandjean (ed.), *Pierre Julien 1731-1804* (Le Puy-en-Velay, 2004).
Schlanger, Judith E., 'Le peuple au front gravé (1793)', in *Les Fêtes de la Révolution. Colloque de Clermont-Ferrand (juin 1974)*, ed. Jean Ehrard and Paul Viallaneix (Paris, 1977), p.387-95.
Schnapper, Antoine, 'Les académies peintes et le "Christ en croix" de David', *Revue du Louvre* 6 (1974), p.381-92.
Schnapper, Antoine and Arlette Sérullaz, *Jacques-Louis David 1748-1825* (Paris, 1989).
Scott, Katie, 'Under the sign of Venus: the making and meaning of Bouchardon's *L'Amour* in the age of the French Rococo', in *Manifestations of Venus: art and sexuality*, ed. Caroline Arscott and Katie Scott (Manchester, 2000), p.69-89.
Scott, Katie and Genevieve Warwick (ed.), *Commemorating Poussin: reception and intrepretation of the artist* (Cambridge, 1999).
Sears, Elizabeth, *The Ages of man: medieval interpretations of the life cycle* (Princeton, NJ, 1986).
Seelig, Lorenz, *Studien zu Martin van den Bogaert gen. Desjardins* (Munich, 1980).
Seneca, *Epistulae morales, in Letters from a stoic* (London, 1969).
Sennett, Richard, *Flesh and stone: the body and the city in western civilization* (London, 1994).
Sewell, William H. Jr, *Work and revolution in France: language and labour from the old regime to 1848* (Cambridge, 1980).
Seznec, Jean, *Essais sur Diderot et l'antiquité: the Mary Flexner lectures delivered at Bryn Mawr College, Pennsylvania* (Oxford, 1957).
–, *La Survivance des dieux antiques. Essai sur le rôle de la tradition mythologique dans l'humanisme et dans l'art de la Renaissance*, Studies

of the Warburg Institute, XI (London, 1940).

Sicault, Michèle and Marc Bouloiseau, 'La notion de "peuple" dans la correspondance de Blin de Sainmore avec la grande-duchesse Marie-Feodorovna 1787-1791', *Images du peuple au dix-huitième siècle (Colloque d'Aix-en-Provence 25 et 26 octobre 1969)* (Paris, 1973), p.47.

Sieyès, Emmanuel Joseph (ed.), Michael Sonenscher, *Political writings including the debate between Sieyès and Tom Paine in 1791* (Indianapolis and Cambridge, 2003).

–, (ed.), Roberto Zapperi, *Ecrits politiques* (1985; Brussels, 1994).

Simonsuuri, Kirsti, *Homer's original genius: eighteenth-century notions of the early Greek epic (1688-1798)* (Cambridge, 1979).

Singer, Brian C. J., *Society, theory and the French Revolution* (London, 1986).

Smith, Adam, (ed.), Andrew Skinner, *The Wealth of nations* (1776; Oxford, 1978).

Solkin, David (ed.), *Art on the line: The Royal Academy exhibitions at Somerset House 1780-1836* (New Haven, CT, and London, 2001).

Sonenscher, Michael, *Sans-culottes: an eighteenth-century emblem in the French Revolution* (Oxford, 2009).

–, *Work and wages: natural law, politics and the eighteenth-century French trades* (Cambridge, 1989).

Spitz, J. F., *L'Amour de l'égalité. Essai sur la critique de l'égalitarisme républicain en France 1770-1830* (Paris, 2000).

Staël, Baroness de, *Considerations on the principal events of the French Revolution* [...] *translated from the original manuscript*, 3 vols (London, 1818).

Staum, Martin S., *Cabanis: Enlightenment and medical philosophy in the French Revolution* (Princeton, NJ, 1980).

–, *Minerva's message. Stabilizing the French Revolution* (Montreal, 1996).

Steiner, Deborah Tarn, *Images in mind: statues in archaic and classical Greek literature and thought* (Princeton, NJ, and Oxford, 2001).

Steiner, Rudolf, translated by D. S. Osmond, *The Four temperaments. A lecture given during the winter of 1908-09* (London, 1929; 1949).

Stewart, Andrew, 'The *Canon* of Polykleitos: a question of evidence', *Journal of Hellenic studies* 98 (1978), p.122-31.

–, *Greek sculpture: an exploration*, 2 vols (New Haven, CT, and London, 1990).

Suratteau, J. R., *Les Elections de l'An VI et le "coup d'état du 22 floréal" (11 mai 1798): étude documentaire, statistique et analytique Essai d'interprétation* (Paris, 1971).

Taillasson, J. J., *Observations sur quelques grands peintres, dans lesquelles on cherche à fixer les caractères distinctifs de leur talent, avec un précis de leur vie* (Paris, 1807).

Temkin, O., *Galenism: rise and decline of a medical philosophy* (Ithaca, NY, and London, 1973).

Teysseire, Daniel, 'Lien social et ordre politique chez Cabanis', *SVEC* 267 (1989), p.353-400.

Teysseire, 'Eugénisme et euthanasie chez Cabanis', *Transactions of the eighth international congress on the Enlightenment* (1992), p.272-75.

Theremin, Wilhelm, *De l'Incompatibilité du système démagogique avec le système d'économie politique des peuples modernes* (Paris, an VIII-1800).

Thomas, Keith, *Man and the natural world: changing attitudes in England 1500-1800* (Oxford, 1983).

–, *Religion and the decline of magic: studies in popular beliefs in sixteenth-*

and seventeenth-century England (1971; Oxford 1991).
–, 'Work and leisure in pre-industrial society', *Past and present* 29 (1964), p.50-62.
Thorndike, Lynn, 'De Complexionibus', *Isis* 49 (1958), p.398-408.
–, *The History of magic and experimental science*, 8 vols (New York, 1923-1958).
Toellner, Richard, 'Logical and psychological aspects of the discovery of the circulation of the blood', in *On Scientific discovery: the Erice Lectures 1977*, ed. Mirko Grmek, Robert S. Cohen and Guido Cimino (Dordrecht and London, 1981), p.239-59.
Tulard, Jean, *Le 18 Brumaire: comment terminer une Révolution* (Mesnil-sur-l'Estrée, 1999).

Van de Sandt, Udolpho, 'The Death of Bara', *FMR* 39 (1989), p.51-57.
–, '"Grandissima opera del pittore sarà l'istoria". Notes sur la hiérarchie des genres sous la Révolution', *Revue de l'art* 83 (1989), p.71-76.
–, 'Institutions et concours', in *Aux Armes et aux arts! Les arts de la Révolution 1789-1799*, ed. Philippe Bordes and Régis Michel (Paris, 1988), p.137-65.
–, (ed.), *Rapports à l'Empereur sur le progrès des sciences, des lettres et des arts depuis 1789. V. Beaux-arts* (Paris, 1989).
Veillon, Marie, 'L'iconographie métallique d'Hercule dans la France du seizième siècle', *The Medal* 46 (2005), p.31-40.
Verdi, Richard, *Nicolas Poussin 1594-1665* (London, 1995).
–, 'Poussin's *Eudamidas*: eighteenth-century criticism and copies', *Burlington magazine* 113 (1971), p.513-24.
Vila, Anne C., *Enlightenment and pathology: sensibility in the literature and medicine of eighteenth-century France* (Baltimore, MD, and London, 1998).
Virey, J. J., 'De l'emploi des caractères d'histoire naturelle et de physiologie humaine dans la peinture; par J. J. Virey du Val-de Grâce', *Magasin encyclopédique, ou Journal des sciences, des lettres et des arts*, rédigé par A. L. Millin. VIe année, an VIII-1800, p.159.
–, *Histoire naturelle du genre humain. Nouvelle édition*, 3 vols (Paris, 1824).
Vissière, Isabelle, 'L'emancipation du peuple selon Condorcet', *Images du peuple au dix-huitième siècle* (Paris, 1973), p.205.
Vivanti, Corrado, 'Henry IV, the Gallic Hercules', in *Journal of the Warburg and Courtauld Institutes* 30 (1967), p.176-97.
Vitruvius, translated by Morris Hickey Morgan, *The Ten books of architecture* (1914; New York, 1960).
Vitry, Paul, 'Une maquette du *Citoyen* de Pigalle', *Bulletin des Musées de France* 11 (1929), p.242-43.
Volney, C. F., *Œuvres complètes* (Paris, 1837).
Vovelle, Michel, 'Child heroes of the Revolution', *FMR* 39 (1989), p.51-64.

West, Alison, *From Pigalle to Préault: neoclassicism and the sublime in French sculpture, 1760-1840* (Cambridge, 1998).
Whinney, Margaret, *Sculpture in Britain 1530-1830* (London, 1964).
Wildenstein, D. and G., *Documents complémentaires au catalogue de l'œuvre de Louis David* (Paris, 1973).
Williams, Elizabeth A., *The Physical and the moral: anthropology, physiology, and philosophical medicine in France, 1750-1850* (Cambridge, 1994).
Williams, Helen Maria, *Sketches of the state of manners and opinions in the French Republic, towards the close of*

the eighteenth century. In a series of letters, 2 vols (London, 1801).

Winckelmann, J. J. translated by. G. Henry Lodge, *The History of ancient art*, 2 vols ([s.l.] 1881).

Wrigley, Richard, *The Origins of French art criticism: from the ancien régime to the Restoration* (Oxford, 1993).

–, *The Politics of appearances: representations of dress in revolutionary France* (Oxford, 2002).

Index

Adam, 37, 43, 44, 178
Aesculapius, 106, 115
Agrippina, 94
Alembert, Jean Le Rond d', 35, 44, 198
Amaury-Duval, 229, 232
Anacreon, 121
Angiviller, Charles Claude de la Billarderie, Comte d', 142, 143, 149
Apollo, 106
Apollo Belvedere, 22, fig.6 (25), 40, 95, 98, 108, 115, 153, 172, 212, 224
Aristophanes, *Frogs*, 211
Aristotle, 52, 56
Athens, 121
Attenborough, David, 15
Audran, Girard, 100, 103

Babeuf, Gracchus, 192, 228
Bacchus, 106
Bailly, Jean Sylvain, 153
Bara, 166, 167, 168, 170
Barère de Vieuzac, Bertrand, 139, 170, 182
Barnave, Antoine Pierre Joseph Marie, 17, 151, 153
Bedlam, 136
Belvedere Antinous, 22, fig.8 (27), 29, 37, 40, 95, 110, 115
Belvedere torso, 108, fig.20 (109), 110, 196, 220
Bewick, Thomas, 2, 7, 8, 9, 10, 11, fig.1 (12), fig.2 (13), 14, 16, 38, 205
Boeotia (Greece), 71
Boerhaave, Herman, 62, 63, 79
Boissy d'Anglas, François Antoine de, 190, 191, 192, 197
Bonaparte, Napoleon, *see* Napoleon
Borghese gladiator, 22, fig.9 (28)
Bordes, Philippe, 153, 162, 163, 167
Bordeu, Théophile de, 46
Bouchardon, Edmé, 17,
Love making himself a bow from the club of Hercules, fig.4 (19), 20, 22, 23, 29, 30, 32, 33, 38, 42, 96, 99, 105, 110, 111, 120, 164, 176, 180
Bourdieu, Pierre, 87
Brotier, Gabriel, 98
Brown, Stephanie, 171n
Buffon, George Louis Leclerc, comte de, 10, 13, 14, 33, 35, 39, 43, 46, 64, 142
Burke, Edmund, *Philosophical inquiry into our ideas of the sublime and beautiful*, 74, 75, 76

Cabanis, Piere Jean Georges, 1, 4, 71, 198-218 *passim*, 225, 233, 234
Cacault, Pierre-René, 183
Calamis, 106
Calas, Jean, 80, 85
Callimachus, 106
Cambacérès, Jean-Jacques Régis de, 215
Camper, Petrus, 95
Campiglia, Giovannovi Domenico, fig.7 (26)
Carmontelle, Louis de, *La Malheureuse famille Calas*, 81, 83
Casanova, Giacomo Girolamo, 63, 78
Cassini, Giovanni Maria, 145, 149
Caylus, Tubières de Grimouard de Pestels de Levis, Anne Claude Philippe, comte de, 23
Celsus, 71, 97
Champagne, 111
Chaudet, Antoine-Denis, 158, 163
Chaussard, Jean-Baptiste (Publicola), 5, 221, 228, 230, 233
Chénier, André, 131, 210
Chénier, Marie-Joseph Blaise de, 131
Chodowiecki, Daniel, *Les Adieux de Calas à sa famille*, 80, fig.14 (82), 84, 85, 86
Chrysippus, 90
Cibber, Caius Gabriel, 134
Cicero, 105

Clodion, Claude Michel, 143, 149
Montesquieu, fig.29 (144), 172
Committee of General Security, 154
Committee of Public Instruction, 154
Committee of Public Safety, 192
Condillac, Etienne Bonnot de, 31, 63, 209
Correspondance littéraire, 38, 81, 111, 113
Crow, T. E., 114
Cullen, William, 200
Cuvier, Georges, 65

Danton, Georges Jacques, 162
Dauch, Martin, 151
David, Jacques-Louis, 13, 114, 141, 150, 166, 182
Catherine-Marie-Jeanne Tallard, 171n
The Death of Bara, 3, fig.37 (169), 171, 172, 180-81, 183
Intervention of the Sabine women, 4, 5, 171n, 221-36, fig.45 (222), fig.46 (231)
Madame Trudaine (*Madame Chalgrin*), 171
Marat, 171, 176
Oath of the tennis court, 3, 137, fig.27 (138), 139, fig.28 (140), 141, 142, 150, 151, fig.33 (152), 154, 155, 157, 158, 163
Triumph of the French people, 3, 158, fig.35 (160), fig.36 (161), 165, 170, 171, 197
De Baecque, Antoine, 137, 151
Defoe, Daniel, *Robinson Crusoe*, 76, 78
Delafosse, Jean-Baptiste, 83
Delamétherie, Jean-Claude, 63, 64, 65, 66, 77
Descartes, René, 58, 63, 69, 87
Deschamps, 197
Desjardins, 58, 59, figs.10-13 (60, 61), 77, 84, 111, 115, 164
De Staël, Germaine, 122, 123, 150, 155, 181
Diadumenos, 90, fig.17 (92), 95, 96
Diderot, Denis, 1, 2, 17, 23, 29, 31, 32, 33, 34, 36, 39, 40, 41, 43, 46, 47, 48, 49, 51, 58, 76, 78, 79, 95, 110, 113, 114, 115, 129, 178, 198, 206
Dijon, 209
Dionysius of Hallicarnassus, 107
Doryphorus, 90, fig.16 (92), 94, 95, 96
Dürer, Albrecht, *Melancholia I*, 116, fig.22 (118)
Dying Gaul, 22, fig.40 (175)
Dying gladiator, 172

Elias, Norbert, 77
Encyclopédie, 22, 35, 41, 44, 45, 48, 62, 96, 157, 198
Espercieux, Jean-Joseph, 182, 183, 184, 187, 188
Estates General, 122
Euripides *Alcestis*, 211
Eve, 178

Farnese Hercules, 22, fig.5 (24), 42, 99, 100, 107, 115, 197, 212
Fea, Carlo, 106, 107
Festival of Supreme Being, 166
Foucault, Michel, 66
Les Mots et les choses, 87
Francavila, Pietro, 59

Galen, 2, 52, 53, 54, 56, 57, 62, 67, 70, 73, 89, 90, 91, 94, 95, 97, 103, 201, 211
Garrioch, David, 31
George III, 158
Gérard, Pierre, 170
Gerle, Dom, 151
Germer, Stefan, 236
Gessner, Salomon, *Death of Abel*, 3, 178-80
Girodet, Anne-Louis, *Une Scène de déluge*, 5, 234, fig.47 (235)
Girondins, 162
Goltzius, Hendrik, fig.5 (24)
Gonzales-Palacios, Alvar, 3, 176
Goodden, Angelica, 33
Gouhier, Henri, 87
Grant, Russell, 78
Grammacini, Gisela, 145, 193, 196
Grimm, Friedrich Melchior, 81, 114, 115, 130

Haller, Albrecht von, 1, 2, 46, 51, 58, 69, 70, 71, 72, 73, 74, 75, 78, 80, 88, 97, 102, 105, 130, 199, 200, 210
Elementa physiologiae, 58, 67

Halperin, David, 66
Harvey, William, 57, 58
Helvétius, Jean Claude Adrien, 46, 47, 48, 49, 51, 65, 81
Hennequin, Philippe-Auguste,
Triumph of the French people, 219
Les Remords d'Oreste, 234
Henri IV, 59, 134, 164
Hercules, 2, 20, 38, 106, 110, 120, 163, 164, 166, 181, 196, 197, 213, 220
Hippocrates, 51, 52, 53, 54, 67, 68, 201, 211, 212
Hogarth, William, 39, 42
Rake's progress: Bedlam, 134, fig.25 (135)
Homer, 68, 108
Hume, David, 127
Hunt, Lynn, 122, 165, 233
Hydra, 164

Ida, 108
Isocrates, 106

Jacobins, 65, 139, 150, 153, 157, 158, 165, 188
Jaucourt, chevalier de, 45, 96, 130, 157
Jones, Colin, 128, 149
Journal de physique, 63
Julien, Pierre, 145,
Dying gladiator, 172, fig.39 (174)
Poussin, fig.31 (147)
Julius Caesar, 64, 65
Juno, 108
Jupiter, 115

Kant, Immanuel, *Observations on the feeling of the beautiful and sublime*, 1, 2, 74, 75, 76, 78, 80, 84, 85, 86, 88, 102, 117, 130, 149, 207
Koepp, Cynthia, 44

Landon, Charles-Paul, 232
Landseer, Edwin, 4
Laocoön, 99, 100, fig.18 (101), 103, 176
Laqueur Thomas, 209
Laréveillèrre-Lépeaux, 228
Lavater, 1, 2, 78, 79, 80, 81, 84, 86, 88, 130
Le Breton, Joachim, 184
Lebrun, Charles, 99, 100
Lebrun, Jean-Baptiste, 182, 184, 187
Le Moine, François, 99
Lenoir, Alexandre, 233
Leonardo da Vinci, *Vitruvian man*, 103, fig.19 (104), 105
Lepelletier de Saint-Fargeau, 162, 166, 170, 181, 193
Livy, 223
Locke, John, 63, 209
Louis XIV, 58, 77, 164, 182, 183
Louis XV, 81, 164
Louis XVI, 122
Louvre, 59
Lucas, Colin, 155
Lucian, 163, 186
Lucius Caesar, 94
Lysias, 106
Lysippus, 95, 98, 99, 100, 102, 105

Mantegna, Andrea, 163n
Manuel, Frank E., 209
Marat, Jean-Paul, 46, 162, 170
Marcus Aurelius, 67
Marie-Antoinette, 123
Mariette, Pierre-Jean, 17, 20, 22, 29, 33, 96, 105, 120
Mars, 20
Masson, François, *Project for monument to Jean-Jacques Rousseau*, fig.44 (195), 219
Maupetit de Mayenne, Michel René, 151, 153, 157
Medici Venus, 22, fig.7 (26), 37, 40, 100, 212
Mercier, Sébastien, 213
Mercure, 23, 29
Mercury, 16, 39
Michel, Régis, 141, 170
Michelangelo di Lodovico Buonarroti Simoni, 56, 236
Mirabeau, Honoré Gabriel Riquetti, comte de, 131, 151, 153, 162
Moitte, Jean-Guillaume, 145, 193
Cassini, fig.30 (146), 197
Jean-Jacques Rousseau, fig.43 (194), 196, 219, 220
Montesquieu, Charles de Secondat, baron de, 143, 144, 145
Montpellier, 199

Moschus, 21
Mozart, Wolfgang Amadeus, 81
Musée Carnavalet, 163

Napoleon, 4, 215, 226, 234
National Assembly, 123, 124, 126
National Guard, 156
Necker, Jacques, 122, 128
Nijmegen, Peace of, 59

Ogmius, 163
Olympus, 108
Opéra, 162, 170, 196
Ozouf, Mona, 166

Pajou, Augustin, 142
Paracelsus, 57
Paris
  Champ de Mars, 213
  Champs-Elysées, 219
  Conciergerie, 81
  Faubourg Saint-Germain, 33
  Faubourg Saint-Honoré, 33
  Faubourg Saint-Marcel, 30, 33, 34, 39, 43, 114, 115, 206
  Notre-Dame, 165
  Place des Victoires, 58, 77, 164
  Pont Neuf, 59, 181, 196
  Tuileries, 128, 156
Parthenon, 106
Phidias, 95, 106
Pigalle, Jean-Baptiste, 3, 111
  Monument to Louis XV, Rheims, fig.21 (112), 115, 128, 130, 134, 145, 164
Pinel, Philippe, 95
Pitt, William, 158
Plato, 40, 52, 56
Pliny the Elder, 94, 95, 96, 97, 102, 107
Plutarch, *Life of Romulus*, 223
Polyclitus, 2, 40, 90, 91, 94, 95, 97, 98, 102, 103, 105, 107, 108, 110
Portique républicain, 228
Poussin, Nicolas, 145, 182, 183
  Summer, 17, fig.3 (18), 183
  Testament of Eudamidas, fig.32 (148), 149, 184, 187
Prix Décennaux, 5
Procé, Marion de, 72
Ptolemy, 54, 55, 56

Quintilian, 90, 106, 107

Rakewell, 134
Raphael, 38
Reims, 111, 113, 128
Ribeiro, Aileen, 157
Richardson, Samuel, *Sir Charles Grandison*, 76, 85
Robespierre, Maximlien, 132, 154, 157, 158, 163, 167, 168, 181, 182, 189, 221
Roger, Jacques, 10
Rome, 149, 176
Rousseau, Jean-Jacques, 49, 192, 196, 219, 220

Saint-Cloud, 216
Saint-Just, Louis Antoine Léon de, 163
Salon, 141
Sanctorius, 57
sans-culotte, 157, 166
Scherf, Guilhem, 11
Seneca, 202
Sennett, Richard, 87
Serangeli, Gioacchino, 170
Sergel, Johan Tobias, *Othryades the Spartan dying*, 172, fig.38 (173)
Seznec, Jean, 49
Shakespeare, William, 56
Sieyès, Emanuel Joseph, 124, 125, 127, 128, 129, 132, 153, 181, 206, 216, 219
Singer, Brian, 129
Smith, Adam, 32, 43, 87, 206
Société populaire et républicaine des arts, 3, 150, 182, 184
Stahl, Georg Ernst, 69, 70
Steiner, Rudolph, 57
Stouf, Jean-Baptiste, *Dying Abel*, 18, 176, fig.41 (177)
Suetonius, 64, 65, 71, 97

Temkin, Owsei, 56
Teniers, David II, *Acts of charity*, 184, fig.42 (185)
Terror, 156, 157
Theremin, Wilhelm, 219
Thermidor, 4, 188, 189, 192, 221
Third Estate, 43, 122, 124, 132, 155
Thouret, Jacques Guillaume, 13

Tourville, Anne Hilarion de Cotentin de, 167
Turenne, Henri de la Tour d'Auvergne, Vicomte de, 167

van de Sandt, Udolpho, 183
van den Bogaert, Martin *see* Desjardins
Van Helmont, Johan Baptist, 57
Van Loo, Carle, 99
Varro, 97, 107
Venus, 20, 100
Vernet, Carle, *Triomphe de Paule Emile*, 163n
Versailles, 121, 122, 164, 183
Vespasian, 71, 99
Viala, 166, 167
Vila, Anne, 209
Virgil, 68
Vitruvius, 94, 102, 110
Volland, Sophie, 114
Voltaire, François-Marie Arouet, *known as*, 80, 111, 115

Ward-Jackson, Philip, 196n
Watelet, Claude Henri, 103
Williams, Helen Maria, 214
Winckelmann, Johann Joachim, 40, 41, 49, 68, 102, 105, 107, 108, 110, 153, 172, 176n, 180, 196
Wrigley, Richard, 157, 168
Wrisberg, Heinrich August, 73

Zeuxis, 153
Zimmerman, Johann Georg, 202